Create a Positive
Health Care
Workplace!

Create a Positive Health Care Workplace!

Practical Strategies to Retain Today's Workforce and Find Tomorrow's

Jo Manion, Ph.D.

Health Forum, Inc.
An American Hospital Association Company
CHICAGO

press

Portions of chapter 8 are reprinted from *Polarity Management* by Barry Johnson, copyright © 1992, 1996. Reprinted by permission of the publisher, HRD Press, Amherst, MA, (800) 822-2801, www.hrdpress.com.

AHA
press is a service mark of the American Hospital Association used under license by Health Forum, Inc.

Printed in the United States of America—07/05

Cover design by Cheri Kusek

ISBN: 1-55648-321-X   Item Number: 088177

Library of Congress Cataloging-in-Publication Data

Manion, Jo.
    Create a positive health care workplace! : practical strategies to retain today's workforce and find tomorrow's / Jo Manion.
        p. cm.
    ISBN 1-55648-321-X
    1. Health services administration.   2. Health facilities—Administration.   3. Personnel management.   I. Title.
    RA971.M34675   2005
    362.1'068—dc22   2005046243

This book is dedicated to:

My husband, Craig (once again), for his love, support, and encouragement. This work could not have been done without his unwavering belief in me.

My big sis Jeanne, who has taught me much about positive workplaces, but primarily that we are each responsible for making our own workplace a good place to be.

And finally, to all of my health care colleagues out there in organizations who are trying, every single day, to make their departments and organizations positive, healthy places to work in the face of difficult challenges in today's business environment.

Contents

About the Author
and Contributors

Jo Manion, Ph.D., RN, CNAA, FAAN, is a speaker, accomplished author, and senior management consultant who offers practical and creative approaches to organizational and professional issues. Since the early 1990s, she has worked with organizations and individuals engaged in creating effective cultural change, developing leadership capacity, and transforming organizational structures. Her focus is on creating positive workplace environments with high-impact retention strategies.

As a widely published author, she has written books on organizational innovation and intrapreneurship, creation of team-based health care organizations, and leadership. The second edition of *From Management to Leadership* is scheduled for release in the summer of 2005. She also coauthored *Nature's Wisdom in the Workplace: Managing Energy in Today's Healthcare Organization.*

She has published dozens of articles and book chapters on current issues in health care and is a frequent contributor to *H&HN OnLine.* Dr. Manion is a fellow in the American Academy of Nursing. After growing up in the Midwest, she earned her undergraduate and graduate degrees from Marycrest College and the University of Iowa. In addition, she has a master's degree and doctorate in human and organizational development from the Fielding Graduate Institute in Santa Barbara, California. She makes her home with her husband and their two dogs in the Orlando, Florida, area.

Sharon H. Cox, M.S.N., RN, is principal consultant and sole proprietor of Cox & Associates, a health care consulting and training company in Brentwood, Tennessee. As a registered nurse and nurse manager, she worked for twenty years in both clinical and administrative positions in academic health centers. She has also worked for twenty years in consulting and staff development for organizations nationwide. Cox is a member of the editorial board of *Nursing Management* magazine and coauthor of *Core Skills for Nurse Managers* (published by HCPro in 2004). She holds a master of science degree in nursing from the Medical College of Georgia in Augusta.

Mary G. Jenkins, M.A., is vice-president for organizational learning and development at Genesys Health System, Grand Blanc, Michigan. Before joining Genesys in 2002, she worked as a consultant for General Motors, Kodak, Shell Oil, the U.S. General Accounting Office, and other clients. She was also a member of the original startup team for Saturn Corporation, where she played a leading role in the design of its unique human resource systems. Jenkins is coauthor of *Abolishing Performance Appraisals: Why They Backfire and What to Do Instead,* and she is a contributor to *Managing Human Resources in the 21st Century: From Core Concepts to Strategic Choice* (published by South-Western College Publishing in 1999). She holds a master's degree in labor and industrial relations from Michigan State University in East Lansing.

List of Figures and Tables

Preface

WORKFORCE shortages, both current and impending, are reported to top the list of the health care executive's concerns in this and future decades. Creating a positive workplace culture is a key factor in attracting good people to an organization as well as in retaining them. The composition of the workforce is changing significantly from years past. "Our economy is rapidly changing from a money economy to a satisfaction economy" (Seligman 2002, p. 165). What Seligman is referring to is the recognition that beyond a certain safety net, money no longer is the primary motivator for most employees. Although this is especially true in times when jobs are abundant, the trend over the past twenty years has moved in the direction of employees' being more motivated to remain with a job because of the work experience rather than the monetary rewards of working. Thus, the organization with a strongly positive work environment has the competitive edge in attracting and retaining high-quality employees.

In contrast to the current exhortation that the manager is the chief retention officer, this book recognizes that maintaining a vibrant workforce is a responsibility shared by both managers and employees. Having strong, savvy leaders who understand and embrace their role in both recruiting and retaining employees is crucial. However, it is not enough. As the illustration on the next page shows, a positive work environment is possible only through the action of all key stakeholders working in partnership.

In fact, a primary working premise of this book is that the possibility of a positive work environment only exists when there is an active and dynamic state of interdependence among the organization, its leaders and managers, and its employees. And that healthy state of interdependence is characterized by positive adult-to-adult relationships among all members of the organization, with employees and leaders alike owning the responsibility for their own performance, knowledge and skill development, career progression, and morale.

Three Factors Important in Creating a Positive Workplace

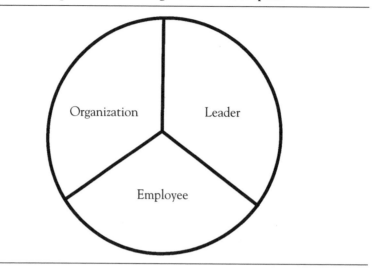

To say that the manager is the chief retention officer for the department implies that he or she is primarily or even solely responsible for creating a culture of engagement that retains high-performing employees. Although an individual leader may achieve a high level of success independent of a supportive organization or participating employees, the sustainability of such success is short term at best. In the same way, an individual employee may not be able to influence an entire organization, and yet to ignore the possibility of an individual's influence is to fly in the face of our own experience and historical events. However, when all three aspects of the system are working in concert, remarkable *and* sustainable results can be attained. A positive and supportive organizational culture coupled with effective leaders and engaged employees is the absolute best-case scenario. Indeed, it could be argued that the presence of any one of these factors alone increases the likelihood that the other two will develop.

With this said, I have chosen to write this book primarily from the perspective of the leader's role with the belief that much of what is offered here is also completely applicable to the individual employee. Some interpretation and application may have to be done by the reader; however, by and large, the concepts are appropriate for an individual focus. Although in some cases the application of the concept is made directly to the organizational level, this book is not primarily focused on the organizational scale as much as it is on the individual

Influence and Interdependence of the Organization, Leader, and Employee

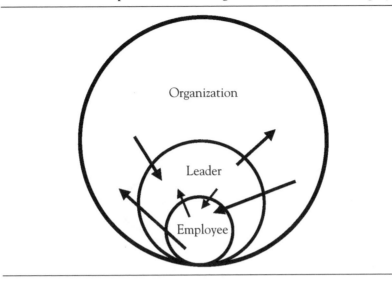

scale. Clearly, to create and support positive workplaces, an overhaul of organizational culture in health care organizations must occur. Although this is clear in many places throughout the book, this work is not intended to be a true organizational development book in that context. Questions at the end of each chapter offer conversation points for discussion about the organization, for the leader/manager, and for the individual employee.

For all of the emphasis on, and importance of, retention and the current focus on the quality of the employee's experience of the workplace, remarkably little evidence-based practice exists that clearly tells us which strategies are most effective. Instead, the literature reports almost any intervention that someone thinks is a good idea. The net is cast broadly in the hope of success, rather than offering targeted interventions that have been demonstrated to be effective. This book is an attempt to provide a more focused view of strategies that are based on the evidence provided through research. Although the emphasis is on an evidence-based approach, the suggestions and strategies offered are immanently practical and applicable in any health care setting.

The first section of the book contains four chapters and represents the foundation upon which the initiatives and interventions in the remainder of the book are based. Chapter 1 focuses on introductory material; it asks and attempts to answer the question, "Where should we put our energies: recruitment or retention?" It explores the high cost of turnover in its many aspects, with a special emphasis on the hidden cost of losing good people.

Chapter 2 explores the reasons people work. An historical review of work and its importance to us as humans is presented. Drawing from the psychological, sociological, and organizational development literature and research, this chapter summarizes briefly what we know about the intrinsic motivators, that is, those internal forces that cause us to do what we do. For some readers, this brief description will be a review of familiar concepts that serves as a reminder of that knowledge. For others, it is the organizational context of this chapter that will be helpful, and for yet others, the information presented may be new. The value of this chapter is that it serves us as a guidepost in evaluating our workplaces. Although intrinsic motivators are those forces within the individual that compel action, an effective leader understands these concepts and uses leadership interventions to create an environment that increases the likelihood that these forces will be acted upon.

Chapter 3 presents a summary of what we know about organizational commitment. This chapter is included because of the recognition that although the intrinsic motivators are what get us to work, what keeps us there is yet another important aspect to understand. Although the intrinsic motivators are closely linked to a person's organizational commitment, these concepts are separated into two chapters for ease of presentation and assimilation. Again, understanding what evidence-based practice has taught us about employee commitment is a foundational step in evaluating your own work environment. Chapters 2 and 3 give the manager and individual employee the ability to assess their workplace and target their interventions rather than using the shotgun approach (trying everything in the hope that something will hit the target).

The fourth chapter is considered foundational because it sets the stage for moving forward into the second part of the book. The goal of a positive work environment is to ensure that the people who are there are happy. This chapter offers a brief review of the remarkable field of positive psychology, highlighting the recent research findings that shed light on the creation of a positive work environment. The business case for happiness at work is examined, and the results of a study of health care workers who report experiencing joy through their work is shared. The chapter concludes with a discussion of the techniques that have been documented and demonstrated to induce lasting happiness in people.

The second section focuses specifically on strategies that have been found to be related to a positive work environment. Chapter 5 begins this section by reviewing the results of a research study conducted in order to understand more fully what first-line managers actually do to create a culture of retention in their organizations. The examples and stories from the research participants offer vivid and rich suggestions for those interested in creating a culture of retention. The findings suggest a variety of organizational ramifications and specific direction for the leaders to whom these managers directly report. The chapters included in the rest of the book are based on these findings.

Chapters 6 and 7 present strategies that directly flow from this study and from what is known about the intrinsic motivators and organizational commitment. Creating healthy working relationships and nurturing a sense of community within the workplace are well-documented strategies with a long-lasting impact. For managers and employees who are naturally talented in the area of relationships, these chapters serve as a review and checkpoint. For those who experience some difficulty with relationships or who are interested in improving their relationships in the workplace, these chapters are essential. Although the chapters emphasize the basics of a healthy working relationship, work from the field of emotional intelligence is also explored. Emotional competencies of both individuals and work teams or work groups are examined. Chapter 7 addresses the relationships within groups of people. Important concepts of team are presented, and the developmental process of community creation is reviewed. Specific strategies that can be used to enhance the formation of a vibrant, healthy sense of community are addressed.

Getting results is the focus of the next two chapters. Chapter 8 presents strategies for getting results, including actual techniques such as problem solving and appreciative inquiry. Models of shared decision making used in health care organizations today are also briefly examined. General principles are offered rather than a specific, cookie-cutter approach.

Chapter 9 discusses the basic principles for creating an innovative work environment. In too many health care organizations today, people with good ideas are meeting almost insurmountable resistance. Our finest employees often give up when it comes to getting a good idea heard and implemented. A positive work environment is considered to be one that is responsive, dynamic, and continuously improving. Yet, there are many structural and philosophical barriers to getting good ideas implemented. This chapter offers suggestions on how such barriers can be addressed.

The final chapter on specific strategies is chapter 10, Influencing Performance. Exemplary managers and high-performing employees simply do not tolerate poor performance from others, nor do they settle for "work-arounds." Instead, they deal with performance issues, each in their own way. The concept of positive discipline is presented as well as other basic techniques for dealing with shortfalls in performance.

Each chapter concludes with a brief summary and a list of questions suggesting ramifications for the organization, the manager, and the employee. Considering these ramifications is challenging because they require thoughtful reflection and honesty with oneself. There is a lot of spin in today's health care organizations. We know what people are looking for, and it is an easy matter to design an advertising campaign that attracts individuals to our organization. Meeting the promises implied is quite another story. Organizations that are good at spin may do well in the short run because they are able to attract new employees. However, keeping employees is quite another story. This book is written for health care organizations and professionals who are serious about undertaking the challenging work of creating or maintaining a positive work culture and environment.

Acknowledgments

A S IN ANY WORK of this magnitude, it is impossible to acknowledge everyone who had an impact on my ideas and work. There are, however, several noteworthy contributions by others that I would like to acknowledge.

First, I would like to acknowledge my long-time friend and mentor Sharon Cox. Not only did she contribute to the writing of two chapters in this book, she has also long been a friend of mine. We share many similar philosophies and approaches, and I know that she could have written most of this book herself! In addition, she has always been a champion of others, and I have been privileged to be one of those to whom she has lent support and given encouragement over the years. Thank you, dear friend.

Second, I would like to acknowledge the contributions of my research participants. I have learned so much from them. They gave of their time and ideas unstintingly and helped me not only to learn, but also to recapture my own enthusiasm and excitement for the work that we do. They are certainly the joyful part of any research project!

Third, I would like to extend my thanks to all of the teachers who have imparted their knowledge, given me guidance, or provided me with opportunities over the years, including those who have served a formal teaching role in my life as well as the many authors who have shared their knowledge with me. Others gave me learning opportunities either through my work or through writing for publication. All of these experiences have blessed me with a richness of perspective and understanding that I might not otherwise have had. Thanks to you all.

And, finally, I would like to thank Richard Hill, editorial director for AHA Press. His insight, gentle suggestions, and challenges have all helped this work develop. Thanks for being the one to bring this book out!

Create a Positive
Health Care
Workplace!

I

Foundations for Understanding
Engagement in the Workplace

THE FIRST PART of this book introduces the key concepts behind the creation of positive workplaces and explores the challenge of recruiting and retaining a vibrant health care workforce. Part I also presents key concepts that will help us understand the complex issues surrounding intrinsic motivation and the meaning and purpose of work. In addition, the first four chapters of this book review the historical literature on the subject of work as well as recent research in psychology and organizational development.

Specifically, chapter 1 discusses health care workforce shortages. Chapter 2 explores the meaning of work, and chapter 3 examines commitment as both a personal issue and an organizational challenge. Chapter 4, the last chapter in part I, introduces the idea of finding happiness and joy through our work and in our workplaces. Chapter 4 also explores the new field of positive psychology and offers specific interventions to help employees find happiness in their work and workplaces.

1

Considering Workforce Issues

Jo Manion

Never before have organizations paid more attention to talent. . . .
Keeping it. Stealing it. Developing it. Engaging it.
Talent is no longer just a numbers game; it's about survival.
—Beverly Kaye and Sharon Jordan-Evans (2002)

TODAY, building and maintaining a vibrant workforce are inextricably linked to, and embedded in, the strategic focus of virtually every health care organization. No health care organization can achieve its strategic imperatives without the full partnership of engaged, talented, and skilled employees. And with workforce shortages already evident today and certain in the future, simply attaining a highly performing workforce itself has become a strategic imperative.

In recent years, escalating shortages of health care workers have received the attention of every professional association, regulatory agency, health care consulting practice, and major health care system. Report after report has outlined the extent of shortages among clinical professionals as well as support staff. Although shortages vary by geographical area, state after state reports high vacancy rates that represent unfilled positions that are likely to remain difficult, if not impossible, to fill. Topics related to workforce shortages fill the agendas of professional meetings and are the subject of seminars all around the country. All of these activities attest to the level of anxiety and concern that health care leaders and executives are currently experiencing.

Unfortunately, a potentially dangerous side effect accompanies this ongoing emphasis on the health care workforce problem. It is easy to become habituated to this bad news. At some point, we stop listening because we are certain that we have heard all of the bad news before. It is interesting to speculate on the day in the not-too-distant future when today's high turnover and vacancy rate crisis becomes the norm. Chronic workforce shortages seem to be our future if only because of colliding demographics as baby boomers, a large portion of our current workforce, reach retirement age.

To believe that we can solve the workforce shortage once and for all is probably short-sighted to the point of being delusional. At one recent hospital association annual meeting, I overheard a conversation during which one hospital executive proudly told another, "We've got the nursing shortage licked. We don't have any open vacancies. The shortage is over for us." The hospital executive in question really should have gone back and looked carefully at his demographics before congratulating himself. Of course, sometimes we are just telling ourselves such things in an attempt to find some measure of comfort in what has become an environment fraught with seemingly continual and often insurmountable challenges.

The health care industry is not alone in facing workforce challenges. McKinsey & Company conducted a yearlong study involving seventy-seven companies and almost six thousand managers and executives. The conclusion: "The most important corporate resource over the next 20 years will be talent: smart, sophisticated people who are technologically literate, globally astute, and organizationally agile" (Fishman 1998, p. 104). In the McKinsey & Company review of the changing workforce, it is clear that the supply of qualified workers is decreasing at the same time workforce demands are increasing. "The search for the best and brightest will become a constant, costly battle, a fight with no final victory. Not only will [organizations] have to devise more imaginative hiring practices, they will also have to work harder to keep their best people" (Fishman 1998, p. 104).

Recently, in preparation for a research project, I reviewed the healthcare research literature on workforce shortages. The review is not included here for two reasons. First, anyone reading this book has probably read the same studies and reports and already knows their content and conclusions. However, I do refer to pertinent findings to support chapter content. Second, I simply do not have the heart to write such a review. Some people might have found it fascinating and exciting reading, but I doubt that such people are the ones who would read this book. Spending energy rereading and synthesizing what must surely be self-evident to most of us seems futile. Instead, I will summarize a couple of major observations as they pertain to workforce issues and then offer some ideas about the concept of retention.

Basic Conclusions

Here are the conclusions from the massive literature on workforce shortages that I believe are important in meeting the challenge of workforce development and maintenance:

1. At various times, critical shortages of key workers in healthcare have occurred. The shortages will likely continue to plague us and even worsen in the future. In the recent past, shortages have been quantitatively documented in several of health care professional groups, including nurses, pharmacists, radiology technicians, physical therapists, and information technology managers. The degree of the shortages varies by location and is often cyclical in nature. The impending loss of baby boomers from the workforce is likely to significantly affect health care organizations in many ways that are unrecognized at this time.

2. Creating a positive work environment is important regardless of the existence of workforce shortages. A positive work environment directly affects the quality and level of service provided, the productivity of employees, and the financial well-being of the organization. During times of workforce shortages, a positive work environment becomes a competitive edge that makes an organization even stronger and more viable.

3. Many reasons for the shortages have been suggested, and several have been very well documented. However, the decreasing size of the generational cohorts means that fewer people are available for recruiting. In addition, the declining attractiveness of health care as an career opportunity is significant. The problem is multifaceted and complex.

4. Not all health care organizations experience workforce shortages in the same way. Many health care organizations recognize that the only substantial difference between them and their competitors is the skills, knowledge, commitment, and abilities of the people who work in the organization. These organizations act accordingly and treat their employees well. Unfortunately, there are just as many organizations that follow a philosophy that regards employees as easily replaceable units who should consider themselves lucky just to have a job. As Stanford professor Jeffrey Pfeffer said, "Loyalty isn't dead . . . but toxic [organizations] are driving people away. There isn't a scarcity of talent—but there is a growing unwillingness to work for a toxic organization"

(Webber 1998, p. 154). Pfeffer went on to say that organizations short on talent probably deserve to be. Sounds a bit harsh, but perhaps he has a point.

The Cost of Turnover

Turnover is an issue even during times when employees are plentiful and every position in the organization is filled. Turnover occurs when an employee leaves his position and must be replaced. Turnover is always an expensive proposition for an organization, although some turnover is to be expected and is even desirable. People who have not been with the organization since the beginning of recorded history can help us see the things we do from a new perspective. Turnover gives us the opportunity to welcome new people who bring fresh and unique ideas to the organization. This opportunity assumes, however, that we are willing to listen to them.

Occasionally, the loss of a particular employee or manager may even make us want to celebrate. We have all worked with disruptive or unproductive people in our careers. Take the case of Agnes. Agnes creates disruption and chaos wherever she goes. She is difficult to work with and is a constant source of complaint. Either Agnes is complaining about something or someone, or her coworkers are complaining about Agnes. When you look at the schedule and see that Agnes is scheduled for the next day, you groan. The knowledge that you will need to deal with her the next day is enough to sink you into a bad mood for the rest of the day. In fact, if you could, you would call in sick rather than face a day working with her. When Agnes finally blows up and resigns in a fit of pique, everyone breathes a sigh of relief. Her manager grabs the resignation letter, immediately copies it, and personally delivers it to the human resources department before Agnes can change her mind. Losing employees like Agnes is a positive kind of turnover.

Undesirable turnover is the loss of people we do not want to lose. Such employees are highly productive, and they often contribute constructive ideas. These are the skilled people who work well with others. You know the people I am talking about. When these people resign, everyone is sorry to see them go. Understanding the ways in which turnover is expensive may encourage us to work diligently to avoid unnecessary turnover.

Financial Cost

The first cost of turnover—the financial cost—is obvious. The financial loss that results from the resignation of a single employee has been estimated to range from 150 to 250 percent of the employee's annual salary. The range is wide simply because there are a multitude of factors to be considered. The most obvious factors include the actual cost of advertising the vacancy and the hours spent reviewing applications and conducting interviews. In addition, the cost of replacement help in the form of expensive temporary employees to cover the position until a new person can be hired must be considered as well as the cost of new employee training and orientation. Regardless of the thoroughness with which costs are captured, even conservative estimates of financial costs are significant for an organization.

A study conducted by the Voluntary Hospitals of America is illuminating (Gelinas and Bohlen 2002). As part of the study, several member hospitals were evaluated carefully on the basis of their actual vacancy rates. For example, in one organization, replacement costs were projected to be 22 percent of total payroll base compensation. The average replacement cost per skilled employee was estimated to be almost $29,000. When these estimates were applied to the organization's actual number of turnovers, it was determined that reducing turnover from 31 percent to 25 percent would result in a cost savings of over $800,000 per year. If the turnover rate could be reduced even further, from 31 to 20 percent, savings would total over $1.4 million per year. This type of case study can be done in any organization by using actual turnover data.

At least three important points should be considered in examining the financial cost of employee turnover. First, a common reaction to proposals for spending money on retention efforts is the refrain: "We don't have the money." The truth is reducing turnover could yield a significant amount of found money that could be used to fund improved retention efforts.

Second, we ought to have a clear idea of just how much turnover is costing the organization. Otherwise we may not be using our resources wisely. For example, in one department over several years, the manager worked hard to keep a key night shift position filled. New employees who began optimistically lasted, on average, less than three months before they resigned. The permanent employees on the night shift had been there for years. Their expectations were quite high, and they purposely created difficult situations for the new people in order to test their abilities. The old-timers were just plain toxic. They complained bitterly about nobody wanting to work with them on the graveyard shift, but they failed to see that they were a large part of the reason why no one stayed. Finally, after years of replacing new employees for this shift, the manager pulled together the cost information and sat down with these long-tenured employees and showed them the facts. She said, in essence, "You are costing this department too much. I can't afford to keep you. If you are unable to accept the next new employee and help him or her assimilate into the department, I am going to have to let you go. I just cannot afford you." They got the message.

In too many organizations today, health care managers do not have accurate or timely information about turnover costs in their department. Very few have specific quantitative data about factors important to retention, such as employee and physician satisfaction levels, the length of recruitment time for open positions, or even basic information such as the overall vacancy rate.

The final point in considering the financial cost of turnover is that it is important to have accurate information. We hold many misperceptions about turnover. For example, we know that the more highly paid professionals in the organization represent a higher cost of turnover in terms of cost per employee. For this reason, organizations focus on shortages of registered nurses, licensed pharmacists, and skilled radiology technicians. However, employees who make a lower wage may actually represent a larger turnover cost to the organization because of sheer number of turnovers in these positions. For example, in a long-term care facility, nursing assistants deliver 80 to 90 percent of the direct patient care. Not only are there higher numbers of these workers, the annual turnover rate among these employees is reported to be as high as 99 percent (Riggs and Rantz 2001). Therefore, the total turnover cost for certified nurse assistants can be much higher than that for registered nurses in long-term care facilities. In acute care organizations, turnover among entry-level environmental service and dietary workers can represent a tremendous cost because hospitals employ large numbers of these workers.

Damage to the Brand

Another cost of turnover—damage to the brand—is often hidden, and many people in health care have not even considered this serious issue. Damage to the brand is a business term that refers to the negative impact that a single product can have on a whole line of products when the product fails to meet the customers' expectations.

At a recent state hospital association meeting, John Houck (2003) reported on the results of a nursing retention study. He introduced damage to the brand as a concept that can have significant ramifications for health care organizations. In his study, Houck reported finding that over

30 percent of the nurses who left hospitals during the period of time studied did not take new hospital positions. Instead, they chose positions in another area of health care or opted out of health care altogether. Houck talked about his previous business experience in the clothing industry, and he pointed out that when a new clothing design or product is released, sales figures are closely tracked. Retailers are interested not just in how many of the items are purchased but in how many people repurchase the same item. According to Houck, repurchase rates of 30 percent or less represent a significant problem. Products with low rates of repurchase are quickly pulled from the shelves because the sale of unsatisfactory new products can damage sales for the entire brand.

What Houck was referring to is the thinking that goes on in our heads as consumers. For instance, I may try a new style of Levis®. If they do not fit right or look good or if no one notices them the first time I wear them, I do not say to myself, "Gee, Jo, you didn't make a very good buying decision here." Instead, I say something like, "Boy, Levis just aren't what they used to be. I guess I better start looking around at some other brands and maybe try something different next time."

The concept of damage to the brand has significant ramifications for the health care industry. Take the example of Sarah, a young registered nurse who recently graduated from college. In her first work experience, fresh out of school, she was assigned to work in the telemetry department of an acute care hospital. She was just three months out of nursing school, and she was assigned to work as the night charge nurse with only one other registered nurse, who was also a recent graduate. Was it any wonder that she began thinking about quitting and becoming a florist? She did not say to herself, "This hospital is using new graduates inappropriately." Instead, she said, "Nursing isn't for me. This is too hard. This isn't what I thought it would be."

Everyone tends to generalize on the basis of limited experience and condemn the entire "brand" of experiences rather than just the single negative experience. In Sarah's case, the brand is hospital nursing or even nursing as a whole. Employees' experiences determine the judgments and decisions they make about the organization, the profession, the specialty, and so on. Health care organizations can no longer afford to recruit good people and then provide a negative work experience. If we do, we will be losing far more than one promising employee. In a recent study by Aon Consulting in partnership with the American Society of Healthcare Human Resources Administration, Runy (2003) reports that 64 percent of the health care workers studied think about or have begun to make plans to leave their health care careers.

Loss of Experience, Knowledge, and Connections

When a valued employee leaves an organization, the departure represents far more than a financial loss to the organization. Also lost is experience with, and knowledge of, the organization that can take the organization months and even years to replace. People who have been with an organization have learned the ropes, both the formal and informal ways to get things done. They know who to talk to about a problem, and they know how to navigate the ins and outs of a complex work situation. They have learned from their mistakes in order to gain this hard-won, tacit knowledge.

Experienced employees who have tenure in the organization also have formed relationships and connections both within their immediate work group and within the larger system. These relationships often help them to accomplish needed results. When such connections and relationships are severed, reestablishing them takes a significant amount of time. When turnover occurs frequently, those employees who remain in the organization often become more cynical and less inclined to form new attachments to the replacement employees.

For example, I was invited to one organization where I conducted a series of retreats for employees in women's services. The department was experiencing very high turnover rates, approaching 40 percent annually. During the retreat, several long-term employees made the comment that a pact had been established among the more seasoned, tenured employees. They had become quite tired of continually orienting new people and trying to get to know them only to have them resign within their first few months on the job. The long-term employees had decided that they were not going to talk to any of the new employees until they had been there for at least six months. It was just too exhausting to try to form a new relationship before they were certain that the new person was likely to stay. Furthermore, the long-term employees felt demoralized, and so they had decided to stop having going-away parties for departing employees. The effect of the pact on the new employees was evident in their comments: "No one talks to us." And, "Sally just had her last day, and she's been here for 20 years, . . . and no one even brought in doughnuts." Their natural conclusion: "No one cares about each other here."

When employees come and go frequently, building connections and satisfying, productive relationships becomes exhausting. In another organization, I was asked to help develop a plan for strengthening the relationship between the senior vice president and the employees in his departments, which were experiencing problems related to trust and openness. During the assessment, I discovered that the vice president was the fifth to whom these people had reported within the past five years. Is it any wonder that employees were hesitant to trust and extend themselves in relationship to this person? Forming relationships takes a lot of energy and a willingness to extend yourself. Continually reforming and reestablishing similar relationships over and over again begins to feel like a no-win situation for most of us, and we become unwilling to make the investment.

Impact on Remaining Employees

The last hidden cost of turnover we will discuss is the sense of rejection that those who remain in the organization often experience. Especially when the individual leaving is a valued, strong colleague or leader, the individual's choice to leave can feel like a personal rejection. The person has chosen to take another opportunity and is basically saying, "I can do better elsewhere." If this happens too many times, we may begin to question our own commitment to stay. A few years ago, I was conducting interviews of people around the country for an article I was writing. One senior-level executive said to me, "I want to work in a system people want to come to, not a place where they are leaving." He was referring to the exodus of good people he had watched over the years, which he found very demoralizing to him personally.

This felt rejection can also influence how managers respond to the employees who resign. When a valued employee's resignation is perceived as a personal rejection, managers and coworkers alike feel hurt and even betrayed, especially when they have worked hard to help the person develop their skills and abilities over time. In some cases, the manager may have worked very hard to create opportunities and meet the person's needs, and it can be difficult for the manager to rise above his or her personal disappointment and concern about finding a replacement. Unfortunately, how the manager responds may determine whether the employee will consider returning to the organization in the future.

During the past several years, it has become evident that many people are disappointed in the reality of their new jobs after they have left an organization for a better opportunity. Savvy recruiters and managers stay in touch with employees who have left and make it clear that they will be welcomed back if they want to return. Some organizations have even reinstated full benefits at the level they were at the time of resignation when employees return within a certain period of time. Managers and work groups have found a variety of ways to keep in touch with people. Some managers actually include former employees on their holiday greeting card lists, or they telephone them periodically to simply say hello. In other cases, being invited to alumni events that highlight the kinds of things that are going on in the department or organization serves to keep former employees informed of changes. Including them in holiday parties or department get-togethers is another way to encourage a continued sense of connection. Increased attention is being given to the recruitment of former employees as a viable recruitment strategy.

The alternative to letting people know that you are still interested and care about them as a potential colleague is that former employees believe that the manager and the organization no longer care about them. Such feelings can create ill will in the community and make it more difficult to recruit high-quality people.

Consider this true-life example. A young pharmacist named Tom interviewed at two organizations. One was a small, community hospital, and the other was a large, tertiary medical center. Tom chose the smaller organization because of the work he would be doing. When he told the recruiter at the large medical center of his choice, the recruiter became very angry with him. She simply could not believe that he would choose the smaller organization. Within about two months, Tom realized that he had made a mistake. He was not doing the work he had been promised but instead had been assigned a different job. He was very disappointed. When he was encouraged to recontact the recruiter from the larger organization, he refused, saying, "You just don't know how angry she was. I couldn't possibly call her back." This young man, a doctor in pharmacology, is quite unlikely to ever consider the larger organization again because the recruiter reacted to Tom's decision in a very negative way because of her own personal disappointment.

In a study that examined nurses' perceptions of factors prompting them to leave their jobs, several nurses referred to being treated poorly by their managers when they resigned. In these cases, the managers' negative actions or comments remained vivid in the memories of the study participants, for example:

- "No manager from my department said good-bye to me. They never acknowledged it was my last day after 18 years of employment. I left thinking I made the best decision I could."
- "I remember the day I told my manager I was quitting. She asked me what was I going to do and when I told her, she replied, 'When

or if you do come back, you'll work nights and every weekend'"
(Cline, Reilly, and Moore 2003, p. 52).

Rerecruiting some of your best former employees has tremendous advantages. When highly skilled individuals leave for other opportunities but years later remember the support they felt during the resignation process, they are more likely to consider returning to your organization. Such employees are often better for their time away, because they have gained new perspectives and different experiences. In this way, returning employees may even be considerably more valuable than when they left. Even when they are not interested in returning to the organization, they may refer other colleagues to the organization.

Employees play a significant role in recruiting former employees as well. Coworkers often keep in touch with their former colleagues. The more positively they continue to speak of their workplace, the more likely the former employees are to consider returning at some point in the future. Employees can also let their departing colleagues know when new positions open up, and thus they can serve as a trusted bridge between the former workplace and the former employees.

Psychological Resignation

"Resignation is not just a behavioral act; it is also a state of being" (Manion 2000, p. 25). Probably the most dangerous form of turnover is that which occurs when the individual leaves emotionally and psychologically and yet remains physically. A person does not have to resign officially for turnover to occur. Managers sometimes deceive themselves when they look at low vacancy rates and conclude that they do not have a turnover problem. Most managers and work groups understand this concept because they have experienced it.

Employees who resign psychologically are often referred to as on-the-job retired. When employees are not fully engaged but have instead psychologically retired from their jobs, their level of productivity plunges. They come to work late or not at all, and the other members of the team must carry heavier workloads to meet the team's goals. Having even 10 or 20 percent of the employees in a work group working below speed creates tremendous morale problems for the rest of the employees.

Thus, turnover may not be adequately addressed just by filling vacant positions. Recruitment efforts need to emphasize finding high-quality employees who are likely to remain committed and engaged in their work and full participants in the workplace. Good managers and savvy employees understand that they must continually re-recruit talented applicants and encourage optimal performance among all employees. In other words, keeping talented and dedicated employees is just as important as recruiting new ones.

Recruitment versus Retention

Recruitment and retention are closely linked. Making sure that all of your recruitment practices work well will yield little if the new recruits leave within a few months of joining your organization or department. In fact, finding good people and convincing them to give you a try but then letting them move on within a relatively short period of time simply increases the level of cynicism and demoralization in the system. And it takes a great deal of energy and effort that ultimately feel nonproductive.

Of course, your recruitment efforts need to be top-notch in a competitive labor market. Many organizations have stepped up their efforts in this area and have enjoyed increased success. However, we cannot assume that all is well. Kalisch (2003) conducted an extensive study of recruitment processes and systems in 122 acute care hospitals throughout the United States. The findings were appalling, especially considering the competitive nature of the talent pool in health care. Example after example of just plain poor practices was found (Kalisch 2003). It is worth examining Kalisch's results here, at least briefly.

Kalisch identified a total of thirty markets. Ten qualified nurses participated in the study and played the role of potential employees. The nurses were coached extensively on a standard procedure for applying and interviewing at the hospitals. One of the ten nurses applied to, and interviewed with, each of the 122 hospitals in the study.

The study results showed that problems within the recruitment process were widespread and began with the preinterview contacts. The preinterview problems ranged from no response to letters and inquiries to cases of extensive telephone tag. The overall quality of the letters and brochures provided by the hospitals was rated as fair to poor. Such communication problems create issues because applicants base their decisions on whether to interview at a given organization primarily on the quality, nature, and timeliness of letters, telephone contacts, e-mails, and brochures and other printed materials.

The interview experiences of the nurses also left a lot to be desired. The problems began with the directions to facility, the parking experience, the physical appearance of the facilities, and the helpfulness of the information desk personnel. Additional problems concerned the welcomes received by the applicants as well as waiting times, testing requirements, interview lengths, and interview environments. A few examples are described here to indicate the degree of problems encountered.

"In 55 percent of the interviews, the recruiter was expecting the candidate but no interviews had been set up with the managers of the units being considered. . . . [For example,] one critical care applicant flew from one end of the country to the other to interview in a well known medical center only to have no one available for the interview" (Kalisch 2003, p. 472). In another instance, "Even though I had a prearranged interview, when I got there, the secretary didn't know who I was. She paged the recruiter once but refused to do it again or to call anyone else to see me. This was despite me telling her I was from 2500 miles away!" (Kalisch 2003, p. 472). Another applicant was told by a nurse manager that she had no time to interview her and the applicant would need to wait for the assistant manager. She waited sixty-five minutes.

Other applicants reported receiving a similar reception. They were often left to wait in an area where they were able to see or hear the person with whom they were supposed to interview. "I sat there 20 minutes waiting and watching the recruiter sip coffee. There was no apology offered for being late." Another said, "I could hear her on the phone talking about last Saturday's date and this was 25 minutes after my interview was to start" (Kalisch 2003, p. 473). And unfortunately, these were not the only problems. At some organizations, the candidates' applications and resumes were misplaced, interviews were shortened to as little as five minutes, interview environments were negative, and postinterview follow-up was lacking. Shockingly, 91 percent of the organizations provided no interview follow-up at all.

Kalisch's study offers insight into potential problem areas, and the results of her study should jolt you into realizing that you cannot assume that your organization's recruiting practices are effective. You need to ask some difficult questions so that you can evaluate your organization's recruitment efforts. You can start by asking new hires about their experience during the recruitment process, but you should also devise a way of following up with the candidates who did not select your organization to find out what they experienced when they contacted your recruiter.

Fortunately, problems in the recruitment process can be fixed when they are recognized and the importance of their impact is appreciated. The National Association for Health Care Recruitment (NAHCR) is a very positive source for this kind of information. (The organization's web site address is www.nahcr.com.) The NAHCR also provides workshops for recruiters as well as other helpful resources such as handbooks and toolkits. The NAHCR will offer a credentialing exam for recruiters in the future.

Conclusion

This chapter explores employee turnover as a key challenge in today's health care organizations. The costs of turnover are considered, with emphasis given to the hidden costs such as potential damage to the brand; the felt rejection and lowered morale experienced among managers and coworkers; and the organization's loss of experience, knowledge, and connections. The concept of turnover extends to individuals who may not physically leave but separate psychologically. And finally, a challenge is offered to evaluate carefully your organization's recruitment practices to ensure you are maximizing your efforts to attract high-quality candidates. Once you have considered the impact of current and future workforce shortages, you can go on to creating a more positive workplace for your employees.

Conversation Points

Organizational Perspective

1. Does the organization provide managers with accurate, department-specific data on a timely basis? Do the data include vacancy and turnover rates and the average length of time a position is open before it is filled?
2. Are new employees tracked to determine their length of employment so that problem areas can be illuminated? Are there any "revolving door" departments, shifts, or positions?
3. How are managers being held accountable for their turnover levels? What are some of the valid reasons for turnover?
4. How much does turnover cost the organization financially on an annual basis?
5. Is your human resources department adequately resourced for recruitment efforts? Has an assessment of the recruitment process been performed? Do you know where the problems are? What is the success rate on a long-term basis?

6. Do managers and recruiters have a process for matching a potential employee's strengths with the open position? Is job fit an important issue that is considered? Are managers skilled in behavioral questioning?

Leadership Issues

1. Do you have accurate, timely data on turnover, cost of turnover, and vacant positions for your department? Do you know how long it takes you to replace employees?
2. When an employee resigns, do you meet with the person to determine the issues and reasons?
3. How do you make new employees feel welcome and encourage their assimilation into the work group? Do you have regular points of contact with new employees to assess their progress?
4. How strong is the orientation program in your department? Do you meet regularly with new employees to determine how they are doing?
5. Are there any problems in your recruiting and interviewing processes that need to be fixed?
6. Have you clearly identified the skills and strengths needed for each of the positions for which you typically interview candidates? Do you use behavioral questioning to determine fit and suitability of a potential applicant?
7. Do you take steps to stay in touch with former employees? Do you take any action to recruit former employees for open positions?
8. Have you been tolerating any employees who have resigned psychologically rather than dealing with their lack of performance?
9. How are current employees included in the interview process?

Employee Challenges

1. Do you know what the recruitment process is in your department?
2. How actively do you or your coworkers participate in interviewing or meeting with potential applicants?
3. How do you support and encourage new employees?
4. Do you participate in the orientation of new employees?
5. Do you keep in touch with departing coworkers and continue to talk positively about the workplace? Do you have any role in helping to bring former employees back to the organization?

2

Understanding Why People Work

Jo Manion

To have a firm persuasion in our work—
to feel that what we do is right for ourselves and good for the world
at exactly the same time—
is one of the great triumphs of human existence.
—David Whyte (2001)

WHEN MANAGERS are asked about why people work, 89 percent of them answer, "for the money" (Kaye and Jordan–Evans 2002). Whether these managers were giving us a quick, flippant answer to an age-old question or whether they truly believe that the people they work with are working primarily for the money, we may never know. What we do know, however, is that when managers believe that employees work mostly for the extrinsic rewards they receive (the salary and benefits), this belief influences them in a variety of ways. Because managers have little or no influence on what employees in the organization are paid, this belief can inadvertently absolve the manager from any responsibility for substantially influencing the attitudes and behavior of their employees. In other words, such managers develop a mindset based on the premise that "it's not my problem if people here aren't motivated." Starting from this negative viewpoint leads supervisors and managers to take little positive action to influence the employees with whom they work.

On the other hand, when people in management positions are encouraged to think more deeply about the reasons why people work, they quickly come to see that the answer to the question, "Why do people work?" is considerably more complex than it first appears. A full investigation of the meaning of work in the lives of people reveals a multitude of reasons why people work. And, in fact, when employees are really working in a particular organization only because of the money, the chances are pretty significant that they are going to be less committed and productive than their counterparts who have deeper reasons for working. In short, research has clearly documented that money is not the primary reason why people work (Atchinson 2003).

The first step to creating a positive workplace is to build a full understanding of the reasons why people work. An appreciation of the complexities and subtleties of this issue informs leaders and employees who are trying to create a positive working environment. In fact, it is virtually impossible to create such a positive environment unless you think well beyond the extrinsic motivators on the job. This chapter explores the question of why people work and examines the research in the area of intrinsic motivation.

Meaning of Work

Why do people work? What is the meaning of work in our lives? Throughout the centuries, these questions have been considered by the great thinkers of the time. The answers they suggested were influenced by various theological and philosophical perspectives, as well as by the societal issues and social structures of the day.

There are a variety of historical viewpoints of why humans work. Contemporary perspectives are represented in the publications of Meilaender (2000), Naylor (1996), Erikson and Vallas (1990), Applebaum (1992), and Amott and Matthaei (1991).

Work Is an Essential Element of Life

Meilaender is editor for *Working: Its Meaning and Its Limits*, which represents the work of a group of scholars interested in the ethics of everyday life. He and his colleagues met over a five-year period under the auspices of the Institute of Religion and Public Life at the University of Notre Dame. Meilaender notes that the group read, wrote, conversed, argued, and continually sought ways for deepening their own understanding of the "meaning of human life as ordinarily lived" (Meilaender 2000, p. v). This work led to the publication of several anthologies covering various aspects of everyday life. The anthology entitled *Working: Its Meaning and Its Limits* (2000) provides an in-depth examination and historical perspective on work and the meaning it has held for individual humans over the centuries. (See figure 2-1.)

Meilaender presents four main categories that capture the meaning of work over the centuries. The four categories include work as cocreation, work as necessary for leisure, work as dignified but irksome,

Figure 2-1.   The Meaning of Work as Categorized in the Literature

Work is an essential element of life
  Work as cocreation
  Work as necessary for leisure
  Work as dignified but irksome
  Work as vocation

Work is a way to fulfill individual, emotional, and psychological needs
  Need for self-identity and self-esteem
  Need to contribute to society
  Need for independence from the control of others
  Need for social relationships
  Need for achievement, competence, and accomplishment

and work as vocation. The anthology includes a variety of readings, essays, Biblical passages, stories, and poetry that illustrate each of the major categories. The readings and other written materials add richness and depth to this work and serve to illustrate the four categories.

Work as Cocreation

Work can be understood as cocreation. The first book of Genesis in the Old Testament of the Bible is used to illustrate a mandate to participate with God in the care of His creation. Meilaender quotes an excerpt from Dorothy Sayer's essay, "Why Work?" which describes this sentiment well (Meilaender 2000, p. 43):

> Work should be looked upon not as a necessary drudgery to be undergone for the purpose of making money, but as a way of life in which the nature of man should find its proper exercise and delight and so fulfill itself to the glory of God. That it should, in fact, be thought of as a creative activity undertaken for the love of the work itself; and that man, made in God's image, should make things, as God makes them, for the sake of doing well a thing that is worth doing.

Thus, from a Christian perspective, work is not something that a person does to live, but instead it is the thing one lives to do. And it should embody the full expression of an individual's faculties, "the thing in which he finds spiritual, mental, and bodily satisfaction, and the medium in which he offers himself to God" (Meilaender 2000, p. 43). In both the Hebrew and Christian ideology, God is portrayed as a worker, laboring six days to make the world and stopping on the seventh to rest (Applebaum 1992).

A citation attributed to Walter R. Courtenay reinforces this notion of work as an act of cocreation with God. "God gave man work, not to burden him, but to bless him, and useful work, willingly, cheerfully, effectively done, has always been the finest expression of the human spirit" (Naylor 1996, p. 36).

Regardless of one's religious beliefs, this concept of work as cocreation is compelling because it seems to correspond to the desire many people express for work that is meaningful and productive. In the literature relevant to the meaning of work in our lives, many of the articles and books are about meaningful work rather than about the meaning of work. It is helpful to differentiate between these two closely interrelated concepts. The relationship exists in that for many people the reason for work relates to their need to have an impact on the world. Meaningful work, work that makes a difference to others, is one source of meaning for them.

Although meaningful work may be one reason or motive for working, it is not the only one. Work has other meanings for humans as well. These other meanings are explored in the following pages.

Work as Necessary for Leisure

The idea that work is necessary for leisure has its roots in classical thinking. For many of the great Greek philosophers, work was important simply because it makes leisure possible. Not only does work make leisure possible, it is through the presence of work that we are able to clearly distinguish work from leisure. Today, we think of leisure as freedom from work, as amusement or time off that refreshes us before we return to work. For Aristotle, in contrast, leisure was the pursuit of silence and contemplation. The contemplative life was thought to be superior; in fact, contemplation was considered the highest form of existence. Our contemporary concept of leisure is very different. For most of us who experience weekends, holidays, and vacations as leisure, nothing could be farther from the contemplative life than leisure. Indeed, many of us return to work every Monday looking for a respite from the hectic pace of our leisure lives.

Work as Dignified but Irksome

The third category of thought about work as presented by Meilaender and his colleagues also has its basis in Biblical teachings. The concept of work as dignified but irksome is first apparent in the book of Genesis. Man, who has fallen into sin, is now condemned to toil for the bread he eats. And his toil is made even more difficult by a recalcitrant earth that brings forth only thistles and thorns. Simply observing ordinary human experience throughout history tells us that work is often burdensome. Over the centuries, humans have enslaved other humans to provide a source of labor. The peasants and serfs of early centuries and the wage earners of early factories certainly were exploited for their labor. The work histories of many groups employed in the secondary labor markets (composed of part-time, seasonal, or temporary employees) are replete with examples of exploitation, physical and psychological abuse, and working conditions that were not just unhealthy but sometimes actually incompatible with life. Even today in the Japanese culture, the word *Karoushi* refers to a sudden death from overwork (Tubbs 1993).

At times, this category of thought also described work as a duty and obligation. However, de Man (1929) found in his research that the Christian theology of the obligatory nature of work is a strong influence only in an indirect and unconscious way. It is not something verbalized in the workers' reports he analyzed (de Man 1929). Quite apart from the theological aspects, de Man did find that, although every kind of working activity contained elements that made it a delight, it also contained elements that make it a torment. He reviewed examples of the words used in various languages that relate work to difficulties and turmoil. According to de Man, these examples were:

> . . . not merely a legacy from the days when the social subordination of the worker made work degrading. Just as in the legend of the Fall, work is a symbol for punishment, so it lies in the nature of things that all work is felt to be coercive. Even the worker who is free in the social sense, the peasant or the handicraftsman, feels this compulsion, were it only because, while he is at work, his activities are dominated and determined by the aim of his work, by the idea of a willed or necessary creation. Work inevitably signifies subordination of the worker to remoter aims, felt to be necessary, and therefore involving a renunciation of the freedoms and the enjoyments of the present for the sake of a future advantage (de Man 1929, p. 67).

Such dignified yet irksome elements fall at opposing ends of the spectrum, but they can be seen in every piece of work. When the aim of work is one chosen voluntarily by the worker, work is seen as a sacrifice. When the aim is one imposed on the worker from an external source, work is more likely felt as punishment. Thus, according to de Man, every worker is both creator and slave. "Freedom of creation and compulsion of performance, ruling and being ruled, command and obedience, functioning as a subject and functioning as an object—these are the poles of a tension which is immanent in the very nature of work" (de Man 1929, p. 67).

Work as Vocation

Work as a vocation, the last category identified by Meilaender (2000), was articulated most clearly during the Protestant Reformation. This category is related to the belief that work is our calling, our vocation. People came to think that God's blessing sanctified their work and gave significance to it. Thus, no matter how menial their work might be, anyone could glorify God by doing his or her work joyfully and with dignity. "God gave man work, not to burden him, but to bless him, and useful work, willingly, cheerfully, effectively done, has always been the finest expression of the human spirit" (Walter R. Courtenay as quoted in Naylor [1996, p. 36]). Clearly, the idea of experiencing joy through work is a major construct in religious teachings and remains a contemporary message as well.

The idea of work as a calling is a powerful affirmation of daily life. Thinking of work as a vocation emphasizes that "work is a social activity contributing in some way to the good of all" (Meilaender 2000, p. 12). Applebaum points out that with Luther and Calvin we saw the beginnings of our modern-day work ethic, starting with "the concept of calling as a Christian duty, and the admonition to be successful in commercial enterprise, something which was looked down upon in the ancient and medieval world" (Applebaum 1992, p. 582). Interestingly, this new Protestant work ethic took two different directions. On the one hand, it promoted hard work and business enterprise while stressing thrift and business success. On the other hand, it stressed the need for respect of the working man, common ownership of land, and the redistribution of goods and services so that none would suffer. The first direction seems to support capitalism, whereas the second seems to support socialism.

The idea of work as vocation is often thought of in our contemporary world as social obligation. Dick Richards (1995a) examines our need as humans to bring passion and commitment to our work and to create workplaces that not only honor, but support these qualities. He addresses the meaning of work in terms of a sense of social obligation:

> All work creates something. Artfulness demands that we engage with the process of the work and with its product. The meaning of the work resides in the meaning of what we create. . . . We have a chance to work artfully when we believe that our work makes the world a better place (Richards 1995, pp. 35–36).

Work Is a Way to Fulfill Individual, Emotional, and Psychological Needs

Although Meilaender's work has provided a useful overview, there is another category of thought related to why people work. In our contemporary world, for at least part of the population, the meaning of work revolves around the desire to satisfy inherent human needs and motivations. "Work, if it has great significance for our lives, tends to be symbolic, having value for us because it helps to fulfill some human need other than work" (Naylor 1996, p. 46). This idea is a common theme in contemporary discussions and examinations of the meaning of work.

In 1994, Brian Dumaine wrote an article titled "Why Do We Work?" for *Fortune* magazine. In it he notes that if you ask people why they work, many people say it is to make money. Yet, he asks, if that is entirely true, how do you account for people continuing to work after winning the lottery or after having made enough money to retire? He notes that when Robert Weiss, a research professor at the University of Massachusetts, "asked people in a survey whether they'd work if they had inherited enough to live comfortably, roughly eight out of ten people said yes" (Dumaine 1994, p. 196).

More and more people today, especially among the baby boomers, "are looking to their work to satisfy some deeply individualistic, emotional and psychological need" (Dumaine 1994, p. 196). This is a recurring theme in the literature. In today's world, work is probably the most important single factor in status and self-respect for the individual, according to Applebaum (1992), who has studied the concept of work in ancient, medieval, and modern times. "The kind of work one performs, one's occupation, and one's employer are all indicators of the type of power and income which one can command and, with that, the type of consumption goods one can command" (Applebaum 1992, p. 286).

The idea that our work fills personal, emotional, and psychological needs is supported by the findings of de Man (1929), who in 1926 read seventy-eight autobiographical reports from workers in Germany. Although we might think these participants are worlds apart from people living in the year 2005, many of the themes and motivations identified are similar to our thinking today. The following needs are often fulfilled by contemporary work: a sense of self-identity and self-esteem; a capacity to contribute to wider society; a need for independence from the control of others; a need for social relationships; and a sense of achievement, competence, and intellectual accomplishment.

Self-Identity and Self-Esteem

A recurrent theme in the literature is the importance of work in forming individual self-identity. When de Man (1929) published his *Joy of Work*, he reported many examples and excerpts from the workers' autobiographies that illustrated this point:

> A smith (case 49), a man endowed with vigorous artistic impulses, says: "How much I had identified myself with the work I turned out, became clear to me whenever I had to hand it over. I felt that it really contained a part of my personality, and I was often on the verge of throwing up my job at the factory and of returning to handicraft" (de Man 1929, p. 38).

De Man went on to note that there was a wide tendency to associate a high valuation of one's occupation with a high valuation of one's self.

This is no less true today, and many of us define ourselves by the job or position we hold or the professional status we enjoy. Our identity is closely tied up with our work. The danger, of course, is when the job or work ends. In today's tumultuous business environment characterized by downsizing and layoffs, mergers and acquisitions, identifying oneself too closely with the organizations we work for can be quite risky.

In *Working*, Studs Terkel (1972) quotes an unemployed, forty-five-year-old construction worker expressing his frustration and discouragement: "Right now I can't really describe myself because . . . I'm unemployed. . . . So you see, I can't say who I am right now. . . . I guess a man's something else besides his work, isn't he? But what? I just don't know" (Terkel 1972, p. 44).

McKenna found this out the hard way. While she was writing *When Work Doesn't Work Anymore: Women Work and Identity*, her husband discovered that his job had been restructured off the organizational chart. "With a tap of the delete key much of who he was and much of what he cared for was wiped away. . . . I knew . . . that it was going to take a while for him to sort out the man and the work. It had been a long time since he'd had to" (McKenna 1997, p. 224).

Self-esteem is closely related to self-identity. It refers to the value we place on ourselves. Multiple authors identify the positive effects work has on an individual's self-esteem (Amott and Matthaei 1991; Applebaum 1992; Aptheker 1989; Bookman and Morgan 1988; de Man 1929; DeChick 1988; Erikson and Vallas 1990; Gould, Weiner, and Levin 1997; Greiff 1999; Grossman 1990; Hesse-Biber and Carter 2000; Josselson 1996; McKenna 1997; Naylor 1996; Schuster 1990;

Seiling 1997; Spencer 1982). There is significant evidence that working increases a woman's sense of well-being (Hesse-Biber 2000), and why should it be any different for men? Warren Bennis, a well-known leadership scholar, notes that "work really defines who you are. So much of a person's self-esteem is measured by success at work" (Dumaine 1994, paragraph 9).

In his book, *Joy: 20 Years Later*, Schutz's description of joy closely relates to his own self-esteem. Although Schutz's work is based on personal experience rather that on systematic research, the connection with joy and self-esteem is worth noting here:

> Joy is the feeling that comes from the fulfillment of my potential. Fulfillment brings to me the feeling that I can cope with my environment; the sense of confidence in myself as a significant, competent, lovable person who is capable of handling situations as they arise, able to use fully my own capacities, and free to express my feelings. Joy requires a vital, alive body, self-contentment, productive and satisfying relations with others, and a successful relation to society (Schutz 1989, p. 11).

Contribution to Society

The desire to make a difference, to be part of something bigger than oneself, and to contribute to the wider society has been identified by many investigators as a driving factor in finding meaning in the workplace today. This idea is related to Meilaender's (2000) concept of work as cocreation. Based on his research, Terez reports that virtually all people have a driving desire to make a difference (Terez 1999). "Believing your work can make a real difference in the world has motivated many people over the years" (Dumaine 1994, paragraph 17). This theme is found in several of the studies examining workers' experiences of joy (Worthington 1994; DiSciullo 1997). "As a therapist, she experiences joy in seeing her clients growing and developing skills to handle their life better" (DiSciullo 1997).

Independence from the Control of Others

Independence from the control of others is related to increased competence as well as to earning capacity based on the work (Hesse-Biber and Carter 2000; McKenna 1997). Especially for women, who in prior times were completely dependent on their husbands or fathers for their income and financial assets, the ability to earn produces a powerful sense of independence. Independence also increases an individual's sense of personal satisfaction as well.

Independence, however, also has a shadow side. As Durning (1993, paragraph 15) notes:

> Members of the consumer class enjoy a degree of personal independence unprecedented in human history, [and] yet hand in hand comes a decline in our attachments to each other. Informal visits between neighbors and friends, family conversation, and time spent at family meals have all diminished in the United States since mid-century.

In fact, affluence has "broken the bonds of mutual assistance that adversity once forged" (Durning 1993, paragraph 14).

Social Relationships

Work is a key source of social relationships. Schuster (1990) studied gifted women at at the University of California Los Angeles. The women came from a range of socioeconomic backgrounds. In her interviews with the women, Schuster sought to determine what characterized the essence of work for them, what aspects of their careers gave meaning and value to their lives. According to Schuster (1990, p. 204):

> For nearly all the gifted women—regardless of their technical competence, their creative ability, the nature of their work, their income, or their level of "success"—the issue of interactive communication stood out as the most salient characteristic of their work lives. In nearly three-quarters of the interviews, the gifted women described themselves, their achievements, and their sense of professional well-being in terms of relationships.

This observation is supported by the work of several other authors in the same volume. The experience of a woman's relationships in the workplace is central to the meaning that her work has in her life (Grossman 1990). Although there is evidence that women are more relationally oriented than men (Gilligan 1982; Miller 1976), the importance of relationships in the workplace does not seem to be a gender-specific issue. The value of work relationships is further emphasized by Applebaum (1992), who notes that work is still a major arena for social interaction. Even when people do not find satisfaction in their work, they often enjoy the social contacts they make at work.

Achievement, Competence, and Accomplishment

For many people, the value of their work lies in the sense of achievement and accomplishment that accompanies it. Dumaine (1994, p. 204) points out that work is a source of feedback and recognition related to this achievement. "Psychologists say few of us have the inner resources to live without constant and meaningful praise." And, in fact, several participants in DiSciullo's (1997) research identified feedback from their work as a source of joy. McKenna (1997) interviewed many women who focused their expectations for fulfillment and recognition largely on their careers. Greiff (1999) suggests that for many work represents the single most important source of accomplishment and intellectual satisfaction. A sense of capability and competence is also critical, and it is closely related to intellectual stimulation.

Historical Changes in the Meaning of Work

Ample evidence supports the idea that the meaning of work has undergone significant change since the advent of the Industrial Revolution in the mid-nineteenth century. As the United States along with other westernized countries moved away from the predominantly agricultural societies of earlier centuries, the meaning of work in our lives was significantly altered. Similarly, the societal changes that began in the mid-twentieth century with the application of modern computer and communications technologies will continue to affect our understanding of what work means for the foreseeable future.

Emergence of Industrialization and Capitalism

Throughout history, the context and location of work has varied. In the early days, work took place in the home and the community. With the decline of the agrarian age and the advent of the Industrial Age, for the first time in our history work moved into large factories and buildings where people came together to do their work. This remarkable change had many ramifications for society, all of which have been documented elsewhere. With the rise of capitalism and the formation of early bureaucracies, the voices and concerns of Karl Marx and Max Weber became prominent.

Marx believed that work is of prime and absolute importance to humans. "Man's essential activity is his work" (Applebaum 1992, p. 584). Marx argued that work went *beyond* irksome; that is, workers in an industrial society become alienated from their work because capitalism, in particular, dehumanizes the workers' relationship to their work. As workers become objects of work and an instrumental part of work processes, feelings of alienation become inevitable.

This viewpoint was contradicted by de Man, who found that "'mechanised work' and 'work at the machine' are not the same thing. Among those who experience the highest joy in work, . . . most of them are among the far more numerous machine workers, who, feeling themselves to be masters and overseers of the machines, have not the same reason to dread repetitive work" (de Man 1929, p. 112). In his study of German workers, de Man found that although the majority of those he studied were Marxian socialists, their personal experience was quite different from Marxian theory. In fact, for many workers, he found that working in industrial settings and learning the skills needed to master the machinery resulted in increased self-esteem and pride.

Introduction of Scientific Management

As the Industrial Age progressed and the continuing impact of mechanization became evident, so did another major change: the introduction of scientific management techniques. The writings of Frederick W. Taylor, a mechanical engineer, emphasized the importance of productivity and efficiency and were widely applied in business and industrial settings during the early twentieth century. Taylor's principles of scientific management included the following:

- Specialization of work into narrow jobs
- Precise and minute specification of jobs
- Constant repetition of tasks by the same workers
- Lack of a need for any judgment or discretion on the part of workers

With the advent of Taylor's scientific management methods and the institution of assembly-line organization of work, the deskilling of workers began. As work tasks were reduced to simple, repetitive, and monotonous tasks, much of the joy of work (as least in the industrial sector) disappeared. Therefore, although Marxian theory seemed to have been contradicted by de Man's work, an explanation for discrepancy is apparent. De Man was reporting on the early effects of mechanization, when workers' lives were made easier by the machinery and workers gained a sense of mastery that increased their self-esteem. However, as the machines became more sophisticated and easier to operate, monotony set in. Many studies and writings of the day reported widespread dissatisfaction with work in industrial society. Soon work was seen as an "instrumental activity, as a means for acquiring income for subsistence and consumption, and that there [was] little or no satisfaction or meaning to be found in the workplace" (Applebaum 1992, p. 586).

Application of Bureaucratic Organizational Structures

Not only has capitalism and the continual pursuit of material goods affected the meaning of our work, but changes in the structure of the organizations in which work is carried out has also had an impact. In the late nineteenth century, industrialized organizations were characterized by despotic management practices based on nepotism, political favoritism, and institutionalized corruption (Nadler 1997). The bureaucratic model was developed as a reaction to the subjugation and cruel treatment of workers and the subjective decision making that characterized the managerial practices of the early Industrial Revolution (Bennis 1966).

The notion of bureaucracy was first articulated by Max Weber, a German sociologist, around the beginning of the twentieth century. At the time, bureaucracy was considered a radical idea and represented a remarkable advance over the traditional management practices of the time. Precursor structures were based on the arbitrary application of patrimonial authority. Weber believed that a modern bureaucracy "formulated on rational legal precepts was capable of sweeping other forms of organization before it" (Clegg 1990, p. 35).

Weber's bureaucracy was a management design based on formalized procedures, clear chains of command in the management hierarchy, and staffing decisions based on merit and technical expertise. The basic precepts of this design include:

- Division of labor based on functional specialization
- Well-defined hierarchies of authority
- Systems of rules that dictate the rights and duties of employees
- Established procedures for dealing with specific work situations
- Interpersonal relationships characterized by impersonality
- Promotion and selection practices based on technical competence

Meaning of Work in Contemporary Society

The simultaneous convergence of these three factors—capitalism, scientific management, and bureaucratic organizational structure—heavily influenced the way we perceive the meaning of work today. The contributions of Weber and Taylor combined to result in the emergence of a new organizational structure, the machine bureaucracy. This new structure perfectly fed the goals of capitalism. Productivity gains were enormous, and this structure became the dominant design of both industry and large corporations. It has been so prevalent that most managers have "grown up" with this model firmly and completely embedded in their approach to organizational design. Health care workers have been heavily socialized in the model of the professional bureaucracy, which has many of the same characteristics as the machine bureaucracy. The only difference is that the professional bureaucracy is based on a professional model rather than a business model. Over time, however, Weber became extremely concerned about the dehumanizing aspects of the bureaucracy and its impact on the creativity and free expression of the humans who worked within.

The bureaucracy is still the predominant structure in many sectors of society (health care, education, finance, manufacturing, and government, for example). Morgan has traced the proliferation of multinational conglomerates, and he suggests that they are at least one example of the impact of an accelerated pace of mergers resulting in megacompanies that will significantly impact our lives in the future (Morgan 1998).

Clearly, bureaucratic structure has an impact on the meaning we derive from our work. The negative impact of increasingly massive and complex bureaucracies on the average worker is a common and repetitive theme in the current business literature (Waterman 1990; Tushman and O'Reilly 1999; Stacey 1992; Snow, Liprack, and Stamps 1999; Silberstang 1995; Sievers 1993; Seiling 1997; Ryan and Oestreich 1991; Reina and Reina 1999; Pinchot and Pinchot 1994; Morgan 1998; Manion 1995; Hock 1999; Hirschhorn 1997; Helgesen 1995; Gowing, Kraft, and Quick 1998; Gould, Weiner, and Levin 1997; Denhardt 1981; Bowles 1991, 1997; Bennis 1970).

In addition, the attitude that work is only performed for money is still prevalent today and has become a significant issue in health care. McKenna is one of the most eloquent contemporary authors to discuss this subject. In the mid-1990s, she surveyed and interviewed almost 1200 women about their work. Many reported a strong sense of dissatisfaction when they discovered they had basically created a level of consumption expectation that required continued feeding. One individual noted: "We quickly found that going to work also meant *having* to work. Quite apart from whether we wanted to or not—and most of us did—it just was a shock how quickly choice became necessity" (McKenna 1997, p. 27). In other words, the women's additional income raised the standard of living obtainable and soon became an expectation and "need" rather than a choice that provided discretionary funds. Another participant in McKenna's study noted that her dissatisfaction began when she realized that she and her husband both needed to work simply to maintain their standard of living. For many Americans, especially those who exist in one of the labor markets *other* than the upper tier of the primary segment, work is mostly about making a living, although the real living goes on after work hours.

One of McKenna's participants was articulate in describing the impact of increasing bureaucracy on her work life. As a woman in the publishing field, she had a long career marked by increasing success. However, as the years passed, the organization for which she worked became larger and larger through mergers and acquisitions. Jane told this story:

> When I was twenty-two, I worked for the editor-in-chief, who, in turn, worked for the head of the company. Twenty-two years later I was a vice president and editor-in-chief of a seventy-nine-million-dollar division. I worked for a president and publisher who, in turn, worked for a group president who worked for a CEO for the group who worked for a corporate executive vice president who worked for. . . . You get the picture.
>
> [For Jane it signaled the end of the community and therefore the end of communal purpose.] The work became increasingly purposeless. I didn't want to move on to the next level. I liked what I did and was happy doing what I was doing, but I just didn't want to be doing it in an increasingly meaningless way. I couldn't devote enough attention. . . . I really felt I wasn't doing it any better, I was just doing it thinner. I was more spread out (McKenna 1997, p. 33).

Will this trend continue into the coming age of knowledge? Will knowledge workers (those who possess and develop highly specialized technical knowledge) experience less satisfaction when computer programs begin taking over decision making and the synthesis of data and the all-important process of converting data into useful information?

Creation of a Positive Workplace

Throughout time a great deal of thought has been devoted to the question of why people work. The readings were reviewed in this chapter in an attempt to provoke a wider range of thinking on the part of leaders in our contemporary organizations. When we understand the deeper, more compelling reasons people work, we may have more to consider in terms of influencing them in the direction of the organization. This extensive examination may be achieved most practically by considering Ken Thomas's work on intrinsic motivation.

Motivation is what makes us do what we do. It is the underlying energy that compels action in a particular direction. Intrinsic motivators are those forces within an individual that cause the person to act. Intrinsic motivators are of primary importance to leaders in organizations because the motivators exist independent of the leaders' actions. In other words, when an employee is intrinsically motivated to do what needs to be done, the leader's presence is of secondary importance. What we want in our workforce are people who know what needs to be done and want to do it. Such people are going to do the right thing whether the manager is standing there or not. When leaders understand the intrinsic motivators that drive employee performance, they can reinforce these powerful factors by their leadership actions, thus increasing the impact in the workplace.

Thomas, in *Intrinsic Motivation at Work: Building Energy and Commitment* (2000), offers a solid conceptual framework for understanding the intrinsic motivators. He also offers a compelling case for their contribution and importance in today's work world. "The new work role is more psychologically demanding in terms of its complexity and judgment, and requires a much deeper level of commitment. While economic rewards were pretty good for buying compliance, gaining commitment is a far different matter" (Thomas 2000, p. 5). He clearly believes that external motivators (such as money and benefits) are no longer enough to compel workers to act. When intrinsic motivators are present, individuals are more likely to feel energized and vitally connected to their work. Much of the work on intrinsic motivation is further substantiated by recent work in the field of positive psychology, which is discussed in chapter 4.

Thomas (2000) developed a model for creating a work environment that engages employees and taps into their creative potential. His work is based on the premise that a positive workplace leads to increased positive energy and commitment on the part of employee–colleagues. Thomas's work is worth noting here because he based his conclusions on an extensive review of the psychological, sociological, and organizational development literature.

Based on his research and experience, Thomas identifies four things that people find intrinsically motivating. These include meaningful work, choices in carrying out that work, a sense of competence, and the ability to make progress toward reaching desired outcomes. My own research and reading compels me to add another factor, the presence of healthy relationships.

Under this framework, leadership interventions become clear. Managers need to inspire and focus employees on the meaning of their work, create choices for the workers, coach for continual development and competence, and ensure that progress occurs and can be measured. In addition, managers have a responsibility to focus on the quality of relationships in the workplace. (See figure 2-2.)

Application of Intrinsic Motivators at the Organizational Level

The following subsections will examine each of four intrinsic motivators with special emphasis on their application in today's health care organizations.

Focus on the Meaningfulness of the Work

"People have a desire to be engaged in meaningful work—to be doing something they experience as worthwhile and fulfilling" (Thomas 2000, p. 12). For many of us, our work is composed of tasks that serve a particular end or accomplish a specific purpose. When we are clear about what the purpose is, we can make intelligent decisions about the work. Rather than seeing work as a necessary evil or something that costs us in a substantial way, work itself is meaningful and rewarding.

Figure 2-2. **Leadership Strategies Based on the Fulfillment of Intrinsic Motivators**

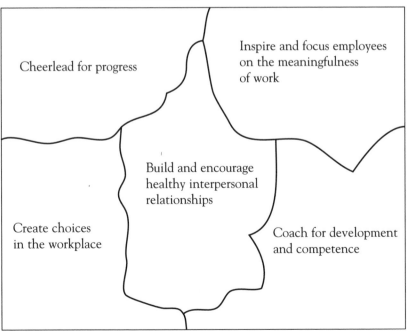

Cheerlead for progress

Inspire and focus employees on the meaningfulness of work

Build and encourage healthy interpersonal relationships

Create choices in the workplace

Coach for development and competence

For example, a second-career nurse was interviewed for a research project and asked about her experience of joy through her work. At the time of the study, the nurse was employed in the outpatient recovery area of a diagnostic center. Over the course of the interview, she casually mentioned that after four years as a nurse, she was nearing the salary level she had reached in her manufacturing job before she entered nursing school. When asked about the higher-paying job in manufacturing, the nurse indicated that she would never return to manufacturing even though the money was better. She was committed to her work as a nurse because she believed she made a difference for every patient she helped. In her words, our world "can live without chrome bumpers for our cars," but it could not survive without someone to care for the sick and injured (Manion 2002). To her, the meaningfulness of her work far outweighed any financial considerations.

Because by its very nature, health care encompasses some of the most meaningful work known to humankind—the care of the sick and vulnerable—it is easy to conclude that health care work is inherently meaningful. Leaders and managers may be tempted to think that no specific action need be taken to enhance the meaning of health care work for their employees. Such an assumption, however, would be counterproductive for several reasons.

First of all, many individuals who work in health care organizations perform such a narrow part of the organization's work that they may not see how their work is connected to the well-being of patients. Examples of such workers include the messengers who deliver patient mail, the maintenance men who paint the walls, the housekeepers who empty the trash, and the collection clerk who handles patient accounts in the business office. Managers can help all types of employees understand the contributions they make to patient care and the importance of their work. In addition, health care workers who work directly with patients can share their stories with those who work behind the front lines as a means of inspiring others.

Second, leaders along with employees must be continually alert to events or situations that indicate that the organization is not living up to its stated mission and values. When organizational decisions and behaviors contradict what employees believe to be the mission of the organization, the resulting dissonance can severely impact the employees' sense of meaning. (This subject will be considered more fully in chapter 3.)

Finally, especially in today's organizations, managers must continually seek to reduce the amount of unnecessary work that creeps into jobs. Few health care workers chose their field because they wanted to spend half of their time documenting and recording what it was that they did. Increased regulation in health care has resulted in an increased focus on paperwork and compliance with arbitrarily established rules, often at the cost of time spent in the delivery of the actual service in the department (AHA 2001). Add to this dissatisfaction the amount of duplicative work, and you can see that we are rapidly reaching the point where health care workers will begin to believe that meaningless requirements have replaced the meaningful work in their jobs.

Create Choices

A sense of choice related to tasks or responsibilities comes along with the feeling that your views, ideas, and insights are important. Choice also involves the feeling of ownership when we feel personally responsible for the outcomes of our behaviors or decisions. "Choice takes on extra importance when we are committed to a meaningful purpose. Then a sense of choice means being able to do what makes sense to you to accomplish the purpose" (Thomas 2000, p. 65).

A manager in today's workplace may have little control over the individual's initial choice to be there, in other words, whether the person must work or not. However, as we will see in the next chapter on organizational commitment, choice is crucial for ensuring that people feel engaged and committed to their work. A freely made choice to work or to be employed in a particular organization is instrumental in employees' feelings of commitment. Beyond this, however, leaders and managers have a great deal of control over this intrinsic motivator.

Shared decision making, empowerment, and delegation are common ways to increase each employee's ability to make choices in their work. Giving people the authority to make decisions that fall within their scope of responsibility and trusting them to do so are important leadership behaviors. Creating a climate characterized by a nonblaming, positive response to mistakes is another way we encourage employees to make decisions and show initiative.

Coach for Competence

"You have a sense of competence on a task when you feel that you are performing your work activities well—when your performance of those activities is meeting or exceeding your own standards" (Thomas 2000, p. 77). Most of us are more likely to enjoy work at which we are good. Seligman (2002) defines authentic happiness as knowing what our signature strengths are and then crafting a life that uses these strengths in all aspects of our lives, including work. In other words, we are more likely to be happy when we are engaged in work that taps into our abilities and is a reflection of our competence.

Csikszentmihalyi (1990, 1997, 2003) has done extensive research on the concept of flow. He defines flow as an optimal experience that is the unintended side benefit of engaging in activities during which we are stretched to our limits by challenges that are worthwhile. It includes both a sense of mastery and a sense of involvement or participation in an event. "Flow is the state in which people are so involved in an activity that nothing else seems to matter; the experience itself is so enjoyable that people will do it even at great cost, for the sheer sake of doing it" (Csikszentmihalyi 1990, p. 4). Competence is an important element of this concept, because flow requires us to stretch but not exceed our abilities. When a task does not challenge us, boredom or apathy rather than flow is the result. But when the challenge exceeds our ability to master it, frustration is the outcome.

The potential ramifications of personal competence in health care work are enormous. The role of the leader as coach is to help followers increase their level of competence, whether technical or interpersonal. Providing opportunities and learning resources, emphasizing individual growth, and ensuring an organizational philosophy of continuous learning are all important.

Selecting the right person for the right work and helping individuals reframe work that does not use their competencies or signature strengths are also crucial. According to Buckingham and Coffman (1999, p. 148), "casting is everything. . . . If you want to turn talent into performance, you have to position each person so that you are paying her to do what she is naturally wired to do. You have to cast her in the right role."

This message is reinforced by Jim Collins's research into why some organizations are able to make the leap from being good performers to exceptional performers while others are not. "The executives who ignited the transformations from good to great did not first figure out where to drive the bus and then get people to take it there. No, they *first* got the right people on the bus (and the wrong people off the bus) and *then* figured out where to drive it" (Collins 2001, p. 41). Furthermore, in determining who the right people are, exceptional organizations place greater emphasis on character attributes than on specific experience or education (Collins 2001; Manion 2004b). It is not that specific skills or knowledge are not important. Exceptional leaders know that skills and knowledge are teachable whereas character traits are ingrained.

Crafting work that fits an individual is another aspect of the manager's role. Loehr and Schwartz (2003) describe their extensive experience in coaching sports athletes as well as corporate athletes (their term for performers in the work world). They share example after example of individuals with whom they have worked who came to them for coaching because they were exhausted and nearly depleted of energy. These people had lost a sense of connection and competence in their work. Sorting through what it is that they are extremely good at is a key aspect of redefining the work so that it engages a person's full capabilities (Loehr and Schwartz 2003; Seligman 2002).

Another potential role of the leader is in creating work environments that are more likely to lead to optimal experience or flow on the part of employees. Flow is also described as engagement. In fact, when we are in flow, we are so engaged that we do not even notice time passing. A quick examination of most health care workplaces reveals multiple barriers to the experience of flow. Endless interruptions, the need to be in constant contact with the rest of the world as evidenced by the preponderance of beepers and cell phones, the never-ending bombardment of overhead announcements, environmental noise, and e-mails are just a few examples of interruptions that break or prevent flow.

An important payoff when employees work with a sense of their own competence is that it leads to the emotion of pride. In an interview about his latest book, *Why Pride Matters More Than Money*, Katzenbach (2003) said that "it's more important for people to be proud of what they are doing every day than it is for them to be proud of reaching a major goal. That's why it's crucial to celebrate the 'steps' as much as the 'landings.' The best pride builders are masters at spotting and recognizing the small achievements that will instill pride in their people" (Byrne 2003, p. 66). Feeling pride is not to be mistaken for acting prideful in the sense of arrogance. It represents the positive emotion that accompanies personal accomplishment.

Recognize and Celebrate Progress

Another strong intrinsic motivator is a sense of progress. A feeling of having made progress occurs when you feel like your activities have had the impact that you intended, when you see that your work is achieving its purpose. Little is more discouraging than the feeling that nothing has changed as a result of our efforts and hard work. When we see progress, we find a sense of momentum and enthusiasm, and the energy to continue our work becomes available to us.

An ancient Greek legend portrays the exquisite torture of a being for whom meaningful work is an inherent part of his nature. According to the legend, as punishment for an offense against the gods, Sisyphus is doomed to push a large boulder up to the top of a hill and then stand aside and let the boulder roll back down to the bottom of the hill. Then his work begins again as he pushes the same boulder to the top of the same hill over and over again for all of eternity.

The research on what brings people joy in their work clearly indicates that seeing results and making progress are essential for most people (de Man 1929; Manion 2002, 2003). The ramifications for health care leaders are multifold. Barriers to progress within our systems need to be analyzed and removed. For too many years we have tolerated the same problems in our systems. Implementing an effective process improvement approach is not just the latest consulting fad or organizational culture change; it is crucial if employees and managers alike are going to have the tools to make both incremental and substantial changes in our systems. The responsibility for true process improvement must be shared by both employees and managers. (Chapter 10 explores approaches for getting results and making progress.)

Systems for measuring progress are also critical to support this motivator. Without such systems, managers and employees find it difficult to track their progress and recognize their results. Such accountability systems are notoriously weak in health care organizations. For example, even with the current emphasis and focus on the leader's responsibility in recruitment and retention, few health care managers have access to department-specific measures of vacancy and turnover rates or measurements of satisfaction among patients, employees, and physicians. Yet, department managers are being held accountable for outcomes in areas where measurements are inadequate or so outdated as to be useless.

A final consideration for leaders is how they can recognize and reward progress. Progress that is not recognized goes by unacknowledged. For example, in the late 1990s, a hospital in the Southeast was positioning itself to become part of a larger health care system. In order to appear as financially viable as possible, each segment of the system was asked to make a substantial contribution in the form of reducing their operating expenses. In the organization's large home health agency, the managers were expected to reduce their operating expenses by $1.5 million over the next year. These managers were exceptional leaders who worked closely with their employees in order to achieve this result. The employees were instrumental in designing and implementing a workforce reduction that was well received. In only nine months, a reduction of $1.2 million was achieved.

Subsequently, the two managers were called to a meeting with the system's chief executive officer and chief financial officer to report on their progress. For an hour, the executives badgered, questioned, and basically harangued the two department managers looking for a way to make the remaining $300,000 in cuts. No mention was made of the progress they had achieved, nor were any commendations offered for the exemplary way the initial results had been obtained. You can imagine the level of interest and motivation that these two managers felt when they left the meeting. In fact, both left the organization within six months.

The studies on happiness also support Thomas's conclusion regarding meaning and progress. "Happiness grows less from the passive experience of desirable circumstances than from involvement in valued activities and *progress toward one's goals* [italics mine]" (Myers and Diener 1995). These conclusions and recommendations reinforce directly the idea that work has meaning for us because it creates opportunities for achievement and competence.

Celebrating and recognizing progress is not as easy as it sounds. We have natural reservations about celebrating too early, and some of us may believe that we do not have enough time during our busy days to celebrate. However, people pay attention to what we emphasize, and celebrations let people know what the organization considers really important.

Support Healthy Relationships

It is clear that people are more highly motivated to perform in a particular way when they have positive, healthy relationships with others in the workplace. It is very unlikely that employees will go the extra mile for coworkers whom they actively dislike or for whom they feel no respect. Research in positive psychology supports this assertion. (Healthy working relationships are examined more fully in chapter 6.) At this point, it is enough to point out that the establishment of positive relationships and a sense of connection to the people in our work environment lead to a higher level of intrinsic motivation.

Application of Intrinsic Motivators at the Individual Level

Understanding and applying the key intrinsic motivators are essential for every leader who wants to influence individual behavior. Understanding this model is also helpful for individual employees because it can help us make better choices about our work. Most of us work in some form of gainful employment throughout the decades of our adult lives. For some of us, work is just a job, a way to earn money in order to do other things or meet our personal needs. Many people see their work as a career, and throughout the years they continue to accumulate skills and achievements as a result of that work. Seeking promotions and new work opportunities is part of the process. When that upward progress is halted, the enjoyment of work is often lost and careers end. Yet for others, their work is more of a calling, work that is done for other reasons. Such people would do the work and enjoy it even in the absence of more traditional extrinsic rewards such as financial benefits or the recognition and adulation of others.

Throughout our years in the work world, we all reach crossroads that make us wonder whether we should stay with a particular job or move on. Understanding the five intrinsic motivators provides an approach for considering and thinking about the decision.

As shown in figure 2-3, there are specific questions that we can ask to help us decide whether our current work situations continue to meet our needs. Sorting these questions by the intrinsic motivators may help

Figure 2-3.   Using Intrinsic Motivators to Answer the Question: Should I Stay or Should I Go?

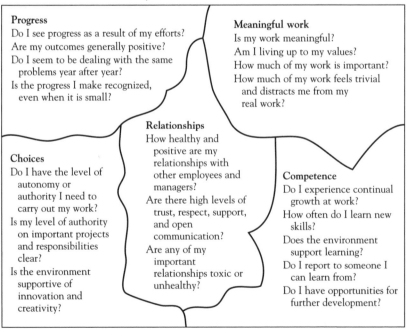

Progress
Do I see progress as a result of my efforts?
Are my outcomes generally positive?
Do I seem to be dealing with the same problems year after year?
Is the progress I make recognized, even when it is small?

Meaningful work
Is my work meaningful?
Am I living up to my values?
How much of my work is important?
How much of my work feels trivial and distracts me from my real work?

Relationships
How healthy and positive are my relationships with other employees and managers?
Are there high levels of trust, respect, support, and open communication?
Are any of my important relationships toxic or unhealthy?

Choices
Do I have the level of autonomy or authority I need to carry out my work?
Is my level of authority on important projects and responsibilities clear?
Is the environment supportive of innovation and creativity?

Competence
Do I experience continual growth at work?
How often do I learn new skills?
Does the environment support learning?
Do I report to someone I can learn from?
Do I have opportunities for further development?

individuals focus on key issues. The answers to the questions range along a continuum, as shown in figure 2-4. Plotting our location on the continuum can give us a visual picture of what our current situations are like. It then becomes easier to determine whether there is a clear pattern or a mix of high and low responses. When you see where my responses are placed, you can ask yourself the following questions:

- Is there anything I can do about the ratings that are low?
- Can I influence these lower ratings in any way?
- Which are within my scope of responsibility?
- Which of these are a high priority for me?

Conclusion

Our understanding of work has undergone change over the centuries. Throughout history, the meaning of work as proposed by the thinkers of the time has revolved around work as cocreation, work as necessary for leisure, work as dignified but irksome, and work as a calling. Today, one of the predominant ways we view the meaning of our work is related to meeting the highly individual, emotional, and psychological needs of each employee. Many answers to the question about why people work are clearly interrelated, and any given individual is likely to identify several factors as motivating. The reasons for working manifest

Figure 2-4. Self-Assessment of Current Job in Terms of Intrinsic Motivators

Where am I?

My relationships are toxic	1 2 3 4 5 6 My relationships are healthy
My work is meaningless	1 2 3 4 5 6 My work is meaningful
Opportunities are scarce	1 2 3 4 5 6 Opportunities are plentiful
Choices are limited	1 2 3 4 5 6 Choices are extensive
Progress is minimal	1 2 3 4 5 6 Progress is frequent and apparent
Work is painful and difficult	1 2 3 4 5 6 Experiencing joy at work is common

differently in each individual, and they are likely to change according to life stage, circumstances, and sociocultural perspective.

Clearly, organizational leaders as well as employees who understand the meaning of work in an individual's life are more likely to use this knowledge to build a strong, supportive work environment. And, when the workplace fails to support any of the five intrinsic motivators (the need for meaningful work, choice and autonomy, competency, progress, and healthy working relationships) are missing, it is clear that what is left to motivate us is *only* the financial rewards of working. To the degree that jobs are interchangeable, if I can easily replace this job with another that is similar, financial rewards are not very satisfying. Atchinson (2003) notes that a common mistake of health care leaders is to try a quick-fix approach for improving employee morale and motivation rather than focusing on the deeper issues.

Conversation Points

Organizational Perspective

1. Does the organization have initiatives that support the intrinsic motivators?
2. Are the organization's actions and philosophies related to employee motivation congruent with each other?
3. Does the organizational culture build on the intrinsic motivators? For example, are stories shared about meeting the mission that inspire others and increase the sense of pride employees feel? Are there organizational structures to enhance employee competence such as a strong educational department, career counseling services, and so on?

Leadership Issues

1. Examine your own beliefs about why people work. Do you have any employees for whom you think the primary motivator is money? Is there anything you can influence in this situation? How can you build on the intrinsic motivators in your department?
2. What is the level of autonomy you expect of employees in your department? Do you transfer responsibility to employees?
3. Do you ask your employees about their individual challenges? Do you know what their aspirations and hopes are?

4. Do employees in your department feel a sense of pride and meaningfulness about their work?
5. How actively do you coach employees?

Employee Challenges

1. What is the meaning of work in your life? Beyond the obvious (it pays the bills), what is the deeper meaning of work in your life?
2. Have you ever worked in a job where you felt like the work was meaningless? Did this make it difficult to go to work? What was the impact on your feelings about the job?
3. Do you feel like you have an appropriate level of decision-making authority for you to do your work well? What could you do if you felt like it was inadequate?
4. Is personal competence a motivator for you? Is it important that you are highly skilled and capable in your work? Think of times you did not feel competent or capable in your work. How did this affect your motivation for going to work?
5. How do you help others in the workplace increase their competency levels? Are you involved in coaching your coworkers?
6. How do you see progress in your workplace as a result of your efforts?

3

Building Organizational Commitment

Jo Manion

*Commitment is the will of the mind to finish what the heart
has begun long after the emotion in which
that promise was made has passed.*
—J. Maxwell (2003)

WHAT KEEPS people at work once they get there? Understanding
the intrinsic motivators helps us to recognize the factors that are
important to employees. Ensuring that individuals are able to fulfill these
intrinsic needs in the workplace increases the likelihood of employee commitment to the organization. Organizational commitment is another area
to explore in understanding how to create positive workplaces. In previous decades, most organizations followed a traditional command-and-
control approach to management in which employees were expected
to do as they were directed without question. At best, compliance was
the outcome. Compliance, however, often is not enough in today's
complex and challenging work environment (Thomas 2000). Today,
the role of leadership requires building a workforce among whom commitment is strong. For this reason, the concept of commitment is
explored thoroughly in this chapter. The more understanding and
knowledge we have about how commitments are made and what we
can to do influence the process, the more likely it is that we will be able
to use targeted approaches for creating a positive work environment.

Leadership is more than influencing others to follow a specific direction; it is creating a desire in the followers to do so (Manion 2005).
Although it is difficult or even impossible to teach people how to build
commitment through reading and classroom work, a thorough understanding of the concept reveals several specific steps that can be taken
by leaders to increase the level of employee commitment.

This chapter is adapted from Jo Manion, Strengthening Organizational Commitment, *The Health Care Manager* 23(4). Copyright © 2004 and used by permission of Lippincott Williams & Wilkins.

Peter Senge (1990, p. 10) describes the importance of commitment shared by leaders and followers when he writes about leading learning organizations: "We have seen no examples where significant progress has been made without leadership from local line managers, and many examples where sincerely committed CEOs have failed to generate any significant momentum." In other words, no leader accomplishes a major change or program initiative alone; it requires a vital partnership with followers, all working in concert to carry out the plan.

In this chapter, I make liberal use of the term *leader* in recognition of the fact that both managers and employees function in leadership roles. Leadership roles are often assumed in organizations without the benefit of managerial authority. In fact, a key way that employee–leaders influence people without the benefit of legitimate authority is through the approaches discussed in this chapter.

Compliance versus Commitment

In the past, when formal managers were considered the primary source of leadership in the organization and the command-and-control methodology was still acceptable, compliance seemed fairly easy to attain. Employees were simply told what to do, and they were expected to acquiesce regardless of their own opinions or ideas. Basically, compliance means conformance. People do what they have been directed or asked to do. There may be very little personal involvement. In contrast, commitment is a personal pledge to a position or issue. It requires giving oneself in trust to the issue or solution. In other words, compliance is a matter of the mind, but commitment is a matter of the heart.

Two factors in today's environment make mere compliance inadequate. The first is the nature of the workforce. A clear majority of today's health care workers are mature and experienced professionals, and they feel more involved in their work than ever. Second, the changes occurring in health care delivery are no longer mere tweaks in the system; they are fundamental, complex alterations to the very way service is delivered. For this deep level of change to be successful, more than mere compliance is required from the individuals who are expected to implement the changes.

Understanding the underpinnings of personal and organizational commitment is crucial for the leaders working in today's health care business environment. Accelerating change, developing organizational challenges and crises, increasing workforce shortages, and mounting environmental pressures make the need for committed and fully engaged employees more critical than ever.

Commitment Defined

Commitment is the act of pledging or engaging oneself. To commit is defined as binding or obligating oneself as in committing to a promise, a certain course of action, or even another person.

Concept of Commitment

A review of the classic literature on organizational development sheds further light on the concept. Brickman and his colleagues studied commitment extensively and report that it is "a force that stabilizes individual behavior under circumstances where the individual would otherwise be tempted to change that behavior. . . . Commitment is whatever it is that makes a person engage or continue in a course of action when difficulties or positive alternatives influence the person to abandon the effort" (Brickman, Wortman, and Sorrentino 1987, p. 2).

We see commitment in the workplace daily when people remain at work despite unpleasant or rapidly deteriorating conditions. All of us can remember days when everything seemed to go wrong and we would rather have been somewhere, anywhere, else. It is our commitment that kept us at work.

The early work of Rosabeth Moss Kanter (1972) included a study of thirty American utopian communities. The purpose of the study was to determine whether their commitment practices were related to their chances of success. Contrary to a prevalent notion at the time that utopian communities existed for people who wanted the freedom to do their own thing, Kanter found a general tendency for the most stable and successful communes to spend more time and effort instilling commitment in their members. In other words, they made an effort to ensure that their members acted in ways beneficial to the community.

Commitment contains a directional element (Trigg 1973). An individual can never just be committed; one must be committed to something or someone. Commitments are not free-floating; they are attached to a person or a thing. There is also a strong evaluative element implied in commitment. In other words, people must believe in the truth and inherent value of that to which they commit themselves. Commitment indicates a belief that an organization or a job is a good one and that it is worth supporting and important in some way. People do not commit to organizations that they believe are trivial, deceitful, or potentially corrupt. They make a judgment about an organization or job in light of their values.

Every individual has certain beliefs, and commitment involves a personal dedication to the actions implied by those beliefs. Therefore, commitment is more than belief; it is a belief strong enough to actu-ally *compel* action. To illustrate this observation, consider the example of membership in a professional association. Members of the profession obviously evidence differing levels of commitment to their profes-sional association. One professional may believe that the association advances the profession, which is of value, but she may choose not to join and support the association. In this case, there would be no action and thus no commitment even though the association's value is recognized. Another professional may join the association and pay dues, but he may not participate on committees and task forces or attend local membership meetings. In contrast, a third professional may choose to become an active member of the association by partic-ipating and contributing in numerous ways. This member would demonstrate a higher level of commitment than the member who merely paid his dues.

The essence of commitment is in the "relationship between the 'want to' and 'have to.' . . . Commitment involves three elements: a positive element, a negative element, and a bond between the two" (Brickman, Wortman, and Sorrentino 1987, p. 6). Therefore, commit-ment is a distinctive and compelling psychological process. The con-nection between the two elements, not merely their joint presence, is critical for commitment. Furthermore, the nature of this connection and bonding determines the nature of the commitment. Negative ele-ments exist in even the most absorbing commitments, for example, the spouse who nurses her partner through a devastating and lengthy ter-minal illness; the manager who spends inordinate amounts of time at work, often at the expense of his personal relationships; the highly skilled surgeon who made heavy sacrifices to learn her skills and puts herself at risk on a daily basis in the exercise of those skills. Similarly, a positive element can be present in even the most alienated commit-ment. "People who stay with a job or marriage after the life has gone out of it may no longer have the reason that initially drew them, but they still have reasons, they still have something of value that they do not wish to lose. . . . Thus the pension the person derives from the job, or the reputation and security from the marriage, become more valu-able" (Brickman, Wortman, and Sorrentino 1987, p. 7). In other words, the investment made in the commitment has become more important than the original reason for the commitment.

> People experience commitment in at least two different ways. If the neg-ative element is salient, persistence is the manifestation. If the positive element is stronger, enthusiasm is manifest. Persistence characterizes

behavior that people continue to enact despite their sense that it calls for them to make sacrifices and resist temptations—they may have to work hard and resist the pleasure of quitting. Enthusiasm characterizes behavior that people enact without ambivalence about what the behavior costs, out of a sense that the behavior itself is meaningful. Persistence in commitment reflects the call of duty; enthusiasm goes beyond the call of duty (Brickman, Wortman, and Sorrentino 1987, p. 10).

The manifestation of commitment is an important consideration for leaders in the workplace. Employees who seem to have lost their enthusiasm may not leave the organization, but their unhappiness may mean that the negative aspects of their jobs have overtaken the positive. Logically, when persistence is all that is keeping the employee in the job, it seems likely that the individual is closer to the next step, severing the commitment. And remember, as pointed out in chapter 1, we can walk with our feet and physically leave, or we can walk with our hearts and emotionally leave a job or organization. Both forms of resignation result in the loss of commitment or engagement.

Interestingly, adversity plays an important role in the formation of commitment (Lydon and Zanna 1990). Without the negative element or adversity and the existence of alternatives that must be sacrificed, a true choice has not been made. Adversity can serve as a catalyst in the development of commitment. It can strengthen and affirm a commitment. For example, researchers have found that romantic love develops more strongly in the face of opposition. The ramifications of this concept in the workplace are addressed more fully in another section of this chapter.

Process of Commitment

Brickman, Wortman, and Sorrentino (1987) describe five stages in the process of commitment. Recognizing these stages may help us understand the process of commitment and the issues related to each stage. Briefly described here, these stages also give insight into the breaking as well as the making of commitments.

Stage 1: Exploration

In stage 1, the level of commitment can be described as exploratory. During this stage, we explore a potential activity or relationship with concern only for what positive elements exist that might make further exploration worthwhile. Commitments at this stage can be considered a precommitment in that they often involve a positive orientation toward the potential object of commitment and significant reflection has not yet occurred. Stage 1 commitment can be characterized as positive and somewhat superficial. For example, recall the early stages of a job search or the exploration of a possible promotion.

Stage 2: Testing

Stage 2 can best be described as a testing phase. By this point in the process, some negative events have been encountered, and we need to assess our willingness and ability to accommodate these events. We may have been involved in testing the environment, for example, to determine the willingness of a manager or coworkers to make concessions and contribute in some meaningful way to the employment relationship. We may test ourselves to determine our ability to solve a problem or accomplish a task or activity. This stage also involves a search for information, but the focus is on the negative and troubling aspects rather than on the positive attributes inherent in the first stage. The focus at this point is external, and the crisis involves encountering unfamiliar and perhaps unexpected events. In other words, in stage 2 we discover that the honeymoon is over. The new job or organization has failed to meet our expectations in some way.

Stage 3: Passion

Passionate describes stage 3. This stage is characterized by the first major synthesis of positive and negative elements as well as recognition of the entire process as a commitment. Commitments at this stage are fiercely positive (with an almost complete denial of negative features), and we are highly self-conscious (Brickman 1987). The individual at this stage of commitment development is sometimes experienced by self and others as fanatical, with compliance to behavioral actions that are rigid and without regard to their cost. It is almost as though we need a more rigid, positive view in order to remain committed once we have a more realistic view of the negative elements in the situation.

Stage 4: Familiarity

Stage 4 can be characterized as quiet. This stage emerges more slowly as the energy needed to maintain the passion of stage 3 fades along with the ambiguity of the previous stage. The crisis of stage 4 occurs when the object of the commitment is attained and energy must be refocused on sustaining the commitment. Familiarity and comfort, characteristic of this stage, can undermine the effort required to sustain the commitment. As Maxwell (2003, p. 8) says, "Commitment is the will of the mind to finish what the heart has begun long after the emotion in which the promise was made has passed."

The orientation of this stage is intrinsic, with any threat coming from inside the person. The crisis comes in the form of boredom. When we reach this stage in our work commitments, many of us begin looking for new opportunities or new ways to experience the job's challenge again.

Stage 5: Integration

Stage 5 commitment can be described as integral. This level of commitment represents a higher level of integration of both positive and negative elements. Stage 5 integration is more flexible and complex than earlier bonding. The structure supports awareness of both the positive and the negative elements, allowing the entire commitment to flow in and out of consciousness. During stage 5, "individuals have the capacity to treat their commitments in a cognitively simple or mindless way, simply acting out of habit or following a well-known script" (Brickman, Wortman, and Sorrentino 1987, p. 179).

Organizational Commitment

Recognizing the five stages of commitment helps us to understand how commitment is established and what the process of commitment looks like. The stages establish clarity about expected reactions, and this can be reassuring for people who may feel confused by the dynamics of the process.

Perhaps one of the most important reasons to understand the stages of commitment formation is because such an understanding increases our appreciation of the fact that forming a commitment is a process. As a process, commitment is dynamic rather than static, and its characteristics change as it becomes deeper and more strongly affirmed.

Understanding the process of commitment also helps us to see how we can intervene at different stages. For example, at stage 4, the manager can play an important role by working with the employee to find new opportunities to explore or challenges to undertake. It is also beneficial for employees to understand the process of commitment because it may encourage them to seek additional responsibilities and opportunities rather than just leaving a job because it has become boring. Finding win–win solutions based on an understanding of the dynamics of commitment becomes more likely.

Commitment has been studied in numerous contexts, but our focus here is on commitment in the work setting. Organizational commitment can be defined in many ways, with the simplest definition being: organizational commitment is an employee's expressed "intent to stay." Wiener (1982) points out that behaviors resulting in organizational commitment possess the following characteristics: (1) the behaviors reflect some personal sacrifice made for the sake of the organization, (2) the behaviors show persistence, and (3) the behaviors indicate a personal preoccupation with the organization, such as devoting a great deal of personal time to organization-related activities. These characteristics vary in degree depending on the strength of each individual's level of commitment to the organization.

Other elements of organizational commitment include (Kanter 1972; Makin, Cooper, and Cox 1996):

- A strong belief in, and acceptance of, the organization's goals
- A willingness to exert effort on behalf of the organization
- A strong desire to maintain membership of the organization
- Group cohesiveness

Group cohesiveness is the "ability of people to 'stick together,' to develop the mutual attraction and collective strength to withstand threats to the group's existence" (Kanter 1972, p. 67). Job satisfaction as an expression of organizational commitment is clearly linked to the employee's intent to stay with an organization (Kleinman 2004).

Types of Organizational Commitment

Extensive research has revealed that there are at least three specific types of organizational commitment: continuance, affective, and normative. Understanding these different types of commitment enables leaders to have a more significant degree of influence on the level of commitment experienced by employees.

Continuance Commitment

Continuance commitment is based on the employee's recognition that there are benefits in aligning with the system as well as sacrifices or costs. Continuance commitment is based on a cognitive process. The balance between costs and rewards must tip in the direction of rewards for an employee to remain in the system.

Early research on commitment focused on "side bets" (Becker 1960). In the organizational context of employment, the term *side bet* is used quite loosely but can refer to anything of value that the individual has invested—including money, ego, time, and effort—that would be lost or deemed worthless if the employee were to leave the organization. Such investments include contributions to nonvested pension plans, organization-specific skills or status, and any specific organizational benefits that could not be duplicated elsewhere. Thus, it is the threat of a loss that binds the person to the organization.

Employees committed to the organization primarily for financial reasons such as pay and benefits are not as likely to feel commitment to the values of the organization (Mayer and Schoorman 1998; McNeese-Smith 2001; McNeese-Smith and Crook 2003). In fact, they may actually become a liability to the organization because such employees experience higher levels of job dissatisfaction and lower levels of job performance compared to employees who are committed to the organization's values (Meyer et al. 1989).

Affective Commitment

Affective commitment occurs as a result of events that increase the employees' level of emotional connection to their work group and lead to enhanced group cohesiveness (Kanter 1972; Iverson and Buttigieg 1999). Over the years, we have seen that lower rates of turnover have been related to strong emotional and affiliative ties with the work group. Employee friendliness and cooperation are reasons healthcare workers stay with their jobs (Strachota et al. 2003; Kangas, Kee, and McKee-Waddle 1999). When the commitment to relationships within the workplace is strong, emotional ties bind members to each other as well as to the community they form (Barney 2002).

In today's world, a sense of community within the workplace has become increasingly important for many people as it may be the only source of community in which they participate. Chapter 7 explores the concept of community in the workplace more thoroughly.

Affective commitment is based on the strength of positive feelings that increase the emotional bond. It also explains why turnover costs more than money. Turnover ruptures relationships and threatens the cohesiveness of the work group (Barney 2002; Manion 2000).

Normative Commitment

The third form of organizational commitment is based on the recognition that your personal values and beliefs fit with the organization. "Commitment to uphold norms, obey the authority of the group, and support its values, involves primarily a person's evaluative orientations.

When demands made by the system are evaluated as right, moral, just, or expressing one's own values, obedience to these demands is regarded as appropriate" (Makin, Cooper, and Cox 1996, p. 69). When normative commitment exists, employees and work groups are less likely to deviate from rules and challenge authority. Normative commitment is also referred to as moral commitment.

Normative commitment explains at least partially why congruence between an organization's (or leader's) stated values and its actions is so critical. A break in moral commitment occurs when employees perceive that the organization or one of its leaders is acting in ways inconsistent with the organization's stated beliefs or in ways significantly different from the employees' values. We have all seen the effects of such inconsistencies at one time or another. For example, one middle-size community hospital in the Midwest stated clearly that its most important value was providing high-quality *patient* care. Yet, the hospital's employees openly and disdainfully argued that the true value held by the organization was high-quality *physician* care. Employees pointed to numerous and highly visible examples of instances when hospital executives failed to put patients first but instead gave physicians what they wanted instead of giving patients what they needed. For this organization, "Patients First" started as a catchy phrase meant to exemplify the organization's values but eventually became a roadblock to building employee commitment.

Employee Commitment to the Organization

Although the three different types of commitment may lead to stronger organizational support and affiliation, the nature of each of these links to employees is quite different. "Employees with a strong affective commitment remain with the organization because they want to, whereas those with strong continuance commitment remain because they need to" (Meyer, Allen, and Smith 1993, p. 152). As a result, the daily performance and behavior of these two types of employees are different. Those who value and want to remain part of the organization are likely to exert considerable effort on behalf of the organization, but those who feel compelled to stay to avoid financial or other costs may do little more than the minimum required to retain their employment.

Unfortunately, the results of multiple studies reveal that many health care workers are not highly committed to their jobs or to the organizations for which they work (Seligman 2002; American Hospital Association 2003). Fifty-two percent of healthcare workers admit to having a low level of commitment to the jobs they perform and the institutions for whom they work (American Hospital Association 2003). In today's health care organizations, we can find many employees who have "stayed, but left" or who "psychologically resigned" a long time ago. (This subject was discussed in more detail in chapter 1.) Such employees can be easily identified by coworkers because they rarely behave in a manner that exhibits strong affective commitment. In fact, studies have shown that job performance and promotability are negatively related to continuance commitment (Meyer and Allen 1984). In recent research, it has been found that affective and normative commitment lead to positive organizational outcomes (such as lower absenteeism and intention to leave as well as a higher acceptance of change) but continuance commitment leads to greater inflexibility. In terms of rewards and benefits, merely introducing higher wages increased the person's "perception of low alternatives but has no effect on improving the alignment of employee goals with the organization" (Iverson and Buttigieg 1999, p. 327).

Leadership Interventions

When leaders understand the essential differences between the three types of organizational commitment, efforts focused on strengthening affective and normative commitment yield more long-term benefits. Makin and his colleagues (1996, p. 81) sum it up nicely: "In simple terms . . . people stay with the organization because they *want* to (affective), because they *need* to (continuance), or because they feel they *ought* to (normative)." The better leaders understand the process of commitment, the more consciously leadership behavior can be selected that encourages employees to form a commitment. Recognizing commitments made and understanding the dynamics involved in severing or dissolving commitments is also crucial. Otherwise, actions can inadvertently lead to further psychological disengagement of employees from the organization. For example, dissolving a team or closing a service or department may be a wise business decision, but if emotional support is not provided to employees in a way that recognizes the value of their commitment and helps them through this transition, their attachment to the organization as a whole may suffer irreparably.

Continuance commitment is often most emphasized in organizations during times of workforce shortages, exemplified by strategies such as recruitment incentives, salary increases, and benefit improvements. Yet, this form of commitment is weak, and it can actually be harmful. Positive organizational outcomes are more likely attained by focusing on and strengthening affective and normative commitment. These two types of commitment are closely related and more likely to lead to personal *and* organizational commitment.

Approaches for Building Affective Commitment

How can we strengthen our employees' affective commitment to the organization? Affective commitment is based on the employee's emotional and social connections with and within the organization. Studies have shown that a person's experiences during the initial months of employment are perhaps the most crucial in developing affective commitment. Focusing on efforts to ensure that the employee's initial expectations of the organization are met is important. During the early days of employment, a period of tremendous change for the individual, the organization needs to clarify roles and pay close attention to the formation of healthy relationships with new employees.

Still, commitment is influenced by the nature and quality of an employee's work experience throughout his or her tenure in an organization. The work experience is an important socializing force, and it significantly influences the extent to which affective attachments are formed with the organization. Experiences found to influence commitment include the work group's attitudes toward the organization, the organization's dependability and trust, and the individual's perception of his or her importance. In addition, efforts that support the development of healthy working relationships in work groups are crucial in the formation of a strong commitment. Peer relationships are important, but so is the relationship between the individual and the organization's leaders and others with whom interaction is common (such as patients and families, people in other departments, and physicians). (Healthy relationships are discussed in more detail in chapter 6.)

Approaches for Building Normative Commitment

The second form of organizational commitment to emphasize is normative commitment. Building normative commitment involves three essential components, as shown in figure 3-1.

Identifying and working from a foundation of shared values, a common sense of mission, and a mutually held shared vision are three concrete ways we can build normative commitment within an organization. The degree to which these exist and the degree to which each has meaning for the people involved greatly influence the level of normative commitment in the work group or organization.

Figure 3-1.   Steps for Building Normative Commitment

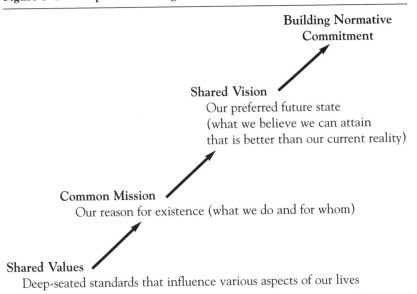

Building Normative
Commitment

Shared Vision
Our preferred future state
(what we believe we can attain
that is better than our current reality)

Common Mission
Our reason for existence (what we do and for whom)

Shared Values
Deep-seated standards that influence various aspects of our lives

Although the concepts behind values, mission, and vision are relatively simple, actually developing and building an organizationwide commitment to shared values, a common mission, and a shared vision are rarely easy. Implicit in each of the three concepts is the need for individuals to possess an extraordinary level of insight into what they find personally important in their work so that they can clearly articulate that insight to others. Sharing personal values also requires a high level of trust, and some employees may not feel comfortable enough to participate fully. Once personal values have been shared, the group or organization must then decide which of the values can be deemed important enough that the entire group can commit wholeheartedly to adopting them as the basis for all of their activities. Similarly, a group process must be followed to develop a statement of the group's essential reason for existing, its mission, as well as a vision for its future that's meaningful to all. Once the group or organization commits to its shared values, common mission, and shared vision for the future, results can be attained through the joint efforts of the people involved.

Deeply held values, a clear sense of mission, and the ability to develop a vision for the future are personal and leadership attributes rather than specific skills that can be developed. Guided classroom activities may help us to clarify our values and beliefs in each area, but such activities cannot help us to develop our belief system when it is absent. Usually forged through life experience and influenced deeply by individual personality and spirituality, personal values evolve over time. Most effective people express their values in both their personal and work lives through their day-to-day behavior.

Shared Values

A system of values shared among leaders and followers and between the individual and the organization is essential to the development of organizational commitment. Values are pervasive, deep-seated standards that affect every aspect of our lives. Values represent our beliefs and determine what we deem to be worthwhile, such as kindness and honesty.

Most people base their behavior on at least two sets of values, the values they hold as individuals and the values held by the groups to which they belong. These different value systems operate simultaneously.

Group values include the values espoused by the families, societies, religions, and organizations to which we belong. Societal values are beliefs generally held by most members of a society. Societal values in the United States include the belief in equality, personal freedom, and democracy. Organizational values are beliefs held to be important by the members of an established entity, such as service to others, intellectual competence, and quality. Family values are beliefs related to what is important within a family unit, such as mutual support, respect, and commitment. Work groups and specialized professions may also share a set of work-related values. For example, physicians and surgeons share a basic value that dictates that they will "first, do no harm."

Alignment of Values

In an individual who experiences a high level of congruence among the different aspects of his or her life, values overlap and are in sync with one another. High levels of energy and enthusiasm for life are the result. Each arena of life supports and reinforces the others. Personal power and effectiveness are at a peak.

Contradiction among values in these different areas creates dissonance, a disturbing experience for an individual. Three choices exist at this point. The individual can take steps to reduce the dissonance, perhaps by redefining the value to make it fit the situation. Another option is to suppress the uncomfortable and possibly painful feelings that arise and deny that there is any discomfort. This happens when we turn our head and pretend not to see a situation that violates one of our values. And, finally, a person can select the third choice and take steps to change that aspect of life in which there are unacceptable contradictions in values. Such changes can be accomplished by addressing or reporting our concerns about the situation or even removing ourselves from the dissonant situation permanently.

Prioritization of Values

Life is about choices. Most of us are continually aware of the values that serve as a foundation for our lives, and we recognize the choices that must be made. Choices, however, are not always seen or experienced with great clarity.

In every society, organization, family, or work situation, the values we state sometimes do not correspond to the values we truly hold. It is easy to let rhetoric drown out the truth. A society may say and believe that it values personal independence but then institute a welfare system that encourages dependence. A health care organization may state that it values service and community when in truth the primary focus of the organization is on its profits and reputation. Recall the hospital with the slogan "Patients First" and how that stated value became a source of great dissonance and dissatisfaction for employees. It takes courage to examine your feelings of discomfort, because it may be only your intuition that is saying something is wrong. An individual who has a great deal invested in the current system may find it difficult to admit that her values are not in alignment with the organization's.

A person of integrity acts in accordance with his or her beliefs. If the values of the organization or group do not match, the individual first assesses the situation to determine whether it can be changed. Action follows, based on a belief and hope that the situation can be influenced. Perhaps leaders in the organization have not recognized the incongruent messages their decisions are sending. Honest feedback and open dialogue about a perceived mismatch between a stated value and an observed behavior need to occur. When nothing changes, the individual's choice becomes clear: stay or leave. "In the work setting, a lack of congruency between personal and organizational values decreases job satisfaction and work productivity and ultimately may lead to job burnout and turnover" (McNeese-Smith and Crook 2003, p. 260).

In some instances, an individual's assessment of the situation results in a decision to stay so that other highly held personal values may be met. It is not uncommon for individuals who value financial security or stability for their families to decide to remain in a job or an organization even though their other values are not congruent. Too many times, individuals remain in a dissonant situation and suppress their feelings of rebellion against the incongruent values. Over the long term, however, they may lose sight of their values and tell themselves that those values are not worth leaving their jobs for.

Courage to choose a different path can also be difficult to find when the conflict is between beneficial values. Which is most important? Which choice will be most true to the beliefs held dear by the individual?

Take the example of Jane, a leader in a health care agency. Jane discovered the difficulty inherent in choosing between two seemingly good values. She strongly valued security and stability and had spent most of her professional career in positions that were relatively safe. Fortunately, the positions also provided her with opportunities to meet two other values she held dear: challenge and achievement. In fact, these differing values were very compatible for most of her years in health care. With every challenge she met and the more she achieved, the higher rewards and greater financial security and sense of stability she attained. As a vice president at the corporate level in a home health agency, she most enjoyed the new projects and service development aspect of her work.

When a new chief executive officer was appointed, Jane gradually became aware that the philosophy of the company had changed significantly since his appointment. Jane's position became responsible for monitoring and ensuring regulatory compliance and advocating with state legislators. Although Jane was highly skilled in these areas, the challenge and sense of achievement she previously enjoyed no longer existed for her in this role. She tried to negotiate a role change so she would be challenged and excited about work again but was unsuccessful. Instead, to make matters more difficult, Jane's salary was increased significantly by the new executive officer, and her sense of financial security became stronger than ever. Her choice was difficult: Would she stay and continue to fulfill her need for security and stability, or would she seek another position full of challenge and the opportunity to grow? After much soul-searching, she resigned and became an entrepreneur. Her new business over the years became far more successful than she had initially dreamed possible. Ultimately, challenge and achievement were more important to Jane than security and stability.

Jane's story illustrates the importance of maintaining our personal values. Values guide our daily decision making and give us a sense of direction in our day-to-day lives. Holding the values of security and achievement simultaneously can lead to a crisis point in a career when situations force an individual to make a choice between remaining in a seemingly secure, well-paying job and seeking a new job with greater challenge. When actions are in accordance with held values, events flow more smoothly.

Results of Shared Values
When values are shared among people, the result is a tremendous feeling of connection and synergy. Achieving such synergy, however, requires that leaders and followers are able to clearly define their values. They must recognize which beliefs are most important in their lives. However, when values are never discussed, a false assumption may be made: either that the values are in agreement or that they differ. Open dialogue about personal beliefs benefits both leaders and employees. When values are shared, people feel united.

The ramifications for a leader who is trying to build commitment to a certain idea are clear. The leader must be absolutely clear about his or her values and how this decision supports those values. When incongruity exists, the leader experiences feelings of dissonance that are reflected to employees in subtle ways. When the path chosen is consistent with the organization's or the leader's values and these values are shared by followers, commitment blossoms. The ability to articulate and communicate clearly is critical for this process to succeed. Not only are the technical skills of communication important, the leader also needs the courage to speak from the heart and share his or her deeply held beliefs regardless of the feelings of vulnerability this may create.

> The challenge we all face is to find ways to use the workplace as a forum in which to express and embody our deepest values. We can derive a sense of purpose, for example, from mentoring others, or being part of a cohesive team, or simply from a commitment to treating others with respect and care and from communicating positive energy. The real measure of our lives may ultimately be in the small choices we make in each and every moment (Loehr and Schwartz 2003, p. 140).

Common Mission

"The first responsibility of the leader is to define reality" (DePree 1989, p. 11). In an organizational context, leaders have the task and responsibility of determining both the purpose and the future of their organizations. Beckhard and Pritchard (1992) note that the turbulence of rapid change forces most leaders to reexamine the very essence of the organization along with its basic purpose, its identity, and its relationships with customers (internal and external), competitors, and other key stakeholders. Mycek (1998, p. 26) asks: "What is the true business of healthcare? Is it the 'high-tech, high-touch' blend of dedicated care-givers and state-of-the-art technology that was prophesied in the late 1980s? Or is healthcare purely a commodity—products and services that are bought and sold at the lowest price, on the spot market?" The questions today are becoming more and more difficult. In addition to defining the organization's mission, leaders and employees also need a clear sense of their own mission or purpose.

Strong leaders and committed employees have a clear sense of mission; they know why they are here and they are clear about their purpose. Mission is a reason for existence: of individuals, projects, teams, and organizations. A clear mission defines purpose and gives direction and focus. It enables an individual to decline opportunities that detract from this true purpose. "It's easy to say 'no' when there is a deeper 'yes' burning inside" (Covey, Merrill, and Merrill 1994, p. 103).

Over time, each individual's mission in life gradually becomes apparent. People grow into their work roles, including leadership roles, by fully experiencing life and learning its many lessons through reading, talking with and listening to others, traveling, learning new skills, and observing the life around them. Fully engaged workers are continual learners who always look for the lesson in a situation, even when it is difficult or painful.

The practice of reflection is growing in popularity today (Taylor 2004). Reflection is a powerful tool that individuals can use to better understand the motivation behind their own actions and reactions and to learn how outcomes are attained and recognize what is really important.

Leadership Mission Statement

Every leader needs a personal mission statement. An individual's personal mission statement may or may not include a leadership mission statement. For some people, these are two different but compatible statements. A leader needs to distinguish between his or her purpose as an individual and his or her purpose as a leader. Mission statements cannot be completed in a one- or two-hour period of time. Writing a meaningful mission statement takes "deep introspection, careful analysis, thoughtful expression, and often many rewrites to produce it in final form" (Covey 1989, p. 129). It means sorting through a great deal of extraneous material to reach the core reason for one's existence and how that purpose is to be achieved. The leadership mission statement usually includes the leader's values, often the means by which the mission is to be achieved.

A strong sense of connection between leaders and followers results when leaders openly share their personal or leadership mission statements. Leaders may feel vulnerable or embarrassed at first, because such statements, to be meaningful, must be very personal statements. However, when leaders sincerely and humbly express themselves, sharing mission statements is a powerful way of making connections with their followers. Even when supporters do not totally agree with or fully value a leader's personal mission statement, mutual understanding can result.

An individual without a sense of purpose is like a rudderless ship buffeted by every strong wind that happens along. People without clear purpose do not make good leaders. Individuals who have no inner sense of direction or understanding of purpose usually find it difficult, if not impossible, to be effective leaders. During periods of rapid change such as the present, it is not enough to simply adopt someone else's purpose because it is politically correct or expeditious to do so. Leaders need a strong inner sense of knowing and a connection to their identified purpose, or it does not serve during stressful times. A point to remember here is that all employees have the potential of moving in and out of leadership roles, regardless of what their formal positions are in the organization. The concepts related to a leader's mission statement apply equally to an individual employee's purpose statement.

Alignment of Missions
Clarity of personal purpose enables us to determine whether our values and goals match those of our organizations. When the purpose or mission of the organization is diametrically opposed to my purpose, I may feel that I will not be able to carry out the organization's mission. For example, assume that I am in a leadership position and I believe that encouraging and nurturing followers to function independently and interdependently is part of my personal mission. However, I work in a bureaucratic, heavily hierarchical organization within which there is no support for empowering employees. It is going to be difficult for me to feel successful or satisfied in my role. Or I may see my primary purpose as developing others, but recent expansions in the scope of my responsibility have made it difficult, if not impossible, for me to serve as a coach for others in the workplace. My primary purpose may no longer be met in this role.

Exemplary health care leaders today demonstrate an abiding sense of personal purpose. Many see themselves as stewards for health care in their communities. Chawla and Renesch (1995) describe this sentiment as a willingness among leaders and managers within health care organizations to become accountable for the well-being of the larger community by operating in service to colleagues, patients, families, and other stakeholders. This enduring sense of operating for the benefit of others and for something bigger than any individual helps create committed partnerships with followers. As described by Robert Greenleaf in the collection of his private writings, *On Becoming a Servant–Leader:*

> The servant–leader is servant first. . . . It begins with the natural feeling that one wants to serve, to serve first. Then conscious choice brings one to aspire to lead. . . . The difference manifests itself in the care taken by the servant—first to make sure that other people's highest-priority needs are being served. The best test, and the most difficult to administer, is: Do those served grow as persons? Do they, while being served, become healthier, wiser, freer, more autonomous, more likely themselves to become servants? And, what is the effect on the least privileged in society; will they benefit or, at least, not be further deprived? (Frick and Spears 1996, p. 2).

Shared Vision

The third approach to building normative commitment among followers in an organization involves the development of a shared vision. In recent years, vision has become a popular concept in management and leadership circles. Everywhere, managers and leaders are exhorted to have a vision. Example after example of governments, organizations, and people for whom vision made a difference are shared. And all are impressive, but Joel Barker, in *The Power of Vision* (1990), raises the question: Does the vision come first, or does the success of an individual, organization, or government lead to a vision? In each instance he examined, the vision came first, and this finding has led him to conclude that "vision has the power to change our lives."

Vision is a crucial attribute of successful leaders. All effective leaders understand vision because of its presence in their lives. It may not be an easily explainable concept, but leaders relate to this idea because they have experienced it. They see the future differently than other people do; leaders see what is possible and dream, while others merely predict. Basically, vision is hope for the future. It is the ability to rise out of the current daily turmoil and see something different for the future.

Developing visions for the workplace is one of the most important functions of leadership. Although the leader's vision of the future may not always be accurate, it is almost always desirable and positive.

The development of a vision for the future is a three-step process. The first step involves describing the vision, the second involves talking about the vision with the others who must help create the new future, and the final step involves putting a structure in place to ensure the realization of the vision.

Step 1: Define and Describe the Vision

A future vision is a picture that the leader has of the horizon. The power of vision is in its expectancy; it is a picture of a preferred future rather than a forecast of a predicted future. A vision is an illuminated look into tomorrow based on what the leader believes is possible. Vision takes imagination and optimism. "It is the ability to see beyond our present reality, to create, to invent what does not yet exist, to become what we are not yet. It gives us [the] capacity to live out of our imagination instead of our memory" (Covey, Merrill, and Merrill 1994, p. 103).

Some leaders seek or rise to a leadership position because they have a vision of what the future could be, and this vision drives and inspires them to lead. Armed with the vision, they find that it becomes a simple matter to put structures in place to achieve the desired future. Sometimes the position comes first, whether it is a formal leadership position in an organization, an appointment to chair a committee or task force, or an election to an office. The individual discovers that he or she has the responsibility and obligation to take the lead in a situation. Sometimes there is a clear mission but only a general vision of the outcomes.

The first step is to develop the vision, but this may be more difficult than it sounds. As in the process of creativity, following a deliberate, intuitive process is valuable. The intuitive process starts with preparation by coming to understand as much as possible through reading anything and everything related to the situation, talking with people, and drawing on past experiences. The second step is to let all information and ideas incubate until a spark jumps forward and brings the leader to illumination, the third step. As the vision becomes clear, it is important to create as much detail as possible. Concrete, specific descriptions of a preferred future help others see the vision more clearly. For example, President John F. Kennedy, when he spoke of America's space program in a State of the Union address, did not say that America would be the world leader in space exploration in the future. Instead, he said that before the end of the 1960s, America would put a man on the moon and return that man safely to Earth. In other words, Kennedy expressed his vision in explicit and definite terms.

To be inspiring, the preferred future must be a stretch, a far reach from the present. Martin Luther King Jr. said, "I have a dream that one day this nation will rise up and live out the true meaning of this creed— we hold these truths to be self-evident: that all men are created equal" (Anderson 1990, p. 11). At the time, in segregated America, this was a tremendous stretch from the reality. Peter Senge (1990) says that once a vision is identified, the greater the distance it is from the current reality, the more creative tension that exists. Creative tension is the pull between the vision and the present. This tension acts like a giant rubber band, pulling us toward a new future. As Senge warns, when a vision seems too difficult, it is better to extend the time frame for achieving the vision than to scale back the vision to fit the time frame available. In other words, settling for less is the first step toward mediocrity.

Step 2: Engage in Dialogue about the Vision

A leader alone cannot achieve a vision. New realities are created when everyone affected by the vision works together. In a successful organization, multiple visions are encouraged in the same way that multiple leaders exist in different areas and on different levels of the organization. The various visions produce more impact when they are consistent and form a cascade of visions in the organization, as illustrated in figure 3-2. Everyone has his or her own vision of the future, and a shared vision is created when people engage in dialogue about the vision. The different visions are discussed, explored, and modified on the basis of information learned from others. A shared vision occurs when two or more people have a similar picture for the future and are each committed to achieving the vision.

In other words, an organization may develop a vision for itself while a specific department within the organization develops a vision that

Figure 3-2.   A Cascade of Visions

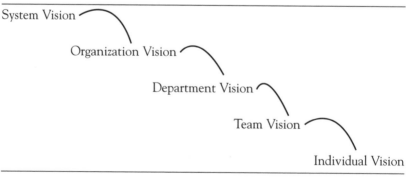

System Vision

Organization Vision

Department Vision

Team Vision

Individual Vision

concretely describes the department's future as it relates to the organization's vision. For example, a health care system may see itself as the premier health care facility in the region, while the cardiovascular department's vision relates to how it feeds or supports the organization's vision.

According to Senge (1990, p. 206), "Today, 'vision' is a familiar concept in corporate leadership. But when you look carefully you find that most 'visions' are one person's (or group's) vision imposed on an organization. Such visions, at best, command compliance—not commitment. A shared vision is a vision that many people are truly committed to, because it reflects their own personal vision." When the shared vision reflects personal visions, a deep sense of caring about the future can evolve. Senge (1990, p. 206) describes such shared visions:

> A shared vision is not an idea. It is not even an important idea such as freedom. It is, rather, a force in people's hearts, a force of impressive power. It may be inspired by an idea, but once it goes further—if it is compelling enough to acquire the support of more than one person—then it is no longer an abstraction. It is palpable. People begin to see it as if it exists. Few, if any, forces in human affairs are as powerful as shared vision.

Shared visions do not happen unless there is plenty of dialogue about the future. Open give-and-take discussions, honest questioning, and stimulating conversations need to happen. Abraham Lincoln is a wonderful example of a leader who understood and applied this concept. "Throughout the [Civil War] Lincoln continued to visit his generals and troops. . . . He always had a kind word for them, frequently telling them his vision of America and how important they were in achieving victory in the cause for which they were fighting" (Phillips 1992, p. 19).

Step 3: Create a Structure for the Vision

Although Martin Luther King Jr. said, "I have a dream" and not "I have a plan," having a dream without a structure in place will not ensure that a new reality can be achieved. To quote the Noah principle: "No more prizes for predicting rain; prizes only for building arks!" The ark in this case is the structure that enables attainment of the desired vision. Some people are great dreamers but are unskilled when it comes to implementing those dreams. Leaders need both skills. "Leaders not only have a vision, they work unusually hard to execute it well. Leaders are implementers, not just strategists; doers, not just dreamers" (Berry 1992, pp. 2–3). Structure includes the steps to be taken to create the future. A person can dream of winning the lottery, but if he or she never purchases a ticket, the dream cannot come true.

Bennis describes vision as the management of attention, and with this simple statement, he captures the power of vision. With a clearly articulated vision and people who believe in it, the vision itself focuses the attention of the visioning community. Attention keeps people focused on the future, hopeful and expectant about its possibilities. Leaders envision "the destination their followers want, they have the superior skill to guide the journey, and they have the belief to drive the group forward in the face of adversity" (Fagiano 1994, p. 4).

Shared values, a common purpose or mission, and a shared vision together produce the ability to influence others. The personal and deeply held values of leaders and followers influence the direction or mission chosen. And where there is a strong sense of mission, there exists the possibility of visions powerful enough to forge a new future.

Common Pitfalls

Leadership interventions for strengthening employee organizational commitment seem relatively straightforward. However, as with any issue dealing with human behavior and interpersonal interactions, hidden pitfalls and challenges need to be considered. Several of the most common pitfalls are discussed in the rest of this chapter.

Mistaking Compliance for Commitment

Effective leaders grasp the difference between commitment and compliance and do not mistake one for the other. Leadership is more than influencing others to follow a specific direction; it is creating a *desire* within the followers to do so. Earlier in this chapter, compliance was discussed briefly. Leaders who also have the legitimate authority of a position may be tempted to rely on giving others direction about the needed actions and behaviors and expecting compliance.

At first glance, it may seem easier to seek compliance rather than to invest in the preparation time it takes to build commitment, as illustrated in figure 3-3. The arrows in the figure represent projects, decisions, or actions that must be implemented. As the figure shows, less preparatory work is needed when the leader simply tells people what to do and people conform. In contrast, a long, intense preparatory period (symbolized by the longer line before implementation) is needed to gain commitment. Preparation includes lengthy conversations, exploration of shared values, refinement of purpose, open sharing of information, collaborative development of the vision and plan, and finally,

Figure 3-3. **Comparing Compliance and Commitment in Terms of Time Investment**

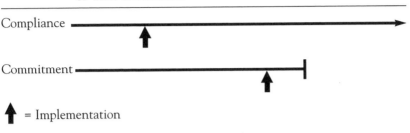

Compliance

Commitment

↑ = Implementation

an internal shift within each person that indicates a deep level of commitment to the outcome.

The paradox, of course, is that when thorough preparation is provided and employees are treated as partners on the journey, the attainment of the desired outcome is actually much faster. In many instances, when mere compliance is sought, leaders find that they have created an open-ended process with no closure because there are always some people who will not comply.

The arrow at the end of the compliance line in figure 3-3 represents the open-ended nature of the situation. Often, leaders must follow up and continually monitor the situation to ensure compliance because people simply have not bought in to the concept and do not support it. Unfortunately, it does not take many of these people within your group to create sabotage and undermining behaviors. And, in too many cases, the resistant behavior may be covert and not readily apparent. In either case, full compliance and, thus, closure are never attained.

A strong leader understands the difference between compliance and commitment and consciously decides when commitment is needed and when compliance is enough. For leaders without formal authority in the organization, understanding the concept of commitment is essential. Without legitimate authority to force people to comply, these leaders often work to build commitment by following the steps outlined in the preceding section.

Failing to Offer Choice in the Work Environment

When leaders understand commitment, the importance of choice is clear. Recall that, according to Brickman, Wortman, and Sorrentino (1987), commitment includes a positive element, a negative element, and a bond between the two. This idea implies that multiple alternatives are to be considered and evaluated. When there is no choice, there can be no commitment because there are not two elements between which a bond can be formed. Choice, then, is essential to the concept of commitment (Waterman 1987). The opportunity to exercise choice is an important construct in American culture. "For Americans . . . making a choice provides an opportunity to display one's preferences and, consequently, to express one's internal attributes, to assert one's autonomy, and to fulfill the goal of being unique" (Iyengar and Lepper 1999, p. 350). As we saw in chapter 2, choice is also one of the intrinsic motivators for work.

Commitment cannot be forced. Therefore, leaders must face the possibility that people may choose *not* to follow them. "If the most competent and trusted people won't commit, the leader should take another look at the cause itself. It may be ill-conceived or stated in a misleading way" (Waterman 1987, p. 299). Research has also demonstrated that people are less open to receiving new information once they have made their choices (Brickman, Wortman, and Sorrentino 1987). Because forcing a choice prematurely is risky, leaders must be comfortable enough to allow employees to come to their decisions about making commitments in their own time. More information is needed to change a decision than to make one. Demanding compliance on a course of action that requires the full engagement and support of employees is hazardous because it may preclude the possibility of ever achieving true commitment.

Probably the most important ramification of providing choice has to do with understanding why emphasizing continuance commitment is so damaging. When salary and benefits levels are high, employees perceive fewer alternatives to continued employment; that is, it would cost them too much to leave the organization. An employee who feels trapped, even by positive circumstances, is less likely to be positively engaged. Although competitive compensation packages are desirable, other rewards such as job variety, promotion opportunities, increased autonomy, and coworker support are probably more effective (Iverson and Buttigieg 1999).

Communicating Insufficient Information

Recognizing that making a commitment involves a rational decision-making process underscores the critical importance of communication. Information is crucial in any decision-making process because it forms the basis upon which the decision is made. Recall the earlier recommendation supporting an open flow of information about the leaders' and employees' individual values and missions as well as the organization's values and mission. Involving employees in the development of a shared vision of the organization's future helps create enthusiasm and commitment. Honest and sincere dialogue between a leader and followers helps further shape and enhance the vision. As Senge (1990) pointed out, only when the vision is shared is true commitment and engagement possible.

How do we get from thought to action? The choices may seem overwhelming. Rational decision making requires accurate information. What are the alternatives? What are the consequences of choosing different alternatives? "The essential conflict between rational thought and functional behavior can be put very simply. Rational thought requires consideration of all available alternatives. Effective action requires the pursuit of one alternative, not necessarily the best one, and the ignoring or suppressing of the others" (Brickman, Wortman, and Sorrentino 1987, p. 51). Decisions must be made and action taken even when compelling arguments exist on both sides of the issue. Being rational requires individuals to choose the better alternative. Thus, a key issue in rationality is whether the individual is aware of the alternatives and his or her reasons for choosing one over the other.

The influence of commitment needs to be respected. "To whatever extent people are rational, they are less so following commitment" (Brickman, Wortman, and Sorrentino 1987, p. 35). When circumstances result in the dissolution of commitments, especially those we have asked people to make, we cannot expect a rapid resolution of the emotions involved. A recent example illustrates this. In a small Georgia community, two hospitals with a long history of fierce competition were set on a course toward merger. The chief executive officers in both facilities worked diligently to gain the commitment of employees, physicians, and the community. Their strongest argument was that this course of action was the *only hope* for the survival of both facilities. People were persuaded that the argument was true, and they became quite committed to the merger. Imagine the difficulties when the merger fell through!

Missing the Opportunity to Escalate Commitment

Another key aspect to understand is the concept of escalation. Escalation is related to our need for self-justification. The concept has been studied widely in social psychology. "Escalation is self-perpetuating.

Once a small commitment is made, it sets the stage for ever-increasing commitments. The behavior needs to be justified, so attitudes are changed; this change in attitudes influences future decisions and behaviors" (Aronson 1995, p. 192). Many savvy telemarketers use the concept of escalation by beginning their sales pitches with questions to which you can only respond positively. They set you up for subsequent positive responses. Thus, when a leader is able to gain even a modest commitment, that commitment sets the stage for more significant commitments later.

Conclusion

Employee compliance with the directions issued by leaders and managers is not enough during these difficult and demanding times for health care organizations. Whether they hold formal or informal authority, exemplary leaders know how to build commitment to action among followers. They also understand the different forms of organizational commitment and how to capitalize on these to create a positive work environment.

In successful organizations, effective leaders focus their efforts predominantly on building affective and normative organizational commitment. Developing shared values, a mission common and relevant to all, and a shared vision for the organization are three specific ways in which a leader can build normative commitment among followers. Affective organizational commitment occurs when healthy relationships and a strong sense of connection exist among people in the workplace. When these two forms of commitment are present, employees do not just comply with the direction set by leaders; they want to follow the recommended path. Together these things inspire passion and provide the energy and courage to create a new reality.

Conversation Points

Organizational Perspective

1. Which form of organizational commitment (continuance, affective, or normative) do you think is the strongest in your organization?
2. Are there times when the organization has not lived up to its stated values, purpose, or vision? How are people treated when

they question incongruities? Do employees feel safe raising issues related to organizational values?

3. How does the organization ensure that all new employees are introduced to the organization's values, mission, and vision?

4. Were all levels of employees involved in creating the vision? Or was the vision developed by a small, select group and then presented to the others?

5. What are the consequences when people do not live up to the organization's stated values? What happens? What is an example of this?

6. Are meaningful conversations occurring on a regular basis about the organization's values, mission, and vision? When was the last time this occurred in a significant way in the organization?

Leadership Issues

1. What are your most important work-related values? What do you stand for? How do you treat your coworkers and colleagues? What do you mean by ethical behavior? How do you want to be known by others?

2. Once you have a list of your important values, identify the specific day-to-day behaviors you engage in that demonstrate how you live by these values. Are there gaps between what you say you value and how you live your life? What values do you say you hold but express infrequently? What values are neglected during periods of high stress?

3. Think of an example when you had to decide which of your values was more important to you. What was the situation, and how did you resolve it? In retrospect, did you make the right decision? Would you change that decision today if you could?

4. What could you do to ensure that you are living by your values on a day-to-day basis?

5. Describe your personal and leadership missions. Why are you here? What do you do, and for whom do you do it? Take some time to reflect, and then write a personal mission statement.

6. What is your future vision? Where do you see yourself in five years? What will you be doing? How will you get there?

7. When was the last time you had a substantial, meaningful conversation with an employee or colleague about organizational or departmental values?

Employee Challenges

1. Think of something to which you are committed. How did your commitment begin?
2. What has kept it strong over time? What are the elements of your commitment? Which is the positive element and which is the negative?
3. Consider your organization's values, mission, and vision. Are your values, mission, and vision congruent with those of your department, service, or organization?
4. Find people for whom vision has made a difference. Ask them to share their story.
5. What is your vision for your future?
6. When was the last time you were involved in a meaningful conversation with someone in the workplace about the values, mission, or vision of the organization?
7. Have you asked your manager or another organization leader what values they hold dear? Are they congruent with yours?
8. What do you do when you see the organization or its leaders or employees behaving in a way that is incongruent with the organization's stated values? Do you speak up or do you ignore it? If you have spoken up and addressed the incongruence, what was the reaction of others?

4

Experiencing Happiness and Joy in the Workplace

Jo Manion

When work is a pleasure, life is a joy!
When work is a duty, life is slavery.
—Maxsim Gorky

EMPLOYEES who experience joy and happiness through their work and in their workplaces are valuable assets in today's health care organizations. Managers and leaders who understand the concepts of positive emotion and are able to apply their knowledge to create a positive work environment are more successful at tapping into intrinsic motivators and building organizational commitment, both among themselves and among their employees and colleagues. This chapter explores recent research from the field of positive psychology and offers concrete, evidence-based suggestions for establishing a workplace in which happiness and joy are key characteristics of the environment.

Positive Psychology

A startling innovation in the field of psychology developed during the late 1990s: the birth of positive psychology. Since the earliest days of modern psychology in the mid-twentieth century, the focus of researchers and practitioners has been on alleviating the misery of people suffering from mental illnesses. Thousands and thousands of research studies have been conducted on depression, anger, fear, hatred, and countless other negative emotions and conditions. Mental illnesses have been examined, defined, and categorized extensively. This research has resulted in tremendous progress in the ability of psychiatrists and clinical psychologists to diagnose and treat clinical depression, schizophrenia, and other serious, debilitating conditions.

However, many behavioral scientists are coming to realize that traditional psychology concentrates on reducing misery but does little to encourage happiness. In other words, even when medications relieve a patient's depression, the person may still be unhappy. Although traditional psychology has made some progress toward understanding the positive emotions, that progress seems almost insignificant in the face of its overwhelmingly negative emphasis.

Positive psychology recognizes that people want more out of life than correcting their weaknesses and deficiencies. People want to live lives full of meaning and purpose, and they want to be happy. The explosive growth of positive psychology during the past decade is primarily due to the efforts of several prominent practitioners and academicians. Several who are notable are Martin E. Seligman at the University of Pennsylvania, Mihaly Csikszentmihalyi at the Claremont Graduate University, and Chris Peterson at the University of Michigan. As noted by Seligman in his book *Authentic Happiness: Using the New Positive Psychology to Realize Your Potential for Lasting Fulfillment*, "the time has finally arrived for a science that seeks to understand positive emotion, build strength and virtue, and provide guideposts for finding what Aristotle called the 'good life'" (Seligman 2002, p. xi).

Work and happiness? Joy at work? For some people, these terms seem inherently contradictory. Yet the truth is how we feel at work and whether we are happy in our work and our workplaces determines to a great extent what our lives are like. Most of us spend the majority of our awake and alert hours at work, and if we are not happy there, we often judge our lives to be unhappy. If your work is unpleasant, tedious, or meaningless to you and others or you feel demoralized, demeaned, or unhappy in your work environment, these feelings will permeate the rest of your life. Although we may try to compartmentalize and segment our lives by telling ourselves "not [to] bring our problems to work" or not to "take the negativity home with you," the reality is that the different aspects of our lives are closely interconnected and intertwined. It is virtually impossible to confine unhappiness to one segment of our lives. It will surface in the other parts of our lives whether we want it to or not.

Csikszentmihalyi, in his book *Good Business: Leadership, Flow, and the Making of Meaning* (2003), explores the relationship between business and happiness in some detail. He points out that "it may seem counterintuitive to argue that happiness and business have anything to do with each other, since for most people work is at best a necessary evil, and at worst, a burden. Yet the two are inextricably linked. Fundamentally, business exists to enhance well-being" (Csikszentmihalyi

2003, p. 21). He goes on to make a historical case supporting this contention. From the earliest of human endeavors, the production and exchange of goods make sense only when those goods improve the quality of the human experience. Good business is not merely related to the generation of monetary profit; it also relates to exchanges that increase and contribute to the happiness and quality of life of humans. Not only does the primary purpose of business seek to improve our lives, but work is also the vehicle through which a measure of happiness may be found. It provides a way for us to apply our strengths and use our positive attributes, and our ability to apply our strengths and attributes is often considered the foundation of happiness. In other words, we are the happiest when we are doing what we do best.

Positive psychology is not just feel-good, pop psychology or "happiology" characterized by easily repeated platitudes. Nor is it the toys and trinkets approach currently popular in many of today's recognition and appreciation initiatives. It is a scientific field of endeavor whose hallmark is research leading to a deeper understanding of the positive emotions. Seligman (2002) sorts the field into three areas: the study of positive emotions, the study of strengths and virtues, and the study of positive institutions.

Study of Positive Emotions

Although the negative emotions have been examined in numerous research studies, prior to the mid-1990s little research was conducted on the positive emotions such as joy, happiness, hope, and satisfaction. Positive emotions include those that are related to the past, the present, and the future.

> The positive emotions about the future include optimism, hope, faith, and trust. Those about the present include joy, ecstasy, calm, zest, ebullience, pleasure, and (most importantly) flow; these emotions are what most people usually mean when they casually—but much too narrowly—talk about "happiness." The positive emotions about the past include satisfaction, contentment, fulfillment, pride, and serenity (Seligman 2002, p. 62).

Clearly all three of these senses of emotion are closely and tightly linked, and although it is desirable to experience positive emotion about all three, it does not necessarily occur this way. For instance, a person might feel proud and satisfied about their work and contributions in the past but still feel quite unhappy with what is happening in the present. And this individual might not feel optimistic about the future. Another person may be quite bitter about the past and yet enjoy pleasure in the present. Still another individual may be positive about the future and yet miserable in the present. These seeming contradictions are apparent in ourselves and our coworkers.

Positive Emotions Related to Past Experiences

Positive emotions related to past experiences include contentment, satisfaction, fulfillment, pride, and serenity. When the three aspects of life are sorted out and we see clearly that there are many examples of individuals for whom the three are separate issues, we can feel very liberated. We can realize that we are not victims of our past, but instead we can exert free will and rise above events in the past to experience our present and our future as we choose.

Positive psychology research has found it difficult to produce evidence of even small effects of childhood events on adult personality, and there is less evidence to suggest that childhood experiences determine adult functioning. According to Seligman:

> The major trauma of childhood may have some influence on adult personality, but only a barely detectable one. Bad childhood events, in short, do not mandate adult troubles. There is no justification in these studies for blaming your adult depression, anxiety, bad marriage, drug use, sexual problems, unemployment, aggression against your children, alcoholism, or anger on what happened to you as a child (Seligman 2002, p. 67).

Clearly, Seligman's viewpoint is different from that held by traditional psychiatrists and clinical psychologists. However, Seligman's research should not be interpreted as suggesting that childhood events do not affect us as adults; it simply has found that traumatic childhood events are not tightly and causally linked to negative adult experiences.

In the same way, in our work world, negative things and even destructive things can happen that are regrettable, but they will affect our futures only to the degree we allow. Instead, what has been found is that we are highly adaptable creatures. When positive or negative events occur, we may experience a temporary burst of mood in the expected direction, but within a short time, our mood settles back into its set range. Thus, emotions, left to themselves, eventually dissipate and we return to our baseline condition.

It should be noted here that it is very common in health care organizations to attempt to measure employee satisfaction levels under the assumption that high satisfaction is related to employment retention and the creation of a positive workplace. However, at best, these measures can give us only a sense of how people feel about the past. Although such information is important, it is only one of the elements that need to be considered. Just as important and as likely to be related to retention is how the employee is experiencing the workplace during the present and how they see their futures.

Positive Emotions Related to Present Experiences

Positive emotions in the present include joy, ecstasy, calm, zest, ebullience, pleasure, and flow. Positive emotions experienced in the present constitute what is often referred to as happiness. From the research, Seligman points out that happiness in the present embraces both pleasures and gratifications. Pleasures are those things from which we derive clear sensory and emotional pleasure, such as having a good massage, listening to favorite music, or enjoying a special meal. Gratifications, on the other hand, are activities that engage us fully, often without any clear emotional content, but because we are immersed and absorbed in them and because we lose our sense of time and consciousness. Reading a good book, mountain climbing, and having a great conversation with someone are all examples of gratifications. The gratifications last longer than the pleasures, they require our key strengths, they demand thinking and interpretation, and they do not habituate easily.

Although pleasures in life increase our perception of happiness, they are not enough. We become easily habituated to the pleasures. For example, the second taste of a creamy, smooth, deep-chocolate truffle is not as marvelous as the first. And with the pleasures, once the pleasure is over, it is over. The good feelings seldom last. Not only do these pleasures fade quickly, but there is sometimes a negative aftermath, such as an addiction to the pleasure that can set up a strong craving. On the other hand, long-term positive feelings often result from gratifications.

This one principle, understanding the difference between pleasures and gratifications, has huge implications for contemporary organizations. Focusing retention efforts on those things that bring immediate pleasure will yield few long-term gains. We will be both surprised and disappointed when people become habituated to such immediate rewards and begin to demand more and more. At this point, it becomes very difficult to emerge from this state of entitlement. Some of these pleasures (gifts, social events, and so on) can be equated with making people happy. Understanding the nature of gratification can help us design initiatives and efforts that focus on more enduring positive emotions.

Positive Emotions Related to the Future

Positive emotions related to the future clearly affect our perception of well-being in the work world. Future positive emotions include faith, trust, confidence, hope, and optimism. Seligman has studied optimism extensively, and he reports that it can be learned (Seligman 1998). He defines optimism very differently than the more common but superficial "glass half-empty/glass half-full" approach. He believes, instead, that we each have a basic explanatory style that includes two dimensions: permanence and pervasiveness. People who are less optimistic and give up easily often do so because they believe the bad events that happen to them are permanent and will continue to affect their lives. This state of mind is different from the state of mind enjoyed by individuals who believe that the causes of bad events are temporary and will pass.

The second dimension is pervasiveness, which is related to whether we see the cause of a bad event as universal or specific. People who adopt a universal explanation for why a bad event occurred are more likely to let it permeate other aspects of their lives. For instance, such people might think, "I lost my job and so I am a bad wife and a bad person." People who assume a specific explanation for the same circumstances might say, for example, "I wasn't skilled enough to perform this job well, and so I need to improve my skills or learn new ones." The job loss would affect their work life but have little impact on their family, personal, or volunteer life.

> People who make permanent *and* universal explanations for good events, as well as temporary and specific explanations for bad events, bounce back from troubles briskly and get on a roll easily when they succeed once. People who make temporary and specific explanations for success, and permanent and universal explanations for setbacks, tend to collapse under pressure—both for a long time and across situations—and rarely get on a roll (Seligman 2002, p. 93).

It is likely that experiencing the positive emotions of the future has a direct impact on an employee's intention to remain in a job within the organization. When there is little faith or belief that the problems on the job are getting better or that the work situation in the future will improve, would the employee not be more likely to consider pursuing other opportunities? We know that work environments characterized by low levels of trust among people are also characterized by less hope for the future. It also seems evident that having less hope or faith in the future would have an impact on an employee's commitment to the organization or the work group.

Study of Strengths and Virtues

The second area of positive psychology is the study of the strengths and virtues. Peterson and Seligman (2004) have published a catalog of the virtues, which is based on a thorough study of the primary writings in all of the main religious and philosophical traditions known to history. The list of virtues is virtually universal across three thousand years and the entire world. The six virtues are wisdom and knowledge; courage; love and humanity; justice; temperance; and spirituality and transcendence. The list of twenty-four strengths describes the traits of human character through which the virtues can be achieved. For example, the virtue of wisdom and knowledge is related to the following five strengths:

- Curiosity/interest
- Love of learning
- Judgment/critical thinking
- Originality/ingenuity/creativity
- Perspective

The virtue of transcendence is related to:

- Appreciation of beauty/awe
- Gratitude
- Hope/optimism
- Humor/playfulness
- Spirituality/sense of purpose

Talents should not be mistaken for true strengths. Strengths must be built and developed; by comparison, talents are more like innate gifts. Although talents can be honed and refined, they cannot be learned. For example, I may learn all I can about music, but if I am tone-deaf (I have limited musical talent), no amount of practice is going to make me a good singer. We make choices about whether to develop our strengths and when to use them.

Every individual has several predominant strengths, called signature strengths. Seligman (2002) believes that we are happiest when we recognize our signature strengths (those that are strongest for us) and use those strengths in our work and personal lives. You can assess your individual strengths by completing the Virtues in Action instrument on Seligman's website (authentichappiness.com).

Study of Positive Institutions

The third area of positive psychology involves the study of positive institutions such as the family, democracy, and free inquiry. In his book *Good Business*, Csikszentmihalyi advances the basic position that business itself is capable of being a positive institution in our lives. Whether businesses can rise to the challenge of being models of virtue is questionable, given the dramatic examples of corporate fraud and corruption over the past decade (Easterbrook 2003; Hammonds 2004). Certainly, health care should be considered a positive institution in our world.

The study of positive institutions is probably the least explored area of positive psychology. However, many books in the popular business press attempt to examine successful organizations and identify their key attributes and characteristics.

Business Case for Happiness

Why should we be concerned about whether people are happy at work? After all, there certainly seem to be more important issues that require our attention in the workplace, such as increasing productivity, ensuring a high-quality patient/customer experience, and establishing effective working relationships, to mention only a few. The truth is that all of these challenges can be better met by people who are happy and who enjoy their work. The business case for happiness is dramatically simple and clear-cut, and it is based on solid research evidence.

The benefits of a workplace characterized by people who are happy seem almost self-evident. These advantages include higher productivity, better outcomes, increased employee retention, healthier employees, and a more positive environment for patients and families.

Higher Productivity

One study measured the amount of positive emotion among 272 employees and followed their job performance over eighteen months. Happier people went on to get better evaluations and higher pay. In a large-scale study of Australian youths across fifteen years, happiness made gainful employment and higher income more likely (Seligman 2002). Myers, in his book *The Pursuit of Happiness*, notes that "compared to depressed employees, those with higher well-being have lower medical costs, higher work efficiency and less absenteeism" (Myers 1992, p. 131). Csikszentmihalyi points out that "a business organization whose employees are happy is more productive, has a higher morale, and has a lower turnover" (Csikszentmihalyi 2003, p. 25).

In trying to determine which comes first, happiness or productivity, researchers induced happiness experimentally in the laboratory and then examined later performance. It turns out that when adults and children are put into a good mood first, they select higher goals, perform better, and persist longer on a variety of laboratory tests, such as solving anagrams. Research conducted by Fredrickson has also found that people in a more positive mood actually think more broadly and can solve problems more readily (Fredrickson 2003). Both of these abilities affect productivity.

Better Outcomes

Positive mood has been directly linked to a range of different performance-related behaviors, including greater helping behavior, enhanced creativity, integrative thinking, inductive reasoning, more efficient decision making, greater cooperation, and the use of more successful negotiation strategies (George 2000; Totterdell et al. 1998). A negative mood moves us into an entirely different way of thinking from a positive mood. When we are feeling negatively, we seem to become critics of each other; negativity engenders a warrior mode of thinking, a win–lose approach to problems. We concentrate on what is wrong and attempt to correct it. Conversely, a positive mood stimulates people into a way of thinking that is creative, tolerant, constructive, generous, undefensive, and lateral. The focus is not on what is wrong but on what is right (Seligman 2002). Patient care outcomes even suffer when employees are unhappy. "Results from a Press Ganey study found that hospitals with the lowest employee satisfaction had the lowest patient satisfaction, and hospitals with the highest employee satisfaction had the highest patient satisfaction" (Strachota et al. 2003, p. 111).

Studies of business teams are fascinating. Losada (1999) studied sixty business teams that were meeting to determine their annual strategic plans. Fifteen teams were considered high performers, twenty-six teams were medium performers, and the remaining nineteen teams were low performers. The performance categories were based on three criteria: profitability, customer service rankings, and the number of positive performance appraisal evaluations received within the team. The planning sessions were videotaped, and all speech acts were coded for three different attributes: whether the act was positive or negative, whether it involved inquiry or advocacy, and finally, whether it was self or other related. The results were astounding. The high-performing teams had the broadest range and widest repertoire of behaviors. They had a significantly higher numbers of positive acts. The low-performing teams had a higher level of negativity, and they lost their ability to question and became stuck in self-absorbed advocacy. They lost their behavioral flexibility all together. The clear conclusion is that the more positive the team, the more effective it is.

Positivity and positive emotions are also related to flourishing, or finding the "good life," and the development of a broad repertoire of skills. Barbara Fredrickson has studied positive emotions extensively, and she has proposed a causal theory of positive emotion (Fredrickson 1998, 2001, 2003). In its study of emotions, traditional psychology has come to conclude that emotions engender thought–action tendencies. For example, anger tells us that our boundaries have been invaded and prepares us to defend ourselves. Fear induces a reaction that brings us to remove ourselves from dangerous situations. Sadness prepares us for loss. The positive emotions have only begun to be understood. Fredrickson's extensive research leads her to suggest that the purpose of positive emotions is to help us to develop our resilience and broaden our repertoire of skills. The positive emotions build and deepen our physical, emotional, social, and intellectual resources. Positive emotions, therefore, clearly produce benefits in the workplace.

Just one example can illustrate this point. When we feel positive emotion, we are more approachable to others and build good relationships with other people, thus broadening our social resources. The impact in the workplace is clear. Improved social resources lead to higher levels of teamwork, cooperation, and supportive behavior. All of these outcomes are desperately needed in today's demanding working environments.

Increased Employee Retention

It is almost impossible to sort out whether higher job satisfaction makes you happier or a happy disposition makes you more satisfied with your job. Clearly, however, these two factors are closely interrelated. Happier people are more satisfied with their jobs, and job satisfaction is clearly linked to employee retention. Engagement and commitment among employees are related to their attitude toward their work and have an influence on retention rates (Buckingham and Coffman 1999; Kaye and Jordan-Evans 1999, 2002).

In addition, happier people form more positive connections with others. Happier people are friendlier and others gravitate toward them. A happier workforce clearly leads to a higher level of affective organizational commitment, as one of the reasons that people stay in their jobs is because they like their coworkers. Employees who are happier are not only looking for settings with is a good work environment; they also help to create that environment.

Improved Employee Health

A great deal of research in positive psychology has focused on the relationship between positive emotions and health status. Although health status does not seem to be directly linked to a person's perception of happiness, there is no question that overall happy people are healthier than unhappy people. "Optimism and hope cause better resistance to depression when bad events strike, better performance at work, particularly in challenging jobs, and better physical health" (Seligman 2002, p. 83). Research studies have also shown that happiness and other positive emotions can actually undo some of the adverse physiological effects of negative emotions, such as the effect of adrenalin released in response to fear or threat. Experiments on nonhuman primates have shown that recurrent emotion-related cardiovascular activity injures the inner walls of the arteries and can initiate atherosclerosis. In empirical studies, it has been found that positive emotions reduced the amount of time the negative emotion had an impact on the cardiovascular reactivity that occurs after negative emotion (Fredrickson 2003).

Positive emotions also seem to fuel resiliency. A study was conducted on students who had been tested for resiliency and optimism shortly before the terrorist attacks on the United States in 2001. The students were interviewed again within days after the September 11 attacks, and more than 70 percent of the participants reported feeling depressed. Yet, those participants who had been identified as resilient during the earlier interviews also expressed strong positive emotions immediately after the attacks and were half as likely to be depressed as those participants who had been identified earlier as being nonresilient. The statistical analysis of the study's results showed that the tendency to feel more positive emotion buffered the resilient people against depression. Resilient participants expressed gratitude about the good things they had learned from the crisis and felt optimistic about the future (Fredrickson 2003).

Study after study has shown that chronic negative emotions, especially anger and depression, correlate with a broad range of disorders and diseases ranging from back pain and headaches to heart disease and cancer. For example, one remarkable long-term study has been widely reported. At the beginning of the study in the 1930s, almost two hundred young Catholic nuns were asked to write a personal essay when they entered the novitiate at the age of twenty. Many wrote about their lives and the reason they chose to become nuns. Their essays were archived and eventually came to light during the 1990s as part of a larger study on aging and Alzheimer's disease. Researchers read the essays and scored them for positive emotional content, recording specific instances of happiness, interest, love, and hope. The findings were quite remarkable: "The nuns who expressed the most positive emotions lived up to 10 years longer than those who expressed the fewest. This gain in life expectancy is considerably larger than the gain achieved by those who quit smoking" (Fredrickson 2003, p. 330). Healthier employees translate to a number of advantages in the workplace, including lower levels of absenteeism, less illness and therefore lower medical benefit costs, and potentially longer tenure on the job because of overall wellness.

Improved Patient Care Environment

It seems almost self-evident that employees who are happier contribute to a more positive patient care environment. Patients quickly and easily pick up on the moods of the people who care for them. Certainly, the quality of interactions among employees in the various departments is also a critical factor in the patient care environment. The research on emotional intelligence clearly documents that emotions are highly contagious from person to person, especially from manager to employee (Cherniss and Goleman 2001; Goleman 1995; Goleman, Boyatzis, and McKee 2002).

Furthermore, some research suggests that happy people are more altruistic than their unhappy counterparts. Happy people are likely to be more giving, not just of money but of time and emotion as well. In laboratory studies, both adults and children who are happy display more empathy and are more willing to donate money to those in need. Although you would think that people who have experienced adversity in their lives would identify with the suffering of others and behave more generously, this assumption is not necessarily true. When we are happy, we are less self-focused, we like others more, and we are more willing to share ourselves and our good fortune. It turns out that looking out for number one is more characteristic of sadness than of well-being (Seligman 2002).

The strong business case for happiness at work is clear. In spite of the corporate scandals in today's world and the apparent increasing negativity in the workplace, many organizations work hard to create an environment that is a challenging and enjoyable place to work. "Contrary to common perception, there are many successful executives who understand that 'good business' involves more than making money, and who take the responsibility for making their firms an engine for enhancing the quality of life" (Csikszentmihalyi 2003, p. 34).

Happiness Defined

Happiness in the workplace is important for a variety of reasons, but just what is happiness? The capacity for happiness refers to the ability to enjoy the good things in life if and when they come your way. Being happy means experiencing pleasure, enthusiasm, and satisfaction (Seligman 2002). As pointed out earlier, happiness can refer to and encompass positive emotions about the past, the future, or the present. "The experience of happiness in action is *enjoyment*—the exhilarating sensation of being fully alive" (Csikszentmihalyi 2003, p. 37). Happiness is far more than temporary pleasure. Pleasure is only one component of a complex concept. As we will see shortly, authentic happiness is a desirable goal that requires a full understanding of positive experiences that go well beyond mere pleasure.

Happiness Set Point

Can we determine or influence our level of happiness? To some degree, the answer is yes. However, extensive research on identical twins has led to the conclusion that every individual has a happiness set point. "Roughly 50% of almost every personality trait turns out to be attributable to genetic inheritance" (Seligman 2002, p. 47). The studies of identical twins separated at birth have been very revealing. The studies report that the psychological makeup of identical twins is much more similar than that of fraternal twins and that the psychology of adopted children is much more like the psychology of their birth parents than like the psychology of their adoptive parents (Lykken 1999). Simply translated, this means that about half of your predisposition toward happiness is genetically determined.

The happiness set point determined by our genetics appears to function much like a thermostat. After a happy or negative event occurs, we return to our previous level of happiness within a short period of time. For example, when a matched sample of twenty-two winners of large amounts of lottery money was studied, it was found that each individual reverted to his or her baseline level of happiness over time. The lottery winners ended up no happier than the twenty-two matched controls who were not winners. On the positive side, this means that after a negative event occurs, the mood thermostat will pull us up out of our misery. Conversely, for those with a lower set point for happiness, even very positive events cannot improve our level of happiness over the long term.

> Even individuals who become paraplegic as a result of spinal cord accidents quickly begin to adapt to their greatly limited capacities, and within eight weeks they report more net positive emotion than negative emotion. Within a few years, they wind up only slightly less happy on average than individuals who are not paralyzed. Of people with extreme quadriplegia, 84 percent consider their life to be average or above average (Seligman 2002, p. 48).

Although 50 percent of happiness is predetermined by our genes, our individual level of happiness can be changed by life events and our own attitudes. Specifically, 40 percent of our happiness is determined by our own interpretation of life events, and only 10 percent is related to actual negative or positive events (Seligman 2002).

Sources of Happiness

Before we examine what brings us happiness, a quick review of the research findings may shatter some commonly held misconceptions about happiness. For example, it is widely believed in modern societies that money brings happiness, and yet the extensive data on how wealth and poverty affect happiness clearly indicate that beyond a basic safety net, more money contributes little to subjective well-being.

> Work is undergoing a sea change in the wealthiest nations. Money, amazingly, is losing its power. The stark findings about life satisfaction— that beyond the safety net, more money adds little or nothing to subjective well-being—are starting to sink in. While real income in America has risen 16 percent in the last 30 years, the percentage of people who describe themselves as "very happy" has fallen from 36 to 29 percent (Seligman 2002, p. 165).

Even among people who live in poverty, levels of satisfaction are high in many life domains. It seems that how important money is to you, more than the money itself, is what influences your level of happiness. "Materialism seems to be counterproductive: at all levels of real income, people who value money more than other goals are less satisfied with their income and with their lives as a whole, although precisely why is a mystery" (Seligman 2002, p. 54). In other words, rich people are only slightly happier than poor people.

Similarly, health is only slightly related to happiness. This finding is probably a tribute to the ability of humans to adapt to adversity. Most of us rate our health positively even when we are quite sick. "Remarkably, even severely ill cancer patients differ only slightly on global life satisfaction from objectively healthy people" (Seligman 2002, p. 58). However, disabling disease that is severe and long-lasting does produce a decline in life satisfaction and happiness for most people. Families that include a member who has Alzheimer's disease also were an exception, and their levels of happiness declined over time.

Although the results of positive psychology research may seem counterintuitive to many people, factors such as educational level, climate, race, and gender seem to have little or no effect on happiness. Similarly, physical attractiveness apparently does not have much effect on happiness (Diener 2000; Diener and Diener 1996; Diener, Sandvik, and Pavot 1991; Seligman 2002).

On the basis of extensive research findings, Seligman has identified three different factors that lead individuals to decide whether they are happy or unhappy. The first is that we experience pleasure in our lives, the second is that we feel engaged, and the third is that our lives are imbued with meaning. Ideally, each of these three elements is present in all areas of our lives: personal, family, and work. (You can evaluate your own level of happiness by completing the Authentic Happiness Inventory on Seligman's website at authentichappiness.com.)

The Pleasant Life

The first of these three aspects, the pleasant life, involves enjoying as much pleasure as possible. Pleasant experiences include short-term, intense sensory experiences such as tasting fresh raspberries, having a hot bath, or receiving a long massage. Because the memory and effects of such pleasures fade quickly, higher scores in this aspect of happiness do not necessarily lead to greater life satisfaction. The effects of pleasurable experiences, however, can be prolonged by techniques such as savoring and mindfulness.

The Engaged Life

Engagement in our activities and pursuits is more likely to lead to a perception that we are happy. In fact, Seligman is very clear on this point. "Authentic happiness comes from identifying and cultivating your most fundamental strengths and using them every day in work, love, play, and parenting" (Seligman 2002, p. xiii). By engagement, Seligman is referring to the idea of flow. Flow is defined as the unselfconscious state you enter when you are totally absorbed in what you are doing. Time passes without being noticed because we are totally engrossed in our task.

Mihaly Csikszentmihalyi (1990, 1997, 2003) was the first researcher to extensively study the concept of flow. Csikszentmihalyi and his colleagues use experience sampling methodology to measure the frequency of flow as well as what leads to flow. In this approach, participants are given beepers that are programmed to beep randomly throughout the day. Each participant records his or her activity and describes what is happening each time the beeper sounds.

Based on thousands and thousands of data points, the research has revealed that the experience of flow depends on several key factors, specifically:

- The activity must require skill.
- The activity must require concentration.
- The activity must include clear goals.
- The activity must generate immediate feedback.
- The individual must experience deep, effortless involvement in the activity.
- The individual must experience a sense of control.
- The individual's sense of self must vanish during the activity.
- The individual's sense of time passing must stop during the activity.

Research shows that flow happens only when you are engaged in a challenging activity that matches your skill level. Unfortunately, flow does not occur when you sit in front of a television set and watch the reruns of *Friends*.

Flow is related to gratification rather than pleasure. In fact, in most flow experiences, people report experiencing little or no emotion. If any emotion is mentioned in connection with the experience, it is usually described in retrospect. Another key point to note is that being in flow is a way to build psychological capital for the future. In other words, it results in growth and further development of our selves.

In one study, Csikszentmihalyi tracked the experiences of 250 high-flow and 250 low-flow teenagers. The results were described in *Authentic Happiness*:

> The low-flow teenagers are "mall" kids; they hang out at malls and they watch television a lot. The high-flow kids have hobbies, they engage in sports, and they spend a lot of time on homework. On every measure of

psychological well-being (including self-esteem and engagement) save one, the high-flow teenagers did better. The exception is important: the high-flow kids think their low-flow peers are having more fun, and say they would rather be at the mall doing all those "fun" things or watching television. But while all the engagement they have is not perceived as enjoyable, it pays off later in life. The high-flow kids are the ones who make it to college, who have deeper social ties, and whose later lives are more successful (Seligman 2002, p. 117).

The results of this study support Csikszentmihalyi's contention that flow is a state that builds psychological capital that can be drawn upon in the future when it is needed.

Dick Richards (Richards 1995a, 1995b) explored the concept of artistry and experiencing joy through work. Finding meaning in our work is directly related to our experience of joy, according to Richards. His examples are closely related to the concept of flow as presented by Csikszentmihalyi (1990):

> You know the experience. . . . Sometimes it happens at work. Your report is due tomorrow. You have thought about it, made many notes, and written a first draft. You have only the afternoon to write the final document. Sitting before your word processor, looking at the blinking cursor, it comes to you. Words and ideas flow. The next idea is there when you are ready for it. The perfect word presents itself when you need it. You get stuck, stand, walk down the corridor for a break and another cup of coffee, and the idea you need is there, as if it were waiting in the corridor for you to fetch it. You skip your break; you forget the coffee. At the end of the day the report seems perfect, and you marvel at what has happened (Richards 1995b, paragraphs 5–7).

Richards is describing the experience of joy, "the kind of joy that ascends during a period of activity that engages the entire self" (Richards 1995b, paragraph 10). He believes that seeking such experiences is part of the artistry of work and that such experiences occur when a person's whole self is absorbed in the activity. It occurs when "we are THERE: body, mind, emotion, spirit" (Richards 1995b, paragraph 12).

As a result of beginning his career as a graphic artist, Richards brings a different perspective to our concept of work. He points out that artists live for the experience of joy in their work. Unfortunately, this is very different from how most people approach their work. When we create emotional distance from our work, rather than being fully engaged in it, the net result is a lack of joy. And "the net result for organizations is a dangerous lack of the very inventiveness, flexibility, and courage they so sorely need" (Richards 1995b, paragraph 19).

The Meaningful Life

The third aspect of happiness is the belief that your life is meaningful. In the context of happiness, meaningfulness means that you are using your signature strengths in the service of something that you believe is larger than yourself. It is a positive focus on something outside or beyond our selves, a larger cause. We know the importance of a clear sense of purpose, both in our lives and in our organizations.

In *From Good to Great* (2001), Jim Collins found that values-driven organizations with a clear purpose perform better in the long run. At the personal level, clarity about your purpose has been an abiding theme in the self-improvement literature for decades (Covey 1989, 1992; Covey, Merrill, and Merrill 1994; Loehr and Schwartz 2003; Thomas 2000). "The search for meaning and purpose is among the most powerful and enduring themes in every culture since the origin of recorded history" (Loehr and Schwartz 2003, p. 131). Purpose is a powerful, enduring source of energy.

In summary, it is quite clear that happiness is a concept of splendid richness. Pleasure is one aspect but not the only thing that brings happiness. Happiness is clearly related to pleasure, engagement, and meaningfulness.

Case Study: Joy at Work*

The field of positive psychology is increasing our understanding of the positive emotions and suggesting concrete, specific interventions that can help increase the amount of happiness in our personal lives. But the research also suggests several approaches to applying positive psychology to the workplace.

The rest of the chapter will go on to pull all of the research findings together with concrete, specific applications for health care organizations. But first let's begin our examination of the implications of applying positive psychology in the workplace by looking at a research project that examined the experiences of health care workers who experience joy through their work. I conducted the study, one of the few to specifically focus on positive emotions in the workplace, in 2000 as part of the research for my doctoral dissertation.

---

*This section is adapted from Jo Manion, Joy at Work: Creating a Positive Workplace, *Journal of Nursing Administration* 22(12). Copyright © 2003 and used by permission of Lippincott Williams & Wilkins.

The decade of the 1990s was tumultuous for the health care indus-try, and many health care organizations experienced significant finan-cial challenges, declining employee commitment, and escalating demands from patients and their families. Every day seemed to bring a new crisis.

I set out to discover what I could about how health care workers experience and express joy in their work. Seeking ways to create a positive workplace, especially during tumultuous and challenging times, I asked twenty-four employed health care workers how they experi-enced joy in their work. Findings from these interviews provided insight into why some people are joyful even during difficult times and how we can bring more joy into the workplace for both ourselves and our colleagues.

Process

The study used a narrative approach and included face-to-face inter-views conducted to solicit accounts of joyful work experiences. The sample was made up of individual health care providers who either vol-unteered to participate or were recommended by their coworkers. All of the participants were credentialed and/or licensed health care providers. They came from a variety of health care facilities, and only individuals who had worked in at least three different employment set-tings were included in the sample.

Twelve women and twelve men in two different age-groups (baby boomers and genXers) participated. Coincidentally, half of the partic-ipants were first-line caregivers and half were managers (supervisors and several executives, including a hospital chief executive officer).

Participants came from California (one), the Midwest (eleven), the Northeast (three), and Florida (nine). Eighteen worked in hospi-tals at the time of the interviews; others were employed by a staffing agency, an association, a leadership institute, a hospice, a community clinic, and a state licensure board.

Questions related to the experience of joy were posed of all partic-ipants. (The interview format is reproduced in figure 4-1.) The inter-views were audiotaped and transcribed later. The data were reviewed using a category content approach, which is a form of content analysis that entails identifying categories and themes as they become apparent through review of the data. The themes and categories were derived inductively from the actual words and phrases of the participants. The assignment of themes and categories was validated by two additional reviewers, who compared the analyses of specific interviews.

Figure 4-1.   Interview Format

1. Would you tell me a little about what you do and where you work?

2. Now, let's talk about joy. What does joy mean to you?

3. When you are joyful, what does it look like to other people?

4. How often would you say that you experience joy through your work?

5. Can you tell me about a time that you felt joy through your work?
   a. Was there anything specifically happening when you felt this joy or that led to the joy?
   b. Is there anything you did that led to feeling this joy?

6. How did you express this joy?
   a. Do you remember how others around you responded to your expression of this joy?
   b. How did you respond to them?

7. Do you think that you do anything, either deliberately or subconsciously, that leads to an environment of joy in your workplace?

8. Is there anything your organization does that helps you find joy in your work?
   a. Are there times when it is hard to find joy in your work?
   b. Can you tell me what is going on during these times?
   c. Have you ever worked anywhere where it was hard to be joyful?

9. How important is it to you that you find joy in your work?

Findings

Analyzing the stories and examples to determine common themes was the first level of interpretation. A deeper level of analysis required hearing each participant's interview as a story of that individual's experience of joy through work. This level of analysis revealed a primary theme expressed by all of the individuals.

Nature of Joy

Participants were not given a specific description of joy. Instead, they were asked to define the term in their own words. Those interviewed described joy from their own perspective and in a variety of ways. Some talked about the experiential component of joy (for example, "having a light and happy heart" and "you're excited about getting up every morning and can't wait to get to work"). Others mentioned the physiological aspects of joy (for example, "you feel warm and fuzzy and glad," "it's kind of a spurt," and "inside I get a warmth, a feeling of excitement"). Others described joy in terms of what brings it about for them ("it's a sense of accomplishment," "when someone says thank-you," and "knowing you make a difference").

For most of the participants, joy was expressed outwardly (through specific behaviors such as laughing, smiling, humming, singing, or having sparkly eyes) and was noticed by other people. The almost universal response of others was positive. Over half of the participants described joy as contagious, noting that their joy led to joy in others. Not all descriptions of joy were of an exuberant nature. There were many examples of joy that illustrated a restrained, quiet, or contented feeling.

On the basis of the participants' descriptions as well as on an extensive review of the literature, the study concluded that joy can be defined as an intensely positive, vivid, and expansive emotion that arises from an internal state or results from an external event or situation. It may include physiological reactions and emotional expressions as well as conscious volition. It is a transcendent state of heightened energy and excitement.

Each of the stories of joy described by the participants was analyzed and coded for factors that were related to the experience of joy. Table 4-1 summarizes these findings. Factors related to joy at work were numerous and experienced differently by each individual. Four general themes were identified: the work itself, people and relationships, the self, and the work environment. Participants mentioned factors related to the work itself most frequently. These work-related factors were categorized into items characteristic of the work or an outcome of the work. The most frequently identified single factor was found in the general theme of people and relationships and was connection with others.

Of all of the various factors, only three were found in every person's stories: (1) the work represented progress, (2) it involved connections with other people, and (3) the work reflected competence on the part of the individual.

Barriers to Experiencing Joy

People were asked about barriers to their experience of joy in their work. The factors most often identified were coworkers (for example, coworkers who displayed negative, nonsupportive, unpleasant, or uncooperative behavior), poor leadership, insufficient resources (such as inadequate staffing or lack of necessary equipment), and unappealing (repetitive, boring, or meaningless) work.

Table 4-1.   Factors Associated with Joy

Factors	Number of Times Mentioned	Number of People Who Identified Item at Least Once (N = 24)
The Work Itself	Total 413	Total 24
Outcome of work		
Represented progress	116	24
Accomplishment	32	14
Achievement	21	13
Characteristics of work		
Appeal of work	89	21
Made a difference	74	21
Helped someone else	37	14
Autonomy	31	16
Was an opportunity	13	8
People and Relationships	Total 341	Total 24
Connection with others	178	24
Recognition	89	19
Appreciation	74	21
The Self	Total 263	Total 24
Competence	129	24
Self-esteem	89	15
Attitudes, values, and beliefs	45	20
The Work Environment	Total 99	Total 23
Social aspects	52	18
The organizational culture	47	16

Organization's Role in Creating Joy

When asked whether the organizations for which they worked did anything that increased their experience of joy, most of the participants indicated that they believed that the organizations did not have an active role in influencing their experience of joy. In other words, the presence of joy is an individual issue. Nonetheless, in the participants' examples, factors were identified that described the organization's role:

- Creation of a positive work environment
- Recruitment and retention of good people (both employees and leaders)

- Provision of adequate benefits and compensation
- Dedication to mission
- Provision of adequate resources

Pathways to Finding Joy at Work

The next step in analysis moved from breaking down participants' stories into factors and instead examined each interview in its entirety. Analyzing the stories revealed four distinct individual pathways to joy: connections, love of the work, achievement, and recognition. Each pathway reflects a major theme of the participants' stories and their primary source of joy through their work.

Connections

The connections pathway to joy is based on the connections made and relationships formed with people in the workplace. Caring for, talking with, relating to, and helping others are frequent aspects identified in this pathway. The *primary* source of joy is other people and relationships. Eight of the participants exemplified this pathway to joy.

Carl, a young director of nursing, demonstrated this pathway when he said, "I definitely like people and caring for them and working with them." Karen initially described joy as "a feeling of well-being . . . surrounded by people you love or care about." Sally and Marie both said that one-on-one contact with others and the opportunity for socialization at work were important to them. Dick and Jake both said that what brought them joy was "working with their peers."

Carl offered several illuminating examples as he talked about his work with patients who had undergone major cardiovascular surgery. In his words:

> I did the heart transplants for quite a while and the by-passes where you work with them for eight hours, trying to recover them, and by the time you got back the next day, they're already shipped out. That's when I started going, "Well, hey, I'm not interacting with them anymore." You dealt with them while you recovered the patient. You got them well through their heart recovery phase, and by the time you got back there on the next shift, they were already gone. For me, **I lost my connection.** That didn't give me joy anymore, if that makes any sense. You start becoming more of a, like a front line factory worker, is what you're doing. **You're not interacting with anybody.**

Most of Carl's conversation about his work in the cardiac recovery unit revolved around the people with whom he worked. He described several of his colleagues in great detail and talked about what a great group they were. He recalled his dismay when the group started to break up and noted that "they're all gone, except for one nurse." He said all of a sudden it was like, "Oh, shoot! I'm the lead guy now! Now I'm in charge! But, hey, I didn't **have any really true connections anymore."**

Karen, a young nurse, worked temporarily at another hospital in their float pool. She tried this work on two separate occasions because the money was so appealing, but she simply could not stay with it. Karen indicated that she did not stay with this job because she had "no relationship with the people . . . [she was] working with." Most of the stories of joy Karen shared throughout her interview were clearly related to a sense of connection with other people. She summed up the joy she felt through her work as an emergency department charge nurse by saying, "A lot of it is **working with other people. The relationships we form** and the fun you get to have with other people, and you really get to know people on a very intimate level when you're working with life-and-death situations."

Love of the Work

A second pathway to joy is through the love of the work itself. Although many other factors were associated positively with their experience of joy, eight of the participants felt a strong connection and identification with the work itself. When they talked about the work they did, they reported that most things about it excited them.

These participants often expressed a deep sense of personal mission. Lana expressed it well: "I feel fortunate that **I get to do what I feel a passion for.**" In several places in Jane's interview she remarked, "I get such joy out of just being a nurse, I love the essence of nursing, this is why I went into nursing, and finally, I realized I really loved being a nurse." All of Jane's comments projected her love and enthusiasm for the work of nursing. Bob, a respiratory therapist, spent the first fifteen minutes of his interview describing his work as an RT in minute detail.

Those who found their pathway to joy through the love of their work often talked about being excited when they woke up just because they were going to work. Alan, a young manager of outpatient surgery, described joy as occurring when you "**enjoy what you're doing.** Means I can't wait to get to work and I'm excited about getting up every morning and going to work." Pam echoed this feeling: "I wake up in the morning, and I'm happy to get up at five o'clock in the morning, even though I'm tired. And I'm happy to go to work. I'm happy to do my day and I'm happy that I've been given this responsibility."

Participants whose experience fell along this pathway shared rich detail about their jobs and expressed enthusiasm about the actual work. Their accounts were vivid in comparison to the accounts of people such as Jake, a young emergency department nurse, who openly declared that nothing about the work itself brought him joy. What brought him joy was working with his peers. Pam, on the other hand, was a good example of enthusiasm and love for her work.

> It's funny, because **I think everything's joyful.** I love watching the cardiac monitors. I like doing the phone calls. I love starting the IVs. I like talking to the patients. I like getting them ready. I like receiving them from surgery. I like giving them their warm blankets, putting them around them, 'cause I can just see them melt, you know? And I like to make them comfortable. Everything, I must say, **it really gives me joy to do all parts of my job.** I [even] love . . . the paperwork.

Achievement

The third pathway to joy is through achievement. For five participants the emphasis in their stories related to accomplishment or attainment of a particular goal. Ellen defined joy as "a job well-done. That I feel good about the work I've completed, that I'm happy to know that I did a nice job for myself or someone else, or completed a project relevant to my work and that made a difference."

John said that joy for him came to him when he realized that "the results of something that you've done, that has truly made someone else happy, then it makes you happy."

Don, senior-level manager, defined joy as meeting management challenges (". . . that's what makes life worthwhile to me"). He provided numerous examples of the improvements and changes he had made over his tenure. His sense of pride and accomplishment was quite evident.

The stories of these five participants were full of accounts of achievements, accomplishments, and positive work outcomes. Melinda described each of her promotions, and Ellen described successful projects that contributed significantly to her organization.

Interestingly, all of these participants worked in management or supervisory positions. Perhaps people who experience joy through achievement are more likely to find their way into management and executive positions, where they have more autonomy, authority, and the specific responsibility for making change happen in their organizations.

It is important to note that for these five people, the world's opinion seemed less important than their internal assessment of their outcomes. Pleasure and pride in the process were not as important as the actual outcome. External trappings of success such as wealth, position, adulation, and awards probably would have made little or no difference to them if they had not achieved positive and meaningful outcomes.

This point was clearly evident during Joyce's interview. Joyce was a chief executive officer of a major health care organization. She began her interview by explaining that she did not feel much joy in her current position. A highly competent and successful woman, she had been promoted to chief executive officer four years earlier. She was considered influential, principle focused, and people oriented and was highly respected by all who knew her. An extremely committed and hardworking professional, she looked back over the past four years of her career and could not see any significant forward progress in her organization as the result of her efforts. She admitted that "spinning her wheels" and the lack of forward progress just "drove her crazy." All of her stories reflected a need for completion and applicability of the results in a useful way. Although the outside world would judge her to be an extremely successful person, inside she felt joyless.

Recognition

Recognition is the fourth pathway to joy, and three of the participants illustrated this beautifully. Recognition has to do with the acknowledgment of others, and in many instances it occurs as a result of expressions of appreciation.

There can be little doubt that warm, genuine expressions of gratitude or recognition of a person's efforts bring joy to most people. And, in fact, twenty-three of the twenty-four participants identified these two factors at least once. For example, Betty said that compliments from coworkers let her know that they appreciated or valued something about her or what she did. The first story of joy that came to her mind when we began the interview was a story about how she had influenced a "grumpy" patient's attitude. In the end, she was recognized for her intervention with a public award.

Although recognition brings most people joy, for these three people it is a *primary* source of joy. After Dan's interview, I was struck by the number of times he talked about appreciation expressed by others. He said, "The most obvious reflections of joy occur when physicians or other staff are complimentary or they recognize a job well done." When asked to share a specific example of a time he felt joy through his work, he shared a beautiful story that drove this point home. He was called into his twelve-hour night shift early, at 3 p.m., to care for a patient who was hemorrhaging severely after an aortic valve replacement. Dan shared in vivid detail the intense work of trying to stabilize this patient throughout a sixteen-hour shift. Around 3 a.m., the patient's condition improved and it appeared that he would survive at least for the near term. Dan went on to say:

> But an incredible thing happened like, at six o'clock in the morning. Three of this man's daughters (pause) three of his daughters and his wife, had somehow, at six o'clock in the morning, they found a thank-you card somewhere, and they got this thank-you card and they said, "Thank you for an extremely good job and we realize just how close, you know, everything was."

It was obvious that receiving a simple thank-you card from his patient's family had the power to move Dan (a tough Vietnam veteran) to tears and a sense of joy. Almost every example of joy that Dan shared was somehow related to recognition or appreciation expressed.

The common theme of this pathway involves being recognized by others in the workplace. Recognition includes receiving compliments, expressions of appreciation, or awards; being given more responsibility; being asked to take on a special project; or being accorded the respect of others in the workplace.

Model of Joy in the Workplace

A model of joy at work was developed on the basis of the interview data, as well as a review of the literature. (See figure 4-2.) Factors in the three thematic areas—the work itself, people and relationships, and the work environment—all provide the stimulus for joy to occur when the necessary internal factors (represented in the theme the self) exist within the individual. The internal factors include self-esteem; attitudes, beliefs, and values; and competence. The person places a value on the particular situation or makes a judgment that the situation is positive and concludes (either consciously or subconsciously) that he or she feels joy. The joy may or may not be expressed externally. When expressed externally (by smiling, laughing, singing, or having "sparkly eyes"), others in the immediate environment react positively with a similar or reciprocal experience. Their expression of joy further reinforces the individual's perception of his or her own joy.

Implications for Managers

The model of joy has several important implications for managers who are seeking to create a more positive work environment. A person's attitude is both necessary and sufficient for joy to be experienced.

Figure 4-2.   A Model of Joy

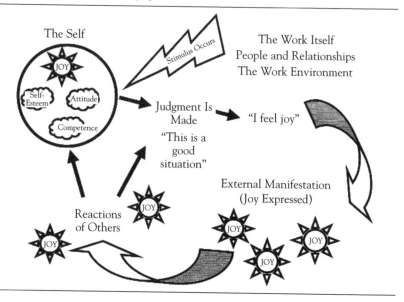

Numerous examples described health care providers who clearly found joy despite a negative or unpleasant situation. This finding suggests that a predisposition toward joy is sufficient for joy to occur. For example, Karen, the young emergency department charge nurse, described several tragic and painful situations in her department during which she felt joyful because she knew she had made a difference for a patient or a family. She chose to feel joyful when others in the same situation might have been negatively affected.

Furthermore, joy often transcends a particular situation; people who experience joy often retain a positive attitude despite current circumstances. A predisposition toward joy is a positive trait that can be sought in job applicants. Positive emotions are important for anyone aspiring to be a leader. Probing behavioral interview questions that focus on what brings the candidate joy at work could shed light on whether the applicant is likely to experience joy in a specific work setting.

Figure 4-3 illustrates the dynamics evident in an interaction between internal factors that affect individuals and external factors in the work environment. The factors that lead to or impede the experience of joy are diagrammed as a force field. Factors such as attitude (identified by eighteen people), competency (identified by all twenty-four participants), and accessibility to a favorable primary pathway are more heavily weighted (as represented by the larger arrows). The

Figure 4-3. Factors Supporting or Inhibiting the Experience of Joy at Work

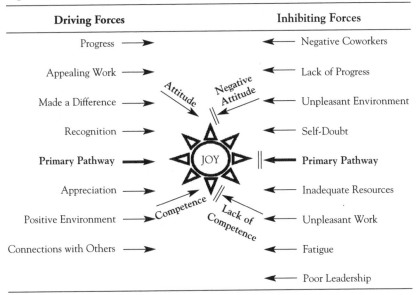

Driving Forces	Inhibiting Forces
Progress ⟶	⟵ Negative Coworkers
Appealing Work ⟶	⟵ Lack of Progress
Made a Difference ⟶	⟵ Unpleasant Environment
Recognition ⟶	⟵ Self-Doubt
Primary Pathway ⟶	⟵ **Primary Pathway**
Appreciation ⟶	⟵ Inadequate Resources
Positive Environment ⟶	⟵ Unpleasant Work
Connections with Others ⟶	⟵ Fatigue
	⟵ Poor Leadership

absence of such necessary factors can actually preclude the experience of joy.

Individual factors (as represented by small arrows) such as progress achieved, appealing work, or the appreciation of others may also lead to joy. These individual factors, however, are not as likely to create the same intensity or sustainability of joyful feeling.

In the same way, inhibiting forces can be significant. For example, incompetence or a negative attitude can lead an individual to feel little or no joy. Lack of accessibility to a pathway may result in a lack of joy as suggested in many of the stories. However, the presence of one or two negative factors does not necessarily rob a person of joy. For example, the person who is predominantly joyful, who has a positive attitude and a job and workplace that match his or her primary pathway, is less likely to feel joyless to a significant level in the presence of one or several impeding factors. No workplace is perfect; likely it is the cumulative effect of impeding factors that drives joy out of the workplace.

The reciprocal relationship between some of these factors is more difficult to map, and yet it is relatively easy to understand. For instance, the factor of competence is related to various triggers of joy. For example, if I am very competent at what I do, I will be more likely to receive recognition for it, know that I make a difference, or see desirable progress as a result of my efforts. These factors, in turn, positively reinforce my sense of competence. Conversely, if I believe I am unable to function in a competent manner because of my lack of training or inadequate resources, I will have trouble experiencing joy. As we saw in an earlier chapter, competence is intrinsically rewarding to people. Understanding this concept can explain employee reactions to changes in policies and practices when the changes have an impact on a person's competence or perception of competence.

From the stories shared by participants in this study, the primary pathway through which an individual experiences joy is necessary and must be present for the person to experience a significant and sustained level of joy. Many participants described work situations in which they had found it difficult to find joy as a result of their inability to access their own individual pathway to joy. For example, Carl "lost his connections" and left the job. Dan was miserable in one position because he was treated with suspicion and dislike rather than appreciation and recognition. Joyce was joyless because she was unable to establish forward progress in her organization. People may experience brief periods of joy in their day-to-day work from individual factors (such as a sincere thank-you, completion of a challenging task, or the knowledge that he or she has helped someone else), but these experiences will not be enough to sustain the individual in the long run.

Implications for Organizational Leaders

Participants in this study experienced joy through their work despite turmoil and challenges in the work environment. Experiencing joy in their work was important enough that they would seek another position if they were unable to find joy in their present jobs. This suggests a direct link to an individual's intent to stay in a job (organizational commitment), which has implications for retention strategies.

The model of joy (figure 4-2) and joy's driving and restraining forces suggests ways leaders can create a more positive work environment. Joy is contagious and transcendent. Study participants provided numerous examples of how joy rubs off on others and creates a reciprocal and reinforcing relationship with those in close proximity. Thus, one person's joy is often shared with others, leading to that second person's experience of joy and, in turn, increasing the original person's feeling of joy.

This finding has major implications for leaders attempting to create a positive environment in the workplace. There is evidence in the literature that the moods or emotions of individuals in a particular work team or group are linked to the moods or emotions of others in the same group (Barsade and Gibson 1998; Bartel and Saavedra 2000). Totterdell has conducted numerous studies that demonstrate that the moods of individual are often affected by the moods of the people around them (Totterdell 2000; Totterdell et al. 1998).

Organizations can use a knowledge of factors that increase the experience of joy as well as a knowledge of the pathways to joy as underlying concepts for making internal decisions. This knowledge can also be very useful in addressing workforce shortages. For instance, if a person is unable to attain his or her primary pathway to joy, the judgment that "this is a good situation" is not made and joy is not experienced on a significant level. Understanding this concept will help leaders appreciate the full impact of organizational change. For example, skill-mix or staffing changes that disrupt relationships may more adversely affect people for whom a connections pathway is important. Changes in work flow that significantly reduce the amount of time spent with individual patients or with coworkers in easy camaraderie can have a negative effect of the development of interpersonal relationships.

For example, one organization implemented a new policy that dictated that employees could no longer use the intranet to transmit information of a personal nature, such as information about baby showers or where friends were meeting over the weekend or who was bringing what to a potluck dinner. The policy change had the greatest impact on those employees for whom connections were an important pathway to joy at work.

In the same way, during restructuring or work redesign efforts, changes that alter the nature of the work can affect those who love the work they are doing. People in the achievement pathway are more likely to be frustrated by meetings that go nowhere, problems that are never solved, and meaningless process refinements that have little impact on end results.

Those who find joy in recognition want that recognition to be sincere, personal, and frequent. For such employees, the annual employee recognition dinner is probably not enough.

Knowledge of the four pathways is helpful for the leader to consider when changes are made. When the potential negative impact on people is appreciated, actions can be taken to recognize and mitigate the potentially damaging effects of the change before the change is made.

Leaders are also instrumental in modeling joyfulness. The participants reported that they purposely monitored their own attitudes and looked for things in the workplace that created a sense of joy. In the words of Lana, "I find things to get joy from." Casey, an emergency department charge nurse, said that she encouraged employees to see the positive side of situations. When complaints were heard about the length of time a patient was held in the department, Casey insisted that they were now that many hours closer to getting the patient transferred.

Strategies for Increasing Happiness and Joy at Work

Joy is a powerful emotion, and when it occurs as a result of our work, life is much more satisfying and pleasant. Most of us spend more of our awake and alert time at work than we do with our loved ones. To experience the potentially positive impact work can have in our lives requires a tremendous amount of engagement and commitment on our part, but that effort promises to bring us fulfillment. In fact, the emotions people feel while they work are likely to reflect most directly the true quality of work life (Goleman, Boyatzis, and McKee 2002).

Each of us is responsible for choosing joy, and this study sheds some light on what we might do to find it. The participants in the joy at work study clearly believed that other people can do little to influence the experience of joy and that choosing to look for and feel joy is an individual rather than an organizational issue. Csikszentmihalyi agrees: "Contrary to what most of us believe, happiness does not simply happen to us. It's something we make happen, and it results from our doing our best" (Csikszentmihalyi 2003, p. 37). Obviously, no one can make you happy against your will, but there are strategies we can use as individuals and as leaders to increase our own levels of happiness and influence the level of happiness experienced by our colleagues and coworkers.

The good news is that there are proven techniques that can be used to achieve lasting improvements in the level of happiness in those who use them. Several are explained in the rest of this chapter. The techniques are organized by time orientation, that is, by whether they affect positive emotions of the past, present, or future. (Figure 4-4 summarizes these approaches.)

Figure 4-4.   Approaches to Increasing Happiness Based on Time Orientation

Appreciation	Pleasure	Mentoring relationships
Gratitude	Engagement	Personal legacies
Forgiveness	Meaning	Optimism
← Past	Present	Future →

Influencing Positive Emotions Related to the Past

The positive emotions related to the past include satisfaction, contentment, serenity, pride, and fulfillment. We can lose or diminish positive emotion about past events when we underappreciate the good things that have happened or overemphasize the negative by holding onto grudges, bitterness, and feelings of injustice. When we understand the value of appreciation and forgiveness, it becomes a relatively simple matter to find ways to begin to mitigate their effects.

Appreciation and Gratitude

Some people have the signature strength of gratitude, and they are very aware of the good things that happen to them and rarely take them for granted. This strength is also evidenced by taking time to express appreciation. Research has found that expressing gratitude and appreciation increases our level of happiness. How can we use this concept in the workplace?

Individual Employees

As individual employees, we can apply this principle in a variety of ways. Letting colleagues, physicians, and leaders know when they have done something you appreciate is important. Few of us can hear too many thank-yous, and you can say thank you in a variety of ways. We often forget that managers and physicians may hear fewer expressions of appreciation than other clinical and support staff. We should never underestimate the power of simple appreciation. An occasional thank-you can really boost the spirits of both the recipient and the giver, and the absence of a sincere thank-you when it is deserved can also have a significant effect. For example, during a recent conversation with the family physician I saw during my childhood, the physician told me about a family whose car was hit by a train. (This event occurred in the 1950s.) The husband was taken by ambulance to one hospital, and the young wife was brought to the small rural hospital's emergency department where the physician worked. The young woman's condition deteriorated quickly, and it was determined that she was in shock owing to internal bleeding. At that time, the hospital had a walking blood bank that had been organized by the director of the laboratory. During the time this young woman was cared for in the small hospital, she received a total of twenty-seven units of blood over a period of thirty-six hours (representing an almost superhuman effort in those days). Neither physician nor hospital staff left her side. Eventually, she was stabile enough to be transferred to a large medical center for treatment. She survived and went on to live a full life. Over fifty years later, this physician still remembers that neither he nor any of the hospital staff ever heard a thank-you from the patient or the family for their extraordinary efforts.

Leaders and Managers

Many effective management and leadership techniques are based on the principle of appreciation. You are probably already using one or more of them without realizing it. Appreciative inquiry is an approach to dealing with problems that begins with recognizing and appreciating what is already going right. Using a forward-focused approach in meetings when the discussion is spiraling downward is another approach based in gratitude. It brings the group back to focus on what is going right and what it is doing well. Simply guiding conversations in the direction of recognizing and appreciating what is good and right is a way of using gratitude. Sending employees handwritten notes of appreciation is another example of this principle in action.

Gratitude works because it amplifies our good memories of the past. In some cases, gratitude flows when we simply pay attention. Too often, however, our attention is focused on immediate problems: the heavy traffic on the way to work, the internet sites your teenage daughter may be looking at, or the heavy workload because John just called in sick. Concentrating on immediate problems and difficulties makes it easy for us to develop a tendency to forget about all of the things that are going well. For instance, you might forget that you got an early start this morning because the weather was clear and the traffic moved quickly; or you might forget that your daughter's grades have improved since she starting using the internet to help with her homework; or you might forget that John's crew works exceptionally well together and will be able to handle the extra work.

Appreciation Exercises

One simple exercise that is based on the value of expressing appreciation is the balancing exercise. It can be used by individuals or groups that are faced with changes in the workplace. The balancing exercise is simple: First, the individual or the leader of the group draws two columns on a drawing board or a piece of paper. Then the individual or group develops a list of the positive things about the change (what they will gain) in one column and the negative things (what they will lose) in the other. If you're working as an individual and find yourself unable to look at the change objectively, you can ask a trusted friend or colleague to sit down with you and share their perspective and thoughts regarding the change. Chances are they will think of things you did not consider. This exercise is powerful because it reminds us that no situation is wholly negative. There are many things to be grateful for, but we tend not to see them when faced with a difficult change, loss, or challenge.

Simply noticing what we are grateful for is an activity that raises our level of appreciation. At least two specific exercises from the field of positive psychology—gratitude visits and everyday blessings—increase the level of happiness among the people who do them. Although the gratitude visit is most often used in the context of the participants' personal lives, it can be modified and used in the workplace. The general idea is to select someone who has been especially kind to you or helpful in some way but whom you have never taken the opportunity to thank. You then write a gratitude letter to that person that describes in concrete terms why you are grateful to that person. Citing specifics and how they affected you increases the impact of the letter. You then personally deliver the letter to the person by reading it aloud. This exercise is especially effective in a group setting when the members of the group are able to discuss their reactions to the letters after they have been read. Seligman uses this exercise in his psychology classes and reports that the exercise results in powerful experiences that affect students for a long time.

This exercise is not easy for many people, because in western cultures we tend to shy away from public or open expressions of gratitude. "We do not have a vehicle in our culture for telling the people who mean the most to us how thankful we are that they are on the planet—and even when we are moved to do so, we shrink in embarrassment" (Seligman 2002, p. 74).

Everyday blessings is another simple exercise to increase the amount of gratitude in our lives. Most of us spend most of our time focusing on how to correct problems, and we remember failures more readily than successes. We tend to ruminate over bad events more thoroughly than good events, and this predisposition reduces our satisfaction levels, elevates anxiety, and deepens depression. Noticing what is going right promotes optimism about the future.

The exercise involves having each individual write down three things, large or small, that went really well that day just before he or she goes to bed. Next to each positive event, the individual then writes and answer to this question: Why did this good thing happen? Over time, this activity has been found to significantly increase participants' perception of their happiness.

Variations of the everyday blessings exercise can be used by managers and employees alike. At the beginning of a shift or workday, participants can quickly share something that went well and why since the last time they met.

One executive uses a similar approach. At the beginning of the week in a quick team huddle on Monday, she asks everyone present to begin by sharing something good that happened the week before. This, she says, starts the entire week off on a positive note even when things promise to be difficult and challenging.

Many managers use another form of this exercise when they end meetings with a key question such as: What has been something good about the time we have just spent together? This is a positive way to end a meeting and is especially useful when the meeting has been especially difficult or negative. The exercise can be done quickly, with each individual sharing one thing they found positive about the meeting. People leave feeling good about their time together.

Forgiveness

Now we have discussed the first way we lose or diminish positive emotions about past events: underappreciating the good things that have happened. The second way is by overemphasizing the negative by holding onto grudges, bitterness, or feelings of injustice. To address these negative circumstances, letting go and forgiveness are approaches that can increase happiness.

Individual Employees

At the individual level, understanding the negative impact of holding onto grudges and grievances is important. Frequent and intense negative thoughts about the past are the raw material that blocks our ability to experience satisfaction and contentment. They make a feeling of peace elusive and serenity impossible. The human brain is wired in a way that gives emphasis to our negative emotions, probably because they are often associated with survival instincts. The positive emotions are much more fragile. The only way out of a negative and hurtful past is by changing your thoughts and rewriting your past, and this can be done through forgiveness and forgetting.

Leaders and Managers

The principle of forgiveness is often called upon during times of tumultuous change in our organizations. Supporting employees through grieving during major transitions helps them to let go of the past and the way things were. Addressing transgressions and betrayals and working hard to reestablish trust among employees and between employees and leaders is another example of this principle at work. Dealing with betrayals in the workplace is important because they can lead to a lack of trust when they are not resolved in a positive way. Our organizations depend on trust in order to function effectively. Betrayal destroys the very relationships the organization needs in order to function (Ciancutti and Steding 2000; Reina and Reina 1999). Building a trust-based organization is crucial in today's health care organizations.

Forgiveness Exercise
The following forgiveness exercise from the field of positive psychology can be used either by individuals or by managers. The letting go of grudges activity was developed by Karen Reivich, coauthor of *The Resilience Factor* (2002). Here is how to do it:

1. Choose a person in your life you know fairly well and have a grudge against. On a piece of blank paper, draw a circle in the center of the page and record a few words that capture the essence of the grudge.
2. Fill the rest of the paper with blank circles, at least fifteen of them. The object is for you to fill each of these circles with a word or phrase that describes something about the person for which you are grateful. Examples include something he or she said to you or did for you or something important about your relationship. Include small or big things, current or past things.
3. Hold the paper at arm's distance and notice how the grudge gets lost in a sea of gratitude.
4. Reflect on how your emotions and thoughts change as you focus on the person now. Are you able to see the person more fully? Do your feelings for the other person change in any way? Did you notice any changes in your mood and how you feel about yourself?

This exercise could be used in coaching individual employees who are holding a grudge. It can also be used with a work group when complaints have been raised about another department or team.

Influencing Positive Emotions Related to the Present

The positive emotions related to the present include joy, ecstasy, ebullience, calm, zest, pleasure, and flow. These emotions are sorted into pleasures and gratifications as discussed earlier in the chapter. The three different aspects to consider are the pleasures, engagement, and meaningfulness. Understanding these three aspects suggests specific interventions in each arena.

Pleasure

Pleasure at work may seem oxymoronic to some people. However, many of us derive pleasure from being at work when the work environment is positive, supportive of our efforts, and conducive to the fulfillment of our intrinsic motivators. An important question to ask is: Is this a good place to work? In other words: Do people experience pleasure here? Are people excited about coming to work? Do fun and interesting things happen when you are here? What is the environment like?

Individual Employees

Years ago I remember having a conversation with a friend who was always telling funny stories about things that were going on at work. She was a radiology technician in a community clinic. At the time, I was studying the meaning of work in our lives, and so I asked her, "What makes your place such a great place to work?" I was genuinely interested in her answer and was shocked at her reply. She said in surprise, "What makes you think it's a great place to work?" I responded that she was always telling such great stories of the fun they were having that I had just assumed it was a great place to work. Her response startled me. She said, "Oh, it isn't a great place to work. In fact, it's horrible. We work long hours and we're underpaid. We have a horrible supervisor that everyone dislikes but no one else would take the job. She comes in late and leaves early. The patients and families all complain about her and her attitude. But you know what? We don't let her rob us of having fun at work. We make it a great place to work. Every day we decide that we are going to have fun and enjoy each other and our time together. It's great!" In other words, she meant that she and her coworkers decided to make it the kind of environment they wanted.

Every of us can create the kind of environment in which we want to work. The work environment does not belong to the manager, and building a positive work environment is not just one person's responsibility. It is the responsibility of every one of us. As an individual, you can decide that you want your department or service to be a good place to work, and your decision may start the ball rolling. We have already seen that positive emotion is contagious. Each of us has a lot more to do with the climate in our work environment than we realize.

Leaders and Managers

One of the first steps in conducting an assessment of any work environment is asking the fundamental question: Is this a good place to work? and then following up with: What can we do to improve it?

Many work groups, departments, and organizations have adopted the FISH philosophy for having fun at work. (The FISH philosophy is based on the customer service concepts followed by the employees at the Pike Place Fish Market in Seattle.) In most instances, employees and managers work closely together to ensure that there is at least a bit of fun in each day's work. Humor and laughter at work can greatly lighten the load of the many challenges that we face. The manager can certainly set the tone for the department in terms of lightheartedness and humor.

Another important factor to consider in an assessment of the work environment is the physical work environment. Is it pleasant? Is it clean and well organized? Or is it cluttered and messy? Is there space for employees to have a break away from interruptions and the typical demands of the department? What is the noise level? Is there adequate lighting, and are there windows that look out on natural settings? Even in an old facility there are things that can be done to make the physical environment more pleasant. Keeping it pleasant should be the responsibility of everyone in the work group.

Engagement

The second aspect of positive emotion in the present is related to our level of engagement. Work is a wonderful vehicle for the experience of flow, and yet many people find it difficult to experience flow in their workplace. According to data collected by the Gallup organization in early 2001, "less than 30 percent of American workers are 'fully engaged' at work, and some 55 percent are 'not engaged.' Another 19 percent are 'actively disengaged,' meaning that they not just are unhappy at work but they regularly share those feelings with colleagues" (Loehr and Schwartz 2003, pp. 5–6). In some instances the work is tedious or repetitive with little challenge.

Individual Employees

Individual employees as well as managers need to consider several issues related to the idea of engagement. One of the first questions to explore is whether the work environment is conducive to a deep level of engagement. In many jobs in today's health care organizations, the physical environment itself is destructive of flow. Many employees carry cell phones so they can be reached (and interrupted!) at any moment, and most managers and many employees are expected to be readily available and responsive to interruptions regardless of what they are doing. The noise level alone in many departments is enough to interrupt flow (Scalise 2004).

Are people being interrupted unnecessarily? If so, is there anything that could be done to minimize the interruptions? One of the time management issues for every work group is that they tend to interrupt each other needlessly. An important activity is for team members to talk openly and honestly about the things they inadvertently do to interrupt fellow team members. When we become more conscious of these things, we can minimize them. Some interruptions are necessary, and we would not want people to feel as though they cannot get help from each other when they need it. However, most of us would be happy to do what we could to make a colleague's day go better. Batching requests and telephone calls, using message boards, and having short but frequent team huddles for communicating information are all examples of simple ways of reducing interruptions. Avoiding interruptions is just another way for employees and managers to express their mutual respect for each other.

One study of nurses observed that during one hour of a typical workday, one nurse worked in eight different locations, changed locations twenty-two times, talked to fifteen different people on twenty-two separate subjects, and spent only one-third of her time delivering patient care (Thompson, Wolf, and Spear 2003). In another unpublished study, nurses were observed during their normal eight-hour work shifts. During this time, nurses averaged 160 separate tasks, with the average task time totaling 2 minutes and 48 seconds. You have to ask yourself how nurses can experience any sense of flow in such work environments? Although the two studies looked at nurses, other clinical professions probably work under similar conditions.

Another way to increase our level of engagement is for each of us to choose to minimize the amount of multitasking that we do. Multitasking is a very popular concept right now, and many of us think we can work effectively on several different tasks at the same time. However, the truth is that we are not able to do multiple tasks simultaneously as the term implies. Instead, we rapidly shift our attention from one task to another and fail to give our full attention to any of them. When we are so inundated with work that our primary mode of working must be multitasking, something is going to suffer. Inevitably, mistakes get made and people feel as though we are listening to them with only one ear. In health care settings, multitasking may actually be quite dangerous for both providers and patients.

Obviously, most people's work requires some amount of multitasking to quickly shift our focus from one area to another. However, each of us must consciously make the decision about when multitasking is an effective way to work and when the task and interactions involved are too important to be given short shrift. Anyone who has developed any kind of listening skills knows the power of simply sitting quietly and listening fully to what the other person is trying to share with you. When you continue to answer the telephone or check your e-mail during a conversation, the message is quite clear to the speaker: I am not important enough to get your entire attention.

Mind-numbing meetings that seem to go on forever can be another source of disengagement. According to Myers (1992, p. 136), one way we can increase the flow in our work lives is by "living more intentionally—saying yes to the things that we do best and find most meaningful, and no to the time-wasting demands." Yet, how many employees feel that they have the option of saying no to meeting requests and other demands on their time?

Leaders and Managers
Flow was discussed in detail earlier in this chapter. A couple of reminders, however, may be in order. "Studies confirm that a key ingredient of satisfying work is whether or not it's challenging. The most satisfied workers find their skills tested, their work varied, [and] their tasks significant" (Myers 1992, p. 133). When we make hiring decisions, we should try hard to match the candidates and their areas of strength with the work they are going to do. We also need to recraft jobs when necessary to increase the sense of engagement for employees who have been doing the same job for a long time. Sometimes adding new responsibilities to jobs can help employees recapture their sense of flow. "To experience flow we need to find challenge and meaning in our work, and to seek experiences that fully engage our talents. Flow comes when we structure work in ways that summon self-forgetful involvement. It . . . takes both individual and managerial effort to accomplish" (Myers 1992, p. 134).

One of the ways managers and leaders can help themselves and their employees increase their experience of flow is through coaching. Understanding what brings engagement and how to increase it is an important part of coaching. We can turn adversity or boredom into enjoyment by incorporating some of the ideas developed by the positive psychologists into regular coaching opportunities. The following process, based on the work of Seligman and Csikszentmihalyi, will help leaders and managers develop a work environment in which flow can be experienced:

1. Identify the signature strengths of every employee and manager.
2. Help employees evaluate how they are using their strengths in their work.
3. Encourage employees to set short-term and long-term goals so that they can monitor their own progress.
4. Look for new ways to use their strengths in their work, and offer them opportunities to do so.
5. Encourage them to pay attention to what is happening. Share conversations about their process and success in using their strengths.
6. Share their enjoyment of immediate experiences.

This approach can be effective for workers in any kind of job. Seligman gives an example of a bagger at a grocery store who was bored and felt her work was mundane and meaningless. She completed her signature strength assessment and discovered that social intelligence was one of her strengths. She decided that a way she could use this strength in her work was to make certain that her encounters with customers were the positive highlight of their day. You can imagine the difference this made in her approach to her work and her customers. In another example, Dr. Seligman was struck by the attitude of an orderly when he visited a severely ill, comatose friend in a hospital. The orderly was changing out the wall hangings in the friend's room and seemed to be enjoying himself immensely. When questioned about what he was doing, his response was, "My job? I'm an orderly on this floor. But I bring in new prints and photos every week. You see, I'm responsible for the health of all of these patients. Take Mr. Miller here. He hasn't woken up since they brought him in, but when he does, I want to make sure he sees beautiful things right away" (Seligman 2002, p. 168).

Csikszentmihalyi's work is also relevant to building engagement. Figure 4-5 illustrates the connection between the level of challenge the task represents and the level of skill we have. When, for instance, our skills are low and the level of challenge is great, as in learning a new piece of equipment or some other technical job requirement, the result may be anxiety. However, when both our skills and the level of challenge are low, apathy is the result. It is only when we have a high level of skill and we are meeting a significant challenge that we can reach flow. In figure 4-6, Csikszentmihalyi shows us the typical kinds of activities research participants were involved in during times when they experienced flow.

Figure 4-5. Relationship of Challenge and Skill in Obtaining Flow (Csikszentmihalyi 1997)

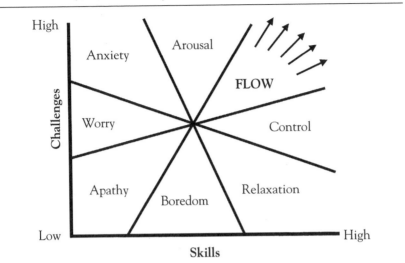

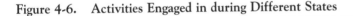

From *Finding Flow: The Psychology of Engagement with Everyday Life*, by Mihaly Csikszentmihalyi. Copyright © 1997 by Mihaly Csikszentmihalyi. Reprinted by permission of Basic Books, a member of Perseus Books, L.L.C.

Figure 4-6. Activities Engaged in during Different States

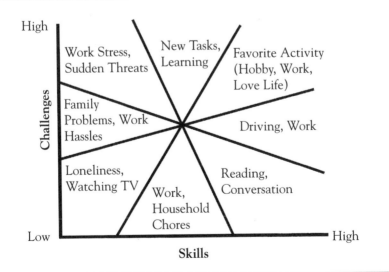

© 2004 Mihaly Csikszentmihalyi. Unpublished figure used with the author's permission.

Meaning

Emphasizing the meaningfulness of our work and that of colleagues is another way to increase happiness in the present. We can affirm each other and reinforce the significance of our work by drawing attention to its importance. Celebrating events such as National Respiratory Therapy Week, Hospital Week, or Nurses Week demonstrates to people that their work is important. Supporting employees in participating in poster presentations and writing for publication is another. Encouraging people to share their stories of when they made a difference is a great way to increase their sense of appreciation of themselves and the work they do.

Finally, doing everything possible to protect people from tasks that do not add value to their work communicates respect for both individuals and their work. Correcting long-standing problems that eat up time unnecessarily is important. A clear example of this was seen in a small Vermont hospital several years ago. An automated clinical documentation system had been installed as part of an electronic patient record. Physicians then became able to retrieve clinical data and laboratory and radiology exam results from their own office and home computers. A handful of physicians refused to use the automated system and instead continued to call the patient care departments to ask the nurses to print off diagnostic results and fax them over to them. This situation was tolerated for two years even though the nurses felt that it showed tremendous disrespect for them and the value of their time and work.

Influencing Positive Emotions Related to the Future

So there are at least three ways of increasing the amount of positive emotion in the present: making certain there are pleasures in the workplace, encouraging engagement or flow in our work, and recognizing and celebrating the meaningfulness of our work. Let us now look at techniques for increasing the amount of positive emotion as it relates to the future. The positive emotions related to the future include faith, trust, confidence, hope, and optimism. At least three different approaches from the field of positive psychology can have an impact on the level of positive emotion employees experience in relation to the future.

Mentoring Relationships

A great deal has been written about mentorship in other resources. Suffice it to say, there are a multitude of mentoring opportunities available in any health care organization. The opportunities can include mentoring around career and job development as well as simply about how to function effectively in a particular organization. Mentoring implies a more formal relationship than simply being supportive of another person. Mentors generally meet with mentees at specific times for the purpose of conversation and idea sharing. Mentoring is a way of producing positive emotion about the future because it is positive action taken in the present but focused on the future. As one manager proudly pointed out, "I have birthed ten managers out of this department."

Personal Legacies

This activity is relatively simple, and yet it demands significant reflection and soul-searching. It involves the individual sitting down and thinking carefully about what it is that he or she would like to leave for his or her colleagues, department, or organization as a result of their involvement there. Unlike writing a will, which often sorts through who receives which material possessions, developing a personal legacy focuses our thoughts on the less-concrete things we will leave behind. For example, perhaps you have been involved in helping create new practices or making changes in the way decisions are made in the department. Or like the manager who had a substantial hand in helping ten employees move into managerial positions, your legacy may be felt for years. Perhaps your contribution is that you taught your colleagues how to have a bit of fun at work and not take themselves so seriously, and the memory of your laughter will become an important part of future department events. The process of writing your legacy helps you to consciously determine what you want to leave behind. This encourages you to focus on behaviors that make your legacy a reality.

Optimism

Optimism is a signature strength that influences positive emotion about the future. Earlier in this chapter, optimism was briefly discussed, and we were reminded that it is based on how we view our world and our perception of whether events that happen are pervasive and permanent or specific and temporary.

At least one way to influence optimism in the workplace is by an activity called "One door closes, another door opens." You can apply this simple activity any time something negative happens. It involves simply asking which door has closed and which has opened; that is, what good things may come from this change? The exercise can also be effective when used in retrospect, because events we see as negative may sometimes have a positive element associated with them.

Conclusion

This chapter explored the role of happiness and joy in creating a positive work environment. Recent findings from the field of positive psychology have been included to give you a sense of the research being done and the ramifications of the findings for our work. Our goal ought to be to have happy employees and coworkers but in the broader and truer sense of happiness. Happy is far more than the immediate enjoyment of pleasure through superficial means, such as materialistic pleasures. Instead, happiness is related to pleasure and a sense of engagement and meaningfulness in one's work. The three together can bring light to the eyes and a smile to the face. Recent research findings on how health care workers experience and express joy through their work were also explored. Specific suggestions for interventions in the workplace to support happiness were identified.

Conversation Points

Organizational Perspective

1. How healthy are employees? Are absenteeism rates climbing, stabile, or declining? What are the most common health problems?
2. Is productivity at a satisfactory level? Do you see a relationship between productivity results and employee morale?
3. How satisfied are employees? Are there opportunities for improvement in organizational practices, policies, and benefits? Do you measure satisfaction levels frequently enough? Does the tool you use measure only positive emotions related to the past, or does it make an attempt to measure positive emotions in the context of the present and the future?
4. Do formal retention efforts focus predominantly on things that bring pleasure, such as gifts and social events? Is the sense of entitlement growing among employees?
5. Are your organization's leaders happy people?
6. What are the signature strengths of key organizational leaders?

Leadership Issues

1. How can you help your followers see the deeper meaning of their work? What kinds of leadership interventions may influence their sense of meaningfulness?
2. Is the work environment a pleasant place? Are there ways you can create more fun within your work group? Are there simple things you could do to increase the sense of pleasure both you and your employees feel?
3. What things in your work environment interrupt people's sense of flow? What can you do about them?
4. Who in your work group is remarkably happy? Unhappy? How do you and others react to them?
5. What can you do to influence the level of positive emotion employees feel about the past? The present? The future?
6. What are your key signature strengths, and how do you use them in your work? Are there any you are not fully using? How can you use your signature strengths in new and different ways? Are there key strengths you need to develop to increase your effectiveness in your leadership role?

Employee Challenges

1. What elements or aspects of your work do you find meaningful? How can you increase your sense of meaningfulness?
2. What brings you pleasure at work? How can you increase the amount of pleasure you feel?
3. How often do you experience a sense of flow at work?
4. What kinds of work or activities are more likely to result in flow for you? How can you increase your experience of flow?
5. Are you happy in your work? What things are affecting your level of happiness?
6. What can you do to find more happiness?
7. What are your signature strengths? How are you using them in your work, and how could you use them in new ways?

II

Strategies and Interventions
for Creating a Positive Workplace

PART I provided foundational information on the complex subject of organizational behavior. Special emphasis was placed on understanding the importance of employees' engagement with their work and commitment to the organization. Chapters 1 through 4 also made a case for focusing on retention programs in addition to recruitment initiatives. The reasons people work were reviewed from both historical and contemporary perspectives. In chapter 3, the issue of personal and organizational commitment was thoroughly examined, and recent research from the field of positive psychology was summarized in chapter 4. It was noted that understanding the emotions of happiness and joy as they relate to workplace productivity and well-being will help managers and leaders develop more positive organization or department environments. And, as employees, this information will give us insight into why we may or may not be happy in our workplace or in our lives.

Part II focuses specifically on the strategies and interventions individuals and organizations can undertake to increase their effectiveness. As in the first four chapters, the suggestions offered in chapters 5 through 10 are meant to apply broadly to individual employees, managers, executives, and organizations. Chapter 5 introduces the various approaches to creating a positive workplace, and subsequent chapters examine specific strategies in more detail.

5

Creating a Culture of Engagement

Jo Manion

We need more than a culture of retention,
we need a culture of engagement and contribution.
It's not enough that you've stayed here for 20 years,
it's "What are you giving? How are you contributing?"
—Jo Manion (2004b)

DIRE PREDICTIONS for the future seem to dominate every discussion of workforce issues in today's health care organizations. Even if your organization or department is not currently facing a shortage of key personnel, given the rapidly approaching retirement of the baby-boomer generation, every health care organization will need to actively take on the challenge of maintaining a vibrant workforce in the near future and for some time to come. The importance of the manager's role in creating a culture of retention began to emerge even before the Health Care Advisory Board exhorted managers to see themselves as chief retention officers for their departments (Advisory Board Company 2000). This recommendation was reinforced by the Gallup Organization's conclusion that employees do not leave their organizations, they leave their managers (Buckingham and Coffman 1999). Other research has also linked the retention of employees to the existence of a positive relationship with their managers (McNeese-Smith and Crook 2003). Today, managers are being held accountable for retaining valuable employees. Yet, retention programs continue to take a shotgun approach to decreasing turnover rates rather than implementing focused and effective strategies. How do managers and leaders actually create a positive work environment and a culture of retention? This chapter presents the results of a study performed to answer this question.

Portions of this chapter are adapted from Jo Manion, Nurture a Culture of Retention, *Nursing Management* 35(4). Copyright © 2004 and used by permission of Lippincott Williams & Wilkins.

The Issue

Identifying the manager as chief retention officer serves to emphasize the importance of focusing on the retention of valued employees. However, assigning titles and responsibilities without an adequate assessment of the capacity of the individual to accept or carry out that responsibility is likely to result in a no-win situation. First-line managers need adequate preparation for the role of chief retention officer and increased capacity through provision of adequate resources. They also need to be delegated appropriate levels of authority for accomplishing meaningful results. Exceptional managers may be successful even without such support, but their success often comes at great personal cost. And for most managers, the situation is likely to lead to a sense of failure and frustration, which can only serve to further escalate the turnover rate for health care managers themselves.

The senior executives to whom the managers report play a major role and have a key responsibility in providing meaningful support for their first-line managers. The truth is that creating a culture of retention and engagement in the organization is a shared responsibility. The manager must work with employees as well as with senior executives and key stakeholders for retention programs to be a successful on the organizational level. But what specific actions can a manager take?

The Study

In 2003, I undertook a qualitative study to determine exactly what successful health care managers do to create a culture of retention. I contacted professional colleagues around the United States and asked them whether they could recommend managers who had successfully created a culture of retention in their areas of responsibility. The participating managers were recommended on the basis of a variety of criteria, which included some combination of low turnover rates; high patient, employee, and physician satisfaction levels; good patient or customer outcomes; and overall positive working relationships among employees. Many of the managers in the study reported having a waiting list of applicants who were seeking positions in their departments.

Interviews were conducted with thirty-two managers from health care organizations throughout the continental United States. The participants managed a number of inpatient and outpatient services including respiratory therapy, pharmacy, radiology, admissions, physical therapy, oncology, perioperative services, critical care, surgery, emergency care, and medicine. About half of the managers were responsible for two or more departments. The span of control ranged from 42 to 170 employees; half of the participating managers had fewer than 75 direct reports and half had more than 75.

To confirm the accuracy of the managers' self-reported information, interviews were conducted with focus groups made up of the participating managers' employees and direct supervisors. There was remarkable consistency in reported behaviors, and it was apparent that the managers' self-reports were accurate.

The Culture of Retention

To begin, participants were asked to describe a culture of retention in their own words. Typical responses included the following:

- It's creating an environment where people want to stay.
- It means people enjoy their work so much and the people they work with that they want to stick around and get involved. Everybody is trying to make it a great place to work.
- It's an environment that meets peoples' needs.
- When they come to work, they enjoy being here, [and] they feel good about being here. They feel safe. They can trust each other [to make sure] that the job will be done and done well.

The results of the study made it clear that the way to create a culture of retention is to create a culture of engagement and contribution. It is this type of culture that makes a workplace people want to work in. It is not enough that an employee stays in the job for twenty years. The employee must continue to be make meaningful contributions throughout those twenty years.

Leadership Strategies

The managers' responses to the question, "What do you do to create this culture of retention?" were recorded, transcribed, and analyzed using a categorical content analysis approach. In other words, the categories and themes emerged from the participants' own words and stories. Over twenty factors emerged, and the factors were sorted into five primary themes: (1) putting employees first, (2) forging authentic connections, (3) coaching for and expecting competence, (4) focusing on results, and (5) working in partnership with employees. These simple and yet powerful interventions are discussed more fully here and illustrated with the participants' words and stories. (See figure 5-1.)

Putting Employees First

The successful managers who took part in the study clearly believed that their job was to put the employees first so that their employees could put their patients or customers first. Typical responses included the following:

- My staff comes first, not the patient first. Because if I make my staff feel valued and respected and good about what they do, then they're going to give the best care in the world.
- I know that if I am looking out for them, they will look out for the department. They know when they need me I will be there for them.
- I put my employees first so they will put the patients first.

Putting employees first may sound simplistic, but it is not always the first thought in our minds. The following example illustrates this point. A critically ill patient was brought into the emergency department of a medium-sized community hospital during the early afternoon. When it became apparent that the patient's death was likely to occur within a few hours, a supervisor called to facilitate the patient's

Figure 5-1.   Major Themes of Effective Managerial Interventions in Creating a Culture of Engagement

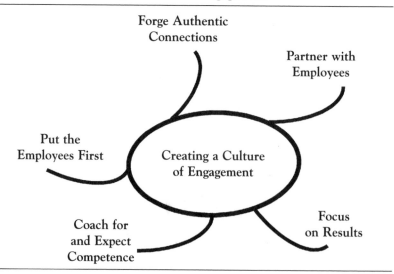

transfer to a nursing unit, where the environment would be more conducive to a peaceful passing for both the patient and the patient's family. The supervisor called the nurse manager of the inpatient department and requested assignment of a room. The nurse manager responded that there were no rooms available and that she would call back when one became available. Surprised that nothing was available, the supervisor waited for about thirty minutes before deciding to go to the department herself to determine whether any beds had become available. She found that there were several suitable rooms to which the patient could be transferred. Somewhat startled, she sought out the nurse manager and questioned her about using one of the empty rooms. The nurse manager surprised her by admitting that she had refused to accept the patient because of concerns for her staff. In her words, "They have had just an awful day. It has been crises and problems one after another all day long, with patients admitted and discharged in a seemingly steady stream. They are exhausted. This close to the change of shift, I just didn't have the heart to ask them to do one more thing." In the supervisor's mind, this case was an example of the nurse manager putting her staff first but to the detriment of a patient. What could she have done then: override the manager's decision and insist that the patient be transferred? A less-often-considered response would have been to ask the question, "What can we do for your staff so that they would be able to accept this patient?" Asking this question could have led to productive problem solving that considered the staff's needs as well as the patient's needs. For instance, it might have been possible to have a nurse from the emergency department stay with the patient and family until the change of shifts had occurred. Alternatively, a float nurse could have been assigned to the patient temporarily.

The specific ways these managers put their employees first included:

- Caring about them as people
- Meeting their needs
- Treating them with respect and high regard
- Expressing appreciation and recognition liberally
- Listening and responding to them
- Providing support

Care about Them

One striking finding was the depth of authentic feeling and caring the participant managers expressed for their staff. This did not mean the manager always liked everything individual employees might do or how they might behave, but the love and caring for them as individuals far transcended any negative incidents. For example:

- It's caring about people and not just their work.
- It's understanding that they have a life outside the department.
- They know I love them. I have fallen in love with my employees!

Managers who were told early in their careers that they should avoid getting too close to their employees, keep their distance, or stay uninvolved and unemotional may find these comments surprising. However, the care and positive regard these managers held for their employees was quite striking, and it was demonstrated through many of the other behaviors the managers reported. These findings support a new awareness of the presence and even the need for strong emotion in our workplaces (Henry and Henry 2004). "We are refocusing on the deep longing we have for community, meaning, dignity, purpose, and love in our organizational lives. We are beginning to look at the strong emotions of being human, rather than segmenting ourselves by believing that love doesn't belong at work, or that feelings are irrelevant in the organization" (Wheatley 1999, p. 14). James Champy, author of *X-engineering the Corporation*, notes that "the caring part of empathy, especially for the people with whom you work, is what inspires people to stay with a leader when the going gets rough. The mere fact that someone cares is more often than not rewarded with loyalty" (Champy 2003, p. 135). Caring in health care organizations is often discussed in relation to patients and their families and only rarely in relation to employees and coworkers. Perhaps it is a need to minimize love in business and work relationships that leads us to uncomfortable feelings of vulnerability (Sherwood 2003).

Meet Their Needs

Another way to put employees first is by meeting their needs. The participating managers reported talking to their employees about how they as managers could do a better job and how they encouraged employees to reveal what was important to them in the workplace. Basically, the successful managers treated employees as though they were their customers.

Scheduling practices were some of the most frequent examples. Using a self-scheduling approach was very common, and this concept was also applied to make it easier for employees to attend classes, facilitate child care, or arrange days off.

However, meeting the needs of employees goes well beyond scheduling issues and extends to understanding each employee's individual situation. Many of the managers' comments supported this idea, for example:

- I try to be responsive to them. If they need to cut down their hours for some reason or another, not letting that be a long process but really making that a very short process for them.
- I try to remember when people are going through stressful times, especially personal [problems], as to what's going on. Undergoing treatment for breast cancer, or a parent that's dying, or a very sick child.

Again, although such simple managerial interventions were common, they fly in the face of the advice most managers receive at an early point in their careers: that managers should not become involved in their employees' lives and that employees and managers should leave their personal problems at home. The managers in the study gave many examples of intervening and assisting employees with personal issues when those issues had an impact on the workplace. However, the managers indicated that they were always careful not to overstep and violate appropriate professional boundaries.

For example, Susan, one of the managers who participated in the study, told the story of an employee we'll call Mary, who had been an excellent worker before the quality of her work began to slip significantly. Mary was a Russian immigrant who had come to the United States after marrying an American man; she was the modern-day equivalent of a mail-order bride. Susan sat down with Mary to discuss the performance problems only to discover that Mary was being abused by her husband. Mary did not know what to do. Susan helped Mary by referring her to the employee assistance program and a support group at the hospital. In her own explorations of the problem, Susan also discovered a local law firm that specialized in this type of case. Although Susan never became personally involved in Mary's problems, she certainly went further than many managers would have. Katzenbach, in *Why Pride Matters More than Money* (2003), notes that "getting involved in the everyday problems of your people may violate the HR rule-book, but it's also the single best way to build an emotional bond with your employees" (Byrne 2003, p. 66).

Listen and Respond to Them

Listening carefully to what employees say and share was identified by most of the managers as essential in how they related to their employees.

Although the managers described using effective listening techniques (such as making eye contact, listening reflectively, and paying full attention), what was most striking about their comments was that when asked how people knew their managers were listening, the managers said that the employees knew because "something changes as a result of [the manager's] listening to them." In other words, people knew they had been heard when there was some follow-up or resolution to their problem as a result of the conversation. It may not have been the answer they wanted, but it was an answer nonetheless.

Atchinson (2003) reports hearing similar comments in his interviews of health care leaders. Contrast this with the admonition delivered to one of the participating managers by an executive: "Just because we haven't done anything doesn't mean we are not listening to you." To the manager who felt frustrated with the organization's lack of response to her repeated pleas for help, nonresponse meant exactly that: that she was not being heard.

Once again, these examples may seem like very simple interventions, and yet the managers in the study went further than just listening when people asked for their help. They often asked probing questions such as: What took you too long to do today? What are you doing that is just plain silly? What is holding you back from doing your best work? What keeps you up at night? What could we change to make your work easier or more fulfilling?

Contrast such authentic questioning with the more typical (and understandable) behavior of wanting to run and hide when you see a troubled employee walking down the hall in your direction. You just know they have more problems or complaints to bring you. Other comments made by the participating managers underscore the value of listening:

- They are the ones with the gems. They will come to you with their problems. You'll know what needs to be fixed, cuz they'll tell you what's broken.
- [When] I address issues they have brought up, it surprises them sometimes.
- I may not have the answer right away because I like to go back and process things, but I always get back to people and they really appreciate that.
- Listening is probably one of the most important things I do. I repeat what they said and then I get back to them on it.

Listening to people is the first leadership intervention presented in the popular book *Love 'em or Lose 'em* by Kaye and Jordan-Evans. The recommendations in that book focus on what we need to do to keep good people. If you are not sure what people want, look them in the eye and ask, "What can I do to keep you? What do you need? What do you want?" (Kaye and Jordan-Evan 1999). The responses to such questions can be powerful.

Treat Others with Respect

Expressing respect and a high level of unconditional regard for others clearly constituted one of the ways the managers in the study treated their employees. For example:

- They have the right to challenge me on any decision.
- I always respect their opinions, and I don't judge them. I listen to what they are telling me.
- I am just in awe of what they do. I am just stunned by it.
- I trust that they are honorable people. If they tell me they need something, I believe it.

One manager told a story about an applicant whom she later hired. The employee told her, "You know, the reason I took this job is because when you toured me in the department, you introduced me to the housekeeper and you not only knew her name, but knew her grandkids by name and told me several things about her. I came here because you clearly respect everyone!"

Show Appreciation and Recognition

Each manager in the study used unique methods for recognizing and appreciating people. Just a few of the methods included:

- Arranging for reports of employees' accomplishments to be printed in a newsletter
- Obtaining funding for employees' attendance at educational events
- Sharing thank-you notes and cards by mounting them on bulletin boards
- Planning department events during national recognition weeks (Respiratory Therapy Week, Hospital Week, Nurses Week, Nurse Assistant Week, and others)

- Displaying evidence of employee accomplishments (such as mounting employee certification plaques on a wall in the department)
- Creating and using recognition and retention "tool kits" with giveaway items such as movie tickets, t-shirts, and discount coupons for the gift shop or cafeteria
- Distributing thank-you notes and special occasion cards
- Taking pictures of employees and posting them in the department
- Acknowledging employees for special accomplishments or service anniversaries at department gatherings

Admittedly, these kinds of activities take time and attention. For instance, if a decision is made to recognize employees by sending birthday cards or employment anniversary cards, managers need to be consistent and send out cards for every employee without exception. What begins as a seemingly simple intervention can become an overwhelming chore over time. Most of the managers in the study undertook such activities in partnership with their employees. Responsibilities were shared so that the burden did not fall too heavily on any one person. For example, some people thoroughly enjoy buying and giving greeting cards, and accepting the responsibility for seeing that everyone in the department gets a birthday card at the right time may be a true pleasure for them. Many of the managers talked about asking a small group of employees to create recognition opportunities for the department.

Support Them

Support is another way that the managers in the study put their employees first and demonstrated their caring. Support encompasses a variety of behaviors, including:

- Advocating on behalf of the employees
- Ensuring the availability of support staff for the department (for example, department-based educators, clinical specialists, social workers, case managers, and pharmacists)
- Creating a nonpunitive environment that treats mistakes as opportunities to learn
- Helping employees deal with irate physicians and patients' families
- Making educational funding available
- Supporting individuals during personal crises and difficult times

Another important way to show support is by recognizing the need to balance your work and your personal life. In a survey conducted by the Families and Work Institute in 2000, a nationally representative group of 3400 employees was surveyed to determine what they considered very important in their current jobs. The second-most important factor identified was a balance between work and life (Barney 2002). When we fail to recognize the importance of work–life balance for employees, we lose a tremendous opportunity not only to demonstrate understanding and compassion, but to provide appreciable help in what has become a significant challenge for most people. "Twenty-seven percent of American workers say their organizations don't understand the tremendous need for work–life balance. . . . People wonder about whether they have enough time to do a good job at work but also do a good job at life" (Anonymous 2002, p. 27).

The past decade has seen a growing appreciation of the various values and needs of employees from different generations. Work–life balance has been identified as a primary concern of genXers, and organizations are being warned that some common practices need to be changed in order to successfully recruit and retain individuals from this age-group. GenXers "think they should have a life. The classic shift–weekend–holiday rotation will not cut it with this group. They are looking for a workplace that offers flexible scheduling, liberal vacations, daycare centers, workout rooms, on-site dry cleaning, florists, and the list goes on. They will pick the job that allows them to get the most fun out of life" (Cordeniz 2002, p. 247). Like it or not, we must face this issue. In addition, many baby boomers are rapidly reaching a time in their lives where they will become more concerned about work–life balance simply because they are tired of working the extra shifts and being on call. After decades of putting up with difficult work schedules, they are ready to call it quits.

Forging Authentic Connections

Taking time to connect with employees is an important behavior. The managers in the study believed that every employee needs to have a personal, individual connection with the manager. Examples of the managers' comments include the following:

- Sharing some of myself with them. Letting them know I care about the same things they care about.
- I take time to connect with my people and listen to them.

A variety of managerial behaviors build the foundation for developing strong connections with employees. Examples include getting to know them, creating a sense of connection and community in the department, hiring the right people, and having fun together.

Get to Know Them

Even managers with a large span of control believe that it is essential to know the people with whom they work, and not just departmental employees but housekeepers, security officers, and any one who comes into the department on a regular basis. Knowing each individual includes understanding something personal about them and calling them by name. One nurse manager described a situation experienced by a patient care technician she had just hired. The PCT had completed an intensive six-month training course at another hospital and then had promptly resigned. When the nurse manager asked her why she had left the first hospital after they had paid for her education, the PCT replied, "After six months they still didn't know my name!" In *Execution*, Bossidy and Charan explain that an essential leadership characteristic is knowing your people as well as your business (Bossidy and Charan 2002).

The managers who participated in the study were not necessarily the most social people at the holiday party, nor did they always join employees for pizza and beer after work. But they took the time to know something special and unique about each individual. For example:

- It's understanding what's important to them outside the institution. That they're human, that they have important lives and need to feel valued.
- I know all of them. I know their names, their families, their dogs, what they like to do.
- I invest time in them, I make rounds, I ask them—what's going on? What's important to you? The investment in them makes them feel wanted. It creates a bond and a rapport.
- I try to have lunch with my staff once a week—not more often because I want them to have plenty of time to talk with each other.
- They need to know who I am. I have pictures of my wife, my kids, my cat on my desk. I let them know who I am.

Several managers described taking note of major events that affected individual employees, such as the loss of a loved one. One manager mentioned that she had lost her sister years ago, and she described how good it made her feel when someone asked her, "How is it going without Marie?" So she keeps track, and on the anniversary date of the loved one's death, she finds the employee and asks: "How are you doing? Are you thinking about your Dad?" And she said, "I don't do it as a strategy. I do it from my heart, and I know it makes a huge impact on them. Because I remembered and they're not alone in their memory." This manager went on to share that she was not the most socially inclined person at the department parties and that she really was more of an introvert. However, it is almost certain that her employees realize that she cares deeply about them.

A pharmacy director who participated in the study reported using a job-shadowing program. He routinely spent a half-day shadowing an employee to stay in touch with both the employee and the work issues that were typical during a shift. All of the managers who took part in the study described their own unique approaches to gathering this kind of first-hand information.

Create a Sense of Community

Many of the managers' stories involved examples of an extraordinary sense of community that had been created in their departments. Examples included employees who rallied together to support a colleague experiencing a tragedy or very difficult times. Several described situations in which an employee had been injured in an accident and was unable to work for an extended period of time. One emergency department put a jar out at the central desk to collect donations, and over $3000 in cash was collected for the individual. Another common example involved coworkers who donated their own vacation or paid leave time to others employees who were experiencing significant difficulties.

In addition, managers who took part in the study described the camaraderie experienced during special occasions such as weddings, graduations, and other life events. In one work group, the young department secretary was planning to move in with her boyfriend. The couple wanted to marry, but they felt that they could not afford a wedding. The secretary's coworkers pulled together and created a beautiful wedding for the couple. The department social worker offered her home for the wedding and reception; two colleagues sewed the wedding dress; another coworker sang and played the music; the department manager (who was also an ordained minister) performed the ceremony for free; other coworkers brought food; and a physician donated a night in the honeymoon suite of a local hotel. The manager laughingly told the young woman, "You're having a nicer wedding than I had!" What a delightful way to celebrate and reinforce our connections at work!

As in other healthy communities, the work environments described by study participants were inclusive rather than exclusive. In other words, no one was deliberately left out, and every attempt was made to include as many people as possible. Anyone in proximity to the department was drawn in, including patients and their families, physicians, and workers from other areas of the organization. An exclusive community is more like a clique, and cliques depend on having narrow membership requirements to maintain their exclusivity. Establishing community is an effective strategy for enhancing retention and is addressed more fully in chapter 7 (Manion and Bartholomew 2004).

Hire the Right People

One way of forming strong connections involves taking care to hire the right people for the department. The importance of careful recruitment practices is a relatively common theme in the business literature. In Jim Collins's words, "you have to get the right people on the bus" (Buckingham and Coffman 1999; Collins 2001). The managers in the study did not emphasize the importance of finding the right technical skills and cognitive intelligence to fill vacancies. They focused instead on the candidates' attitudes, behaviors, and emotional intelligence. The following comments were typical:

- I look for optimism. I look for perky. I look for people who are very comfortable with themselves.
- I look for emotional intelligence. How they deal with interpersonal problems in the workplace, how assertive are they?
- We look for people who are passionate about their work.
- We look for people who really have the energy and the sense of humor that fits with our group.
- We want someone who is going to contribute, participate on committees, be a part of what's going on.

One manager said that her favorite question to ask during selection interviews was, "How has life treated you?" From this, she claims, she can tell a great deal about a person's perception of their lives and whether they have a victim mentality or are optimistic people who do not let events and others get them down. This managerial approach is strongly validated by the recent findings in the field of positive psychology.

The managers who participated in the study also described the involvement of employees in helping select their new colleagues. There were a variety of approaches for involving coworkers in this process, and the managers found employee involvement in hiring to be very effective. Even employees reported that, although technical expertise was important, it was not the key attribute they looked for in a new colleague. More important was the person's ability to fit in well with the work group.

Have Fun Together

Whether it was making cookies or popcorn in the middle of a busy shift or giving a prize to the person who most closely guessed the number of syringe caps in a jar, the workplaces described by the participating managers were full of humor and fun. Several actually reported setting up employee committees whose only purpose was to plan lighthearted activities for the staff. Some described using the FISH philosophy based on the now famous Pike Place Fish Market in Seattle, where fun is considered an important component of everyday work life (Whiley 2001).

In one department, three different employee committees were responsible for fun activities. One committee handled the events and activities that were held in the workplace, such as birthday celebrations, fun contests, and activities that stimulated and brought enjoyment to the staffers. Another committee was responsible for off-site activities, which included summer golf tournaments, picnics, and trips to cultural, sports, and theatrical events. No one was bothered when some employees chose not to participate, recognizing that for some people another night away from their family would not be perceived as fun. However, for many of the young people and singles for whom work represented an important part of their social lives, such activities were considered a real treat. The third committee was responsible for the bulletin boards in the department; they designed the boards along a new theme every month. Their creative ideas delighted everyone who saw them: employees, physicians, patients, and patients' families and friends.

In some cases, managers talked about having to feed the committees ideas in the beginning, but most of the work was accomplished by employees. This is an important point because the staff members felt more ownership when they played an instrumental part in the process.

All of the managers said that it was important to create a positive work environment by making certain that the workplace was fun, but they also said that they made sure that work got done. Comments included the following examples:

- We try to keep it lighthearted in the department. I have a good sense of humor. Employees see that, and it sets the tone for the department.
- I use humor and fun to emphasize the things I think are important. For example, we always celebrate the end of orientation. I take the new employees to breakfast and the preceptors out to dinner.
- We have so much fun at our parties. We started having these little cookouts every month. One of the employees brings his grill and we'll do hamburgers and hotdogs around 6 p.m. so oncoming and offgoing staff can have some. We invite everyone.

Coaching for and Expecting Competence

The third way successful managers create a culture of retention is by focusing on the growth and development, both personal and professional, of the people with whom they work. As noted in an earlier chapter, competence is a key intrinsic motivator for work. Thus, it is no wonder that supporting employee development was identified as a major leadership intervention in the study. Highly effective workers are rarely impressed with glitzy perks and increased fringe benefits. "What keeps them around are extensive training and career-development programs that offer valuable benefits to both workers and employers" (Dobbs 1999, p. 51). Organizations that recognize that their best employees are eager to develop their careers realize that development opportunities are some of the best perks around. The factors in this key theme include setting high standards and expectations, coaching and supporting development, modeling behavior, and managing performance.

Set High Standards and Expectations

The managers who participated in the study set high standards, both for themselves and others, and helped people achieve those standards. Performance expectations for clinical and technical performance as well as for interpersonal behaviors were made clear, and people were held accountable for meeting them. For example:

- My leadership team and I actually look for and create new goals every year so that people are always feeling challenged. So we're always on the cutting edge. You cannot be satisfied with what you did last year.

- I have very high standards and expectations for participating in performance improvement efforts [and] committee work and for practicing their profession in a high-quality way.
- I don't expect anything of them that I wouldn't do myself.

Support Development

The managers in the study talked with pride about having helped develop the skills of individual employees who were later promoted to other positions in the organization. They took pride in the accomplishments of their employees. Coaching is a common approach, but successful managers also employ other strategies, including:

- Supporting attendance at national conferences and educational programs
- Encouraging and helping employees present posters at national meetings or coauthor articles
- Obtaining reference materials for the department
- Implementing strong orientation and development programs
- Encouraging employees to take advantage of tuition reimbursement programs
- Encouraging membership in professional associations

Managers in the study offered the following comments:

- I take a personal interest, finding out what they want to do is important. And then not just delegating and dumping, but really giving them growth opportunities.
- I constantly look for opportunities for them.
- Each employee has particular strengths and it means recognizing those and asking people what they would like to develop. They may like teaching others, or improving their clinical skills, or being charge or a case coordinator. So what kinds of experiences would be beneficial to help them prepare for that role?
- I get them involved in things. First of all I solicit what they are interested in. I ask, "if you're interested in doing other things, let me know." Then when opportunities arise, I ask them.

These successful managers talked extensively about the need to be proactive in identifying people's interests. Opportunities that arise are evaluated and shared with others. The Gallup Organization reported years ago that when employees do not have at least one or two conversations about career planning with their manager every year, they conclude that their manager does not care about them (Buckingham and Coffman 1999).

Model Behavior

An important way the managers in the study coached and developed others was by serving as a role model. They modeled the behavior they wanted to see. Acting as a role model includes living up to the expectations they hold of others, staying positive, using a nonpunitive approach to problem solving, remaining calm in the midst of chaos, and persevering in the face of extreme difficulty. Typical examples of the managers' comments include the following:

- I have faced many situations that would get most people down, but I don't let it. I'm choosing my attitude every day and I want my employees to see that.
- You have to lead by example. We have to help each other. This job is difficult enough as it is. We need to be supportive of each other. If you see someone is sinking and having a really tough day, help them out.
- I try to model the behavior that I think most employees want— they want honesty, they want fairness, and they want to see that I treat everyone the same.

A beautiful example of role modeling was shared by a manager during a conversation. A very unpopular decision had been made in the organization, and employees were quite unhappy and upset about it. Throughout the day a great deal of complaining went on. Early in the afternoon, an assistant manager finally said to her manager, "I simply cannot believe that you are not upset about this." The manager replied, "Oh, don't mistake me. I'm very angry about this decision, but that doesn't mean I have to spew all that negativity out and infect everyone around me! I can control my emotions and not let them infect everyone else." What a wonderful example for others!

Manage Performance

Performance management is a critical element of coaching for competence. Performance management was specifically mentioned by over 80 percent of the managers in the study. The managers recognized and rewarded positive behavior and dealt with problem behavior immediately. They had learned the hard way that managers cannot ignore problems, and they understood that their own credibility with staff would be jeopardized if they ignored performance problems. For example:

- I hold people accountable for their behaviors. We follow a process. It's time-consuming, but you know what? They either comply or move on.
- Here's the bar. It's set right here, and if you don't get up to that bar, then there are consequences. Too many people are afraid to discipline, afraid to counsel, because there are workforce shortages. But the reality is you can't keep bad apples. You really dilute the quality of care and morale in the work group.
- If things have to be addressed, then I address them. It doesn't do any good by waiting for it to go away, 'cause it doesn't.
- When employees bring these problems, they want to see that they are taken care of. They want to trust that something will happen.

A major issue for most of the managers related to their working relationships with the human resources departments in their organizations. Some of the managers reported that the support they received from human resources was exquisite, but other managers indicated that they needed to work around a weak or poorly functioning human resources department that was more a roadblock than a support.

For example, one nurse manager of an orthopedic service was the fifth new manager for the department over a five-year period. When she began in her position, she identified several toxic and dysfunctional employees who acted as highly skilled saboteurs within the department. They not only attempted to block virtually every positive step she initiated, they were also bullies who made life miserable for their coworkers. The manager was on the verge of resigning. She had worked extensively with an organizational development specialist from human resources to initiate team building and begin setting expectations within the department and among employees. The manager had also begun counseling and disciplining the most toxic of the employee bullies, because she was determined to deal with their unacceptable behavior. As a result, she found herself in trouble with the human resources staff, who saw themselves as employee advocates. Roadblock after roadblock was thrown in her way until the internal organizational development consultant sat down with her human resources colleagues and said point blank, "If you don't help her deal with these toxic employees, you are going to be hiring manager #6 for this department and nothing will have changed." The HR staff had been unaware of the extent to which they had become employee advocates rather than organizational advocates, well beyond what would have been appropriate.

It is not uncommon for toxic employees to find a safe and comfortable home in a department where manager turnover is the norm. The challenge is to recognize poor performance and then deal with it appropriately. Threatened lawsuits, fear of aggression, fragile race relations, and workforce shortages are just a few of the reasons managers may be reluctant to deal with poor performance. Yet, when we ignore such problems, the employees we lose are usually the good ones, the ones we wanted to keep, and not the employees with substandard performance or bad attitudes. The best workers simply do not need to put up with a dysfunctional environment; they can and will find another place to work. Even when they do not walk with their feet, they walk with their hearts. Managers and executives lose a tremendous amount of credibility among the decent, hard-working employees in the organization when poor performance is tolerated. (Chapter 10 addresses this subject in more detail.)

Focusing on Results

The fourth group of leadership strategies for creating a culture of engagement involves focusing on results. The managers who took part in the study worked hard to solve problems, and they achieved improvements in their departments, often with the help of the people with whom they worked. Four factors are related to the focus on results.

Solve Problems

Solving problems seems to be an important way that managers gain and maintain their credibility among employees and colleagues. The managers in the study reported that they continually asked for input on what needed to be fixed and then they acted on that information. Some of the bigger system problems took longer and results often took more time, but the managers always gave feedback to their employees on what was being done to address the problems. As a result, employees felt as though progress was being made. Examples of the managers' comments include the following:

- I try to deal with whatever they need in a very timely manner. I try and be responsive to them. They don't have to come back to me again and say, "Whatever happened to . . . ?"

- People know they've been heard when the problem is solved.
- Taking action quickly is crucial. Delay, delay, delay will kill them and the manager's reputation and credibility. If they bring something forward or you see something wrong, take care of it now.

The managers in the study also talked about the importance of establishing trials during implementation of major projects so that the bugs and glitches can be worked out early in the process. Examples of difficult system issues included:

- The speed of patient throughput
- The delays caused by neurology residents who insisted on using emergency department beds to do patient workups
- The conversion of the pharmacy distribution system to a new approach
- The implementation of electronic medical records
- The initiation of work redesign projects

Simpler problems included malfunctioning equipment and insufficient supplies.

Empower and Involve Employees in Decision Making

One of the most influential ways the managers in the study had for getting results involved using empowerment and employee participation in departmental decision making. Many of the managers' stories mentioned exquisite examples of employee involvement and participation and increased levels of autonomy and decision making among staff. Using a department council structure, encouraging and supporting employees' involvement in committees, establishing problem-solving task forces, and delegating responsibility for specific tasks were examples.

- A big role of the leader in this environment of retention is that you start by giving up as much power as possible. I measure my success by how little they need me anymore!
- I want to create more leaders in my department, people that can take the ball and run with it instead of always feeling like they have to come to me. My goal is to get them so self-sustaining that they don't need me anymore.
- Micromanaging kills you. You've got to let go. You think you're going to do it all, but you can't. It will kill you. You've got to have everyone helping you.

The managers also reported instances when employees were empow-ered to deal with interpersonal issues and conflicts, order equipment and supplies without the manager's signoff, make decisions about where floating staff was needed most, determine work schedules, and decide what types of employee education were needed. Contrary to common complaints about the unwillingness of employees to participate in department activities, the successful managers who took part in the study seemed to have little or no difficulty finding people to take on extra responsibilities. The advice they offered for other managers was that if you are planning to promote staff participation, the participa-tion has to be valued and supported. If you ask someone to participate on a committee, for example, but fail to follow through in terms of helping them get the time off to go to the meetings, the result is likely to be frustration.

Provide Adequate Resources and a Pleasant Physical Environment

As one manager said, "It's the little things that tick people off . . . like when you go to get some linen and there's not enough there. Or you go to find a PCA pump and we don't have any." Many of the managers in the study considered it an important part of their jobs to make sure that employees had everything they needed to provide high-quality service. Nothing is more frustrating to employees during times of short staffing than knowing that they waste incredible amounts of time tracking down equipment (Lanser 2001), calling for supplies, or fol-lowing up with coworkers and support staff who have not done their work properly. Addressing such problems requires managers to pay attention to the resource issues employees raise and to take appropri-ate action as quickly as possible.

In a recent study conducted by the Federation of Nurses and Health Professionals, 56 percent of the respondents cited working conditions as the biggest problem with their jobs (Menninger 2001). The suc-cessful managers in this study also talked about improving the physical environment in ways that increased retention. Such improvements can be achieved through structural changes in the department's facili-ties as well as through process changes in the way services are deliv-ered. For example:

- One of the things that draws them to this department when they're being interviewed is the physical environment. That it looks clean. It's organized. It's not outdated.

- I'm a huge gardener, so I bring in flowers and put them on tables and around the department.
- We created a new cardiovascular inpatient department where our open-heart patients stay in the same bed throughout their stay. . . . It's rewarding for the caregivers.
- We created a quiet room. It's beautifully decorated, has music, and an easy chair. [Employees] can go in and put their feet up and relax for a few minutes.

Working in Partnership with Employees

The last theme in leadership interventions for creating a culture of engagement relates to the way managers work with their employees. Most of the managers who participated in the study described using leadership styles based on partnership relationships and the concept of servant leadership. Examples of the managers' comments include the following:

- My job is to facilitate their work. I make a joke about it, but really the truth is that I work for them. They don't work for me. . . . I work for them.
- It's understanding that it's never about me. . . . It's about we. I'm not retaining people, we are.
- All of these things create a sense that I'm working for them and an environment where there's mutual respect between us.
- My job, and I can never forget this, is to provide service to these employees. That's my job. I'm working for them.

These successful managers were quite clear that they alone could never produce a positive workplace environment, but that they must work interdependently with others. They worked together to create an environment in which people felt liberated and were willing to take risks to accomplish innovation and progress. The type of environment the managers described is very similar to a workplace culture of coherence as described in a recent article published by Ponte (Ponte et al. 2004, p. 173): "Developing a sense of coherence depends on the existence of mutual trust, a commitment to the process of working together, and a shared responsibility for practice and professional development." A culture of coherence depends on how individuals perceive their individual place in the department and the department's place in the larger organization. Coherence is a pervasive, enduring, and dynamic feeling of confidence that a person's internal and external environments are predictable, that even when the day starts badly, it is highly probable that things will work out well by the end of the day.

The key factors related to the partnership approach to engagement include high levels of visibility and accessibility to employees, clear boundaries between managers and employees, and open, positive, and direct communication.

Be Visible

Visibility was crucial for the managers in the study. In many cases, visibility was not limited to being present and being seen, but included jumping in and helping out when and where they were needed. Making patient rounds was the most common example in the patient care departments, but visibility also meant being present for employees on every shift. For these leaders, spending most of their time out in their departments was a priority. Most actually scheduled time to be visible. For example, one pharmacy director and his assistant made certain that one of them was in early enough to see people on the night shift and the other was there late in the afternoon to overlap with people on the evening shift.

The way these managers pitched in and helped was unique. Some were still clinically or professionally skilled, while others simply answered the telephone, got coffee for family members, brought food for employees during extremely busy times, helped out with uncomplicated work, or picked up a mop when needed.

- Whenever I can just jump in and help out, that's a good opportunity to be with that employee.
- I spend time out at the desk. . . . I take as much of my work out there as I can. Just to be around the people.
- I make it a point of getting out at least once a day, making rounds and seeing everyone.

One very astute manager noted that presence does not always mean physical presence. "It's getting back to people, following through, answering their phone messages, leaving them a note in their mailbox; even if I don't have the answer, it's staying connected in all of these ways." In contrast, what seemed to have a devastating effect on both managers and employees was seldom seeing their managers or experiencing any sense of their presence in the workplace.

Be Accessible

Accessibility is closely linked to visibility; however, a manager can be accessible without being visible. The managers in the study talked about how important it was for employees to have someone available to talk with about their concerns and issues. Frequently mentioned strategies included having an open-door policy, occupying an office located within the department, being available by pager, responding promptly to voice and e-mails, holding frequent and convenient employee meetings or team huddles, and attending to people. Attending means actively observing, listening, and making a concentrated effort to be present, open, and available (Clarke 1999). Examples from the interviews with the managers for the study include the following:

- I'm out there with them. I tell them, "I'm available. . . . This is what I'm here for. If you need me or need to talk about something, I'm here."
- Things like where your office is are important. What you wear to work. If you come in dressed to work with them or you are in business attire. Wearing the proper clothing sends the message, "if you need my help, I'm ready."
- I post my schedule on the door so people will know where I am at all times. If they want to talk to me and don't know where I am or when I am coming in, it creates a lot of frustration. This way, they know.

Maintain Clear Boundaries

Even though the managers in the study were visible and accessible to employees, they also set appropriate boundaries between themselves as leaders and their employees. Several noted that employees want a leader who clearly is a leader and not their friend. Maintaining a connection while keeping an appropriate distance was an area to which these successful managers gave attention. A significant issue for these leaders was balancing accessibility and visibility with staying focused and protecting themselves so that they were able to put their time where it would make the most difference.

One nurse manager described being told by the chief executive officer that she was not delegating enough. He pointed out that whenever she was in the department, people freely came up to her and asked for her input or for a decision on an issue that did not really need her level of authority. Her initial reaction to his comment was anger and defensiveness. With reflection, however, she came to see that he had a point. To address the problem, she put a note in the department's communication book and asked people to go to the charge nurse with issues first but to feel free to come to her with problems that the charge nurse was unable to handle. The nurse manager made it clear that it was not that she did not want to hear about problems, but (in her words) "you don't ask the general if you want a weekend pass, you go to your commanding officer." She told her employees that her past level of accessibility had made it difficult for her to focus on the bigger problems in the department. The manager was surprised to find that no one on her staff had been insulted by the change or felt that she was distancing herself from them. They understood and were eager to help because they wanted her to continue to act as a strong advocate for them.

Provide Open and Honest Communication

It is no surprise that open and honest communication characterized the relationships between the successful managers and their employees. Participants in the study talked not only about their methods of keeping people informed, but also about their philosophy of communication. For example:

- I don't hide anything from my staff that they need to know. I hold no secrets from them.
- We post data every month to show where we are.
- I approach things from a "no surprise" perspective.

These effective managers talked about the importance of creating a climate in which employees were able to give each other as well as the manager direct feedback about issues, concerns, and even the manager's performance or behavior. The managers believed that when their employees felt liberated, they would hear about problems much sooner than anyone else did. Thus, issues can be dealt with more quickly, which can keep small issues from escalating into large problems.

Open and honest communication is the foundation for all of the leadership strategies for building a culture of engagement. Listening, for example, is one way to put the employee first, and listening is clearly a specific communication skill. In the same way, focusing on results and coaching for competence would be impossible without effective communication skills.

Summary of Strategies

So, in the end, the effective strategies reported by managers who have successfully created a culture of engagement and retention are not complex; neither are they glitzy or expensive. In fact, they can be deceptively simple practices, practices that when authentically expressed can create a workplace in which people want to work. (Figure 5-2 summarizes the interventions discussed in this chapter.)

Jim Collins's research on organizations that make the leap from being good, solid companies to being great companies has helped us understand how we can achieve excellence on an organizational basis. During an interview, Collins was asked whether he could put his finger on what really differentiated good from excellent companies. His response is telling and has application to our research on positive workplaces: "The people in the good-to-great companies did things that seemed so incredibly obvious, straightforward, simple; . . . the comparison companies may have had very smart people, brilliant, but they saw things as complex, and they had elaborate plans and complicated strategies" (Flower 2002, p. 19). In other words, the people in the organizations that never made the leap to excellence were smart

Figure 5-2. **Managerial Interventions for Successfully Creating a Culture of Engagement**

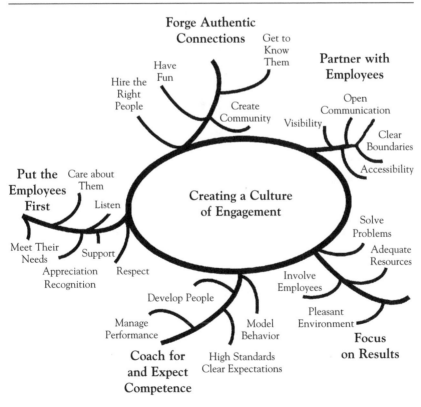

but just could not seem to grab onto simple strategies that would actually work.

The findings in this research study substantiate the foundational work presented in the first part of this book. The major themes that emerged from these data are clearly related to many of the intrinsic motivators as well as to the various forms of organizational commitment. Forging strong connections relates to the intrinsic motivator of healthy and positive working relationships and forms the foundation of affective commitment. The manager's focus on results produces improvements and changes in the workplace, which are clearly related to the intrinsic need we have to see progress as a result of our efforts.

Furthermore, a key way the managers in the study obtained results was by empowering or delegating responsibility to employees along with an appropriate level of authority. Autonomy is an intrinsic motivator for work as well. The theme of coaching for performance and developing people supports the intrinsic motivator of competence. All five major themes as well as the factors within them demand managers and leaders whose behavior reflects the specific values held by the individual. When the managers' values are congruent with the values held by the employees, the possibility of normative commitment emerges.

Organizational Ramifications of Positive Leadership Strategies

It is clear from the findings presented in this chapter that simply expecting more and more from today's managers without providing ways to increase their capacity is a no-win situation for everyone. The participants were asked how their organizations supported them. Although at least half of the participating managers felt a strong level of support from within their organizations, too frequently comments like this one were heard: "It's hard to keep doing this for employees when no one does it for me." When organizations are serious about improving their work environment and reducing costly turnover, at least some of the answers are simple: Provide the same support to managers that the managers are expected to provide to their employees. Complaining that the organization cannot afford to take these steps is shortsighted and ultimately destructive. We cannot afford not to invest in practices that will help organizations keep their best people.

When the managers in the study were asked the question, "What would make your job easier?" the responses were not surprising. The managers asked for adequate administrative support, more visibility from senior leadership, more manageable spans of control, and the cooperation of physicians in retention efforts. Put simply, the managers needed everyone to do what they are supposed to do. They said:

- There is a lack of insight into just how much they've asked us to do. Unrealistic deadlines, meetings, expectations. It's just overwhelming.
- What would help? Having support for some of the mindless details that have to be taken care of.
- Even a day or two a week of secretarial support, 10 to 12 hours, just to help with the paperwork.
- Physicians have to understand that their behavior affects people. Their outbursts, their sarcasm, their flippant remarks. Staff take it to heart.
- If I had any support. I don't feel like I can trust anyone.
- If every department would just do what it's supposed to do.

Support from Senior Leadership

To provide effective support, senior leaders (in this case, any leader to whom managers report directly) should examine the evidence rather than relying on anecdotal experiences or interventions that were effective in the past. As noted earlier, continuing to expect more and more from today's managers without providing ways to increase their capacity is a no-win situation for everyone.

What can senior leaders do to support employee retention efforts? The research suggests the following recommendations:

1. Understand which leadership behaviors make the difference and support managers in implementing those behaviors.
2. Help managers deal with the polarities.
3. Negotiate for a strong supportive role from human resources staff.
4. Remove organizational barriers to getting results.
5. Encourage managers to develop a support network.
6. Listen to what the managers tell you.
7. Encourage managers to learn from each other through appreciative inquiry.

Supporting Effective Behaviors

Although executing many of these simple interventions appears to be within the direct control of front-line manager, too many mixed messages from the organization sometimes make managers reluctant to take action. For example, how can managers ensure their own visibility and accessibility when they are scheduled to spend six to eight hours every day in meetings outside their department? How can managers form authentic connections with their staff when they have a hundred or more direct reports? How can managers put their employees first and focus on results and employee development when they are bogged down with administrative responsibilities such as managing payroll, tracking absenteeism, verifying certifications, filing new policies in binders, and finding information for other departments?

In many health care organizations today, the demands placed on managers border on being unrealistic and overwhelming, and a significant inconsistency exists in the availability of administrative support for managers. Most departments in hospitals employ secretaries who work closely with department managers to support administrative functions; however, patient care departments are a clear exception. Most nurse managers have minimal or no dedicated administrative support even though nurse managers, like their counterparts in other departments, are expected to run multimillion-dollar business operations, manage large numbers of people who often work from multiple locations, and basically deal with one of the most complex organizational systems known.

Each patient care department usually employs a full-time support person, called a unit secretary, to serve as the department's receptionist and coordinator of traffic, support patient care, and provide clerical assistance for the physicians who flow in and out of the department every day. However, most unit secretaries are too busy to provide consistent, dependable administrative support for nurse managers. This issue simply has not been addressed adequately by most health care organizations.

There were numerous examples of nurse managers in this study who, when asked by an executive, "What can we do to make your work easier?" responded by saying, "I need consistent, qualified secretarial support." The answer in almost all of these instances was along the lines of this response: "Nurse managers in this organization will never have their own secretaries." This response may well reflect the reality in most organizations, but if it does, it suggests that organization executives are not listening to what the managers are saying. In the end, they are likely to continue to see a high level of nurse manager turnover at a time when it is critical that every health care manager is able to function at the highest capacity possible. Keep in mind that turnover is not limited to physical departure. How can a person continue to stay committed to an organization that seems to misunderstand and devalue the work they do?

One participant in the study discussed her extreme frustration with this situation. Karen was a second-career nurse who came to the health care field with extensive business experience. Because of her performance and skills, she rose quickly to a management position. At the time of her initial interview during this study, she was the manager of two inpatient orthopedic departments. During her tenure as a manager, she repeatedly communicated her needs for support and felt increasingly frustrated at the lack of response to her requests. Eventually, she resigned, much to the consternation of the nurse executive and the chief operating officer, both of whom recognized that Karen was probably the most competent manager they had. At their request, she met with the chief executive officer to discuss her concerns before she made the resignation final. She challenged the executive directly in his thinking.

"You keep talking about health care as a business and telling us that we have to be good business people. Give me an example of a business where a manager has responsibility for eighty employees, two geographical locations, and a multimillion dollar annual budget but is told that she cannot have a secretary!" The executive was unable to rebut her argument, and he could not think of an example of a business that would organize itself this way. The end result? Karen was given permission to use the unit secretary's services for a specific, dedicated amount of time each week. Was this a satisfactory solution? Hardly. The decision meant a reduction in the amount of support available to the rest of the department. At the end of the year, Karen was given a $10,000 bonus in her paycheck. She was furious and returned the money with the response, "I didn't ask for more money, I asked for help!" Her case became just another example of senior management not hearing what a manager was desperately trying to communicate.

Because effective managers are the key to creating a positive work environment, organizations ought to be looking for anything they can do to increase their managers' capacity. To do so requires conducting a careful review of each manager's activities, implementing up-to-date technological support, and providing consistent administrative support.

Senior leaders need to open-mindedly consider the key factors that lead to a manager's success and then honestly ask themselves whether the organization is providing the resources the manager needs to be successful.

Helping Managers Deal with Polarities

The manager is a bridge between operational and administrative practices in the organization. A bridge is a sturdy structure that provides a path between two widely separated banks. Organizationally, bridges ensure the open flow of energy, information, knowledge, and other resources between the various parts of the organization. To keep this flow moving requires a lot of support. All five of the interventions identified through this study require judgment in their application. We need to recognize that issues such as visibility and accessibility are not problems to be solved but rather polarities to be managed.

For example, within nursing it took years to transition from the "head nurse" in white uniform image to the nurse manager dressed in business clothes who appears more managerial than clinical. Yet, the managers who took part in this study strongly believed that it was better for them to appear for work in clinical uniforms, at least part of the time. For some nurse managers, returning to clinical garb may seem a step backward. Yet, what these managers were saying is that if their primary responsibility is the management of a clinical function, there are some very real requirements for presence, comfort, and ability to fit into a clinical environment, even to the point of occasionally performing clinical services. Balancing clinical and business dress is important, because there is something to be lost in following either approach 100 percent of the time. Whether the manager is a director of nursing, a director of pharmacy, or a director of physical therapy, the same principle holds true.

The interventions all entail polarities to be managed:

- How to get to know employees and forge strong connections without becoming too personally involved
- How to set high standards and expectations and yet know when standards, policies, and practices can be bent to create a more humane workplace
- How to be accessible to staff without becoming fragmented and distracted
- How to support and become involved with people dealing with personal problems without developing or encouraging codependent relationships

All of these challenges are more likely to be met with the support of trusted senior mentors and coaches.

Negotiating a Supportive Role with Human Resources

It is very clear that if first-line managers are to successfully create a culture of engagement, they must be able to manage employee performance effectively. Performance management concentrates on eliminating unacceptable performance. Although some of the managers in the study identified human resources as one of their key supports, many others characterized human resources staff in a much more negative light, with comments ranging from they are no help at all to they are a barrier to effectively managing performance. Many managers also referred to the damaging effects their inability to deal effectively with employee performance issues had on their credibility and the credibility of the organization.

In some organizations, it is not reasonable to expect individual managers to negotiate a positive relationship with human resources alone. Senior leaders, often at the executive level, must insist on an effective working partnership between the manager and the organization's human resources department.

Removing Organizational Barriers for Getting Results

For managers to be credible in the eyes of their employees and physician colleagues, they must be perceived as efficacious in getting problems solved, issues dealt with, and improvements made. Processes in health care organizations must be simplified to enable managers to solve problems. Managers must have not only the skills to resolve issues, but they must also have the authority they need to act. When problems require the intervention of people with higher levels of authority, that support must be readily available. Effective methods of process improvement must be standardized in the organization to avoid the sense of futility that comes from dealing with the same problems month after month and year after year.

Encouraging Managers to Develop a Support Network

A recent study recognizes the importance of social support for coping with stress in the workplace (AbuAlRub 2004). Managers should be encouraged to develop support networks made up of their peers. One manager told of getting together with her peers for lunch every Friday afternoon. After debriefing the week and sharing issues, the attendees leave for home and an early start for the weekend. In other organizations, the encouragement of senior leaders may be needed before managers feel comfortable taking an afternoon away from their departments even though most first-line managers already work significantly more than forty hours per week.

Contrast this with the frustration expressed by some study participants who reported that there was simply no time to keep in touch with their peers, much less talk through issues and provide support to each other. Of even more concern was the finding that in some health care organizations, exemplary managers are finding themselves ostracized by their fellow managers, who are afraid that their colleagues' success makes them look bad in the eyes of other people in the organization.

Listening to Managers

Successful managers in the study reported that one of their most important responsibilities was listening to their employees. In the same way, senior managers must listen to what the managers tell them about their difficulties if the managers are to feel supported. Important to remember is that individuals will not feel as though they have been heard until something is done with the information they communicated. Senior leaders need to ask probing questions to learn what needs to be fixed and where the managers' frustrations lie. In fact, several managers identified feeling supported by behavior that demonstrated that they had been heard:

- I have always been able to say what I needed to say.
- They give me the latitude to be who I am, they want to know who I am.
- I feel supported by my boss, and it's okay to make mistakes. She says, "We trust you in that position to do what you do. Tell me what you need me to do."

Encouraging Managers to Learn from Each Other

Appreciative inquiry is an approach to organizational learning that assumes something is already going right in the organization, for example, that some managers implement effective strategies that lead to employee retention. Finding those who are successful and then encouraging other managers to learn from their practices is a useful intervention. However, it requires finesse and tact to avoid making the successful manager uncomfortable and creating unnecessary tension among colleagues. Treating success as an opportunity to learn and openly discussing what the manager has done that led to success can increase the level of organizational learning in the group. Remember, however, that all managers need not do things in the same way. Finding a unique approach that works for each department is the key to success, because applying cookie-cutter approaches can yield unanticipated negative results.

For example, Joan, a manager who participated in the study, described her anger at the standardized approach used by her organization in response to very poor employee satisfaction ratings. Based on the recommendations of a popular consulting group, Joan received an e-mail telling her that in the future she would be required to "write down who [she] sent thank-you notes to on the staff. It was insulting!" She was furious when she was required to attend a three-hour in-service to learn how to write thank-you notes. Joan's response: "I've been sending people handwritten thank-you notes for years." She added that to make matters worse, within two weeks after the mandatory educational program, she had received handwritten thank-you notes from her executive and her director both. Having never received a thank-you from either of them in the past, much less a handwritten note, it was clear to Joan that she was merely an assignment to them, which just added fuel to her fury.

The sad truth is that we have access to success stories by the hundreds in our organizations, and yet we fail to capitalize on what successful managers already know. Appreciative inquiry is an opportunity to learn from other managers. (This process is discussed more thoroughly in chapter 8.) If our organizations were true learning organizations, we would find ways to learn from our internal successes and perhaps need fewer external consultants to guide us. The trap in relying on external help is our tendency to implement their recommendations without taking into account the unique culture and people in our own organizations.

Conclusion

Developing and retaining good managers is a critical issue in today's health care organizations. The credibility of the manager and his or her capacity to establish effective relationships with employees is a central factor in employee commitment and engagement. It is imperative that we understand which managerial and leadership interventions lead to a positive workplace and that management and leadership practice become evidence based. Once we understand the key strategies available to us, we can encourage first-line managers to adopt effective management practices that lead to employee retention. Specifically, coaching for these skills in our front-line leaders can help them attain higher levels of success and make work more enjoyable for them. Organizations and senior leaders who are serious about improving the work environment and reducing costly turnover in their organizations can use the recommendations outlined in this chapter.

Conversation Points

Organizational Perspective

1. If a research team approached your organization and asked for the names of exceptional managers to participate in a study, how many would you recommend? How many first-line managers have successfully created a culture of engagement and retention in their departments?
2. Most organizations claim that people are their most important asset, and yet the organizations' behavior does not reflect this philosophy. What organizational behaviors and practices do you see that demonstrate the idea that employees should come first (so employees will put their patients or customers first)?
3. Do well-received, positive forms of recognition and demonstrations of appreciation occur on a regular basis in your organization? Are some of the activities celebrated in an organizationwide event, such as an employee recognition night or a summer picnic, as well as at the individual level? Do employees perceive these efforts as authentic demonstrations of appreciation?
4. How are healthy working relationships encouraged in the organization? Do executives and other senior leaders have good working relationships with employees? How much hierarchical thinking and behavior goes on?
5. Are managers listened to when they express concerns? Are they encouraged to be honest about their needs?
6. Is there a concrete, specific plan for the retention of managers?

Leadership Issues

1. Have you created a positive workplace in which a culture of engagement exists among employees?
2. What do you do to demonstrate that you put your employees first? What are examples of concrete behavior?

3. What is the quality of your working relationships with your employees? Do you genuinely care for them? Or is this emotion uncomfortable to feel and express in the workplace?

4. What progress have you been able to achieve in the past four months on problems that make working in the department difficult? Have you seen any substantial improvement in the issues you and your employees are dealing with?

5. How much time during a week do you spend deliberately coaching employees on their development? When was the last time you sat down with each of your employees and had a conversation about their career plans or job aspirations?

6. What level of support do you feel from senior leadership or the organization as a whole? Have you had a conversation with the person to whom you report about your need for more or different support? What was the reaction? What is your next step?

7. What would make your job easier? Have you communicated this information to anyone?

Employee Challenges

1. On a scale of 1 to 10, with 10 being the most positive, how would you rate your work environment? What would it have been three years ago (that is, if you worked there then)?

2. What specific things do you do to help your manager create a positive workplace?

3. Do you put the patient (or customer) first? What are the barriers, if any, to doing so? Do you feel like employees are put first by your manager?

4. What is the quality of relationships within your department? With people in other departments? What could you do to improve those relationships?

5. Do you see any signs of progress in your work area? Are long-term problems being addressed? Do you anticipate changes that will help you do your work more effectively in the future?

6. Do you feel as though you are treated as a partner by your manager? Do you see senior leaders on a fairly regular basis?

6

Building Healthy Relationships
in the Workplace

Jo Manion

Few can walk alone.
—Mary Wollstonecraft

W E EXIST in a web of relationships, the quality of which directly affects the richness of our lives and the degree to which we perceive ourselves to be happy. In chapter 2, the presence of healthy relationships was identified as a motivator, and chapter 3 examined the role of healthy relationships in forming commitment. Although a few people in health care organizations do work primarily alone, they are still immersed in a complex network of relationships in which others rely on them or they rely on others in order to carry out their work. Interdependence is the nature of relationships in any health care organization. For this reason, a primary strategy for creating a positive workplace is the formation and cultivation of healthy working relationships among people.

Simply the range of relationships to be considered makes this a complex issue. The relationships among coworkers in the same work group, among people in the same department on the various shifts, among coworkers in different job categories, and between employees and their manager must be considered. In an earlier chapter, the importance of a positive relationship between the manager and the employee was discussed and identified as being of primary importance in retention. However, the relationships between employees and other key stakeholders such as physicians, vendors, and people from

This chapter is adapted from *From Management to Leadership: Interpersonal Skills for Success in Health Care*, second edition, by Jo Manion. Copyright © 2005 Jossey–Bass Publishers. This material is used by permission of John Wiley & Sons, Inc.

other departments must also be considered as well as relationships among employees, managers, and administrators. Not to be left out, relationships between employees and customers or patients are also critical. Thus, an issue that may seem relatively straightforward can become overwhelming owing to its magnitude.

This chapter explores aspects of healthy relationships among individuals. Chapter 7 explores the importance of group or collective relationships. The impact of teams and the importance of a sense of community in creating a positive workplace are explored. The basic principles of relationship formation remain the same and can be transferred from the individual level to the collective level; however, several additional aspects should be considered when the relationships involve members of the same team. Clearly, the formation of healthy working relationships among individuals often precipitates the development of community within the work group.

Leadership Relationship

The relationship between manager and employees is the relationship most closely examined in this chapter. Because managers play a pivotal role in the creation of a positive workplace, they are the focal point of this chapter. Bear in mind, however, that the principles explored apply to all relationships. You should also note that although both terms—manager and leader—are used, the two terms are not synonymous. Not all leaders are managers; many of the effective leaders in health care organizations do not hold formal management positions. Of course, simply attaining the position of manager does not make a person an effective leader (Manion 1998, 2005). However, for the manager to be fully effective in creating a positive workplace, the basic nature of his or her relationship with employees is that of leader–follower. Thus, the two terms are used interchangeably in the context of this chapter.

Leadership exists only within the context of a relationship. It is an intensely personal experience, a process of relating to another person who ideally becomes a follower. All definitions of leadership include the ability to influence others to do what needs to be done. Leadership is a dynamic interaction between the leader and the follower, and both are changed irrevocably. It was noted earlier in this book that there is increasing emphasis on the importance of the relationship between the leader and the follower for the formation of a positive workplace environment that leads to a culture of engagement and retention.

Research in the area of emotional intelligence clearly demonstrates that the emotions of the leader directly affect the atmosphere and quality of the leader's relationships with others. The emotionally intelligent leader is described as one who is able "to generate excitement, optimism, and passion for the job ahead, as well as to cultivate an atmosphere of cooperation and trust" (Goleman, Boyatzis, and McKee 2002, p. 29). Leaders need competencies in four different domains: self-awareness, self-management, social awareness, and relationship management. Figure 6-1 presents these four domains as well as the competencies that exist within them. Closely intertwined, these competencies form the basis for effectiveness in the workplace.

Emotional intelligence was first described by Mayer, Salovey, and Caruso (2000, p. 396) as "the ability to perceive and express emotion,

Figure 6-1.   Emotional Intelligence Competencies
(Cherniss and Goleman 2001)

	Self (Personal Competence)	Other (Social Competence)
Recognition	**Self-Awareness** Emotional self-awareness Accurate self-assessment Self-confidence	**Social Awareness** Empathy Service orientation Organizational awareness
Regulation	**Self-Management** Emotional self-control Trustworthiness Conscientiousness Adaptability Achievement drive Initiative	**Relationship Management** Developing others Influence Communication Conflict management Visionary leadership Catalyzing change Building bonds Teamwork/collaboration

assimilate emotion in thought, understand and reason with emotion, and regulate emotion in the self and others." The emotionally intelligent individual has a high degree of self-awareness and is able to recognize his or her own emotions. Not only is this self-awareness accurate, but importantly, the individual is able to regulate a response to the emotion. The example used in the preceding chapter of a manager who was confronted by several employees in the department about her seemingly neutral response to a recent administrative decision about which the employees were very angry is a good illustration of this point. They confronted their manager by saying, "We're surprised you aren't angry about this, what's the matter with you?" The leader's response took them by surprise when she replied, "Oh, do not mistake me, I am very angry about this decision, but that doesn't mean I have to spew all that negativity out and infect everyone around me! I can control my emotions and not let them infect everyone else." In her brief words, the employees were given a beautiful role model of an emotionally intelligent leader capable of emotional self-regulation.

But emotional intelligence is not limited to the individual level. The leader also is competent in relationships with others, both in social awareness as well as in relationship management. These competencies build on the personal competencies of recognition (emotional self-awareness, accurate self-assessment, and self-confidence) as well as self-regulation (emotional self-control, trustworthiness, conscientiousness, adaptability, achievement drive, and initiative). The social competencies related to social awareness include empathy, service orientation, and organizational awareness (Cherniss and Goleman 2001). Other authors and scholars have supported the importance of these competencies as well.

The quality and depth of the relationship between the leader and the follower directly affect the abilities of the leader. Without a strong foundation for a healthy relationship, the aspiring leader cannot attain extraordinary outcomes. Although troubled leaders seldom return to the basic components of a healthy relationship when they are frustrated by followers who do not follow, the answer to their difficulties often lies within this basic concept.

Developing and maintaining healthy relationships among people seems like it should be a simple proposition, and yet there are many ramifications for us if we are seeking to do this in our organizations. First, we must share an understanding of what precisely we mean by a healthy relationship. Unfortunately, many of the people with whom we work would not recognize a healthy relationship if it was staring them in the face. Misconceptions abound regarding what comprises a vibrant, dynamic relationship. For some people it means not making waves, going along to get along, and being accommodating to the other person. For others it means not being direct and honest about how they feel in a situation because it may hurt the other person's feelings or the other person may not agree with them. The first step is to be crystal clear about what we mean by a healthy relationship in an organizational context. Figure 6-2 presents a sample of behavioral expectations that clearly address the components of a healthy relationship.

Second, once we are clear about what we mean, then we must clearly say to all employees, "You have two responsibilities to the organization, one is to do the work for which you were hired, at the quality we expect. Second, you are responsible for creating and maintaining healthy working relationships with the other people in this workplace." Too many employees *and* managers believe that healthy working relationships in a work situation are the responsibility of the manager. The manager is expected to deal with interpersonal conflicts, communicate negative or constructive feedback, and generally act as the spokesperson for the department when there are difficulties. In positive workplaces, the creation and maintenance of healthy relationships must be accepted as everyone's responsibility and there must be some consistent level of understanding about what a healthy relationship entails. Once these expectations have been clarified and accepted, then everyone must be held accountable for their own behavior.

Definition of a Healthy Relationship

Although these concepts may seem self-evident, Dr. Phil would not be so popular today if more people understood and embraced the simple elements of good relationships. Those of us who relate comfortably to others often take this talent for forming relationships for granted. There is a naturalness and spontaneity in relationships that result in mutually beneficial outcomes. When a particular situation is not going well, the relationship-centered individual often reflects first on the quality of the connection with the other person to determine potential problem areas. And because this person is already skillful in the relationship arena, the assessment process is not likely to produce undue anxiety. If, however, you are not naturally talented at forming strong relationships, you may feel uncomfortable during this assessment process. The good news is that it is possible to build your relationship-building skills or strengthen them if you already have the innate talent.

Chapter 6

Figure 6-2. Sample Behavioral Expectations

In this organization, we expect the following of all employees:

1. To develop and maintain positive and healthy interpersonal relationships with others in the workplace.
   a. Communicates openly, directly, and honestly with other employees.
   b. Gives both positive and negative feedback in an affirming, supportive manner.
   c. Shares ideas and opinions in a positive and honest manner even if these differ from peers or managers.
   d. Maintains a positive attitude toward others (and speaks positively of others in their absence).
   e. Follows through on commitments and promises made.
   f. Assumes other people have positive intentions.
   g. Shows respect for and values the diverse skills, abilities, and characteristics of other employees.
   h. Expresses appreciation of others.
   i. Shares work-appropriate information openly with others on a need-to-know basis.
   j. Accepts and respects differences (in approach, styles, and personalities) of coworkers.
   k. Has a will-do attitude.
   l. Seeks mutually beneficial solutions when solving problems or resolving issues.
   m. Maintains confidentiality and does not talk about coworkers' sensitive or personal business to others.

2. To work interdependently with coworkers and employees from all departments.
   a. Looks for ways to help others and makes self available.
   b. Works at a steady pace and carries an equitable share of the workload.
   c. Supports the goals of the organization and department by behaving and acting in a manner that helps achieve these goals.
   d. Participates positively and successfully completes any needed cross-training.
   e. Is willing to learn new skills and grows in ability to take on new responsibilities.
   f. Keeps coworkers and manager informed so they can work as effectively as possible.
   g. Focuses on similarities between coworkers rather than using differences to separate and isolate.
   h. Cooperates with others.
   i. Shares responsibility and delegates appropriately.
   j. Does what needs to be done for good patient care or customer service regardless of whose job it is.
   k. Shares knowledge and expertise openly with other people.

3. To participate actively and positively in ongoing department and team processes.
   a. Attends department and team meetings.
   b. Initiates problem-solving activities when issues or problems occur repeatedly.
   c. Supports the department's decisions even when they disagree personally.
   d. Works with coworkers and manager to achieve the department's goals and outcomes.
   e. Works to help the department and organization succeed.

Based on a model I have used over the years, at least three essential elements are needed in a successful working relationship among people: trust, mutual respect, and communication. These three elements are described as essential because the absence of any one of the three can damage or reduce the effectiveness of the relationship. (See figure 6-3.) As you can readily see, the circle would not be complete without all three elements. Each of these elements will be discussed in some detail, with a primary focus on the leader–follower relationships, especially the manager–employee relationship. The concepts apply to all relationships equally.

Trust

According to *Webster's Encyclopedic Unabridged Dictionary*, trust means that you can rely on the "integrity, strength or ability of a person or thing. Confidence implies conscious trust because of good reasons, definite evidence or past experience." The importance of trust in the leader–follower relationship is clear. Without trust or confidence in the person attempting to influence them, people do not follow the leader's direction. In organizations, when the leader also holds legitimate positional authority, the relative health of the relationship can be

Figure 6-3. Three Essential Elements of a Healthy Relationship

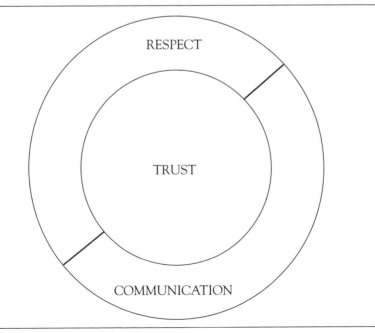

deceptive. People may do what the manager wants, not because they agree or believe in the direction set or the request made, but because they believe they must comply in order to avoid painful or undesirable personal consequences.

Understanding the concept of trust is important for understanding relationships, but it is imperative for anyone aspiring to lead others. Warren Bennis offers a concrete, applicable framework for under-standing trust within the context of a leadership role (Flower 1990). He defines three essential ingredients of trust: competence, congru-ence, and constancy. (See figure 6-4.) Examination of these three com-ponents of trust provides a guide for anyone seeking to more fully understand their personal effectiveness.

Competence

Webster's defines *competence* as the possession of required skill, knowl-edge, qualification, or capacity. The application of this definition in a leadership context is clear. Supporters must believe that the leader has the skill and knowledge to do what is required. "Whenever we step in front of the crowd and say, 'Follow me,' the implication is that we know where we're going and what we want to achieve and that we're

Figure 6-4.   Components of Trust in a Healthy Relationship

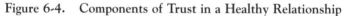

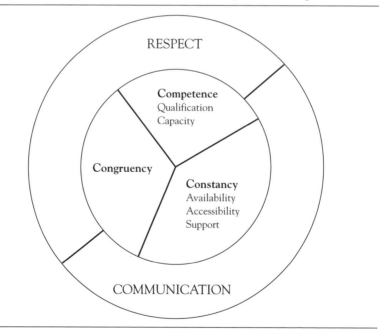

committed to giving our very best efforts" (Melrose 1996, p. 20). Confidence in a leader develops from working with that person and from evidence of the leader's past performance demonstrating competence. Both skill and knowledge are included in this definition. Knowledge alone is insufficient. The leader may know that followers need accurate information and clear communication, but an unskilled leader is greatly hampered if not totally unable to articulate information clearly.

For this reason, changing key leaders in organizations can result in a troublesome situation. It takes time to establish trust and confidence in new leadership. Nevertheless, many health care organizations embarking on major changes choose to alter the managerial and executive structure by eliminating or combining positions. Entire departments find themselves in a new reporting relationship. Leaders in these new positions are then expected to lead their followers through the changes, and yet they are severely disadvantaged because they must first form a trusting relationship. Although this sequence of events may be appropriate, its impact on the time required to change should be carefully considered. In one Midwestern hospital, for example, the chief executive officer routinely changes reporting relationships every couple of years because he likes to keep people off balance, in his words, "to shake things up a bit." What he fails to see is the effect on productivity and the cost in terms of relationships of such frequent changes in leadership.

Qualifications are an interesting factor in competence. In health care there is a notable emphasis on technical expertise as a necessary qualification for managers. Some people simply do not follow an individual unless the person has a particular qualification believed to be important, such as a particular clinical discipline background or a certain academic degree. Whether the qualification actually prepares or enables the manager to function competently is a moot point; from the perspective of the employees, the absence of such qualifications can become a critical issue with significant repercussions. Organizations that have consolidated departments and replaced two or three managers with one manager often encounter significant obstacles when the new manager no longer shares the background or expertise of the employees in the department. Although this is not an insurmountable obstacle, it can take longer for the new manager to establish a trust relationship with employees because of his or her need to prove his or her competence in the face of what appears to be a significant qualification issue.

Capacity issues also influence the level of trust in the leader. When a leader is seen by others as simply having too much to do, too many responsibilities—juggling too many balls—a question of trust may arise. Can this leader handle the current situation? Will it be too much? What if it pushes the leader over the edge? When managers appear frazzled and out of control, employees become uneasy. Personal endurance and a phenomenal capacity for work often go hand in hand with effective leadership. The motto "Never let them see you sweat" may be appropriate but it should not imply that a good leader never lets followers see the reality of a difficult situation.

In one West Coast hospital where significant organizational consolidation of leadership roles was under way, a newly appointed executive had a personality style characterized by spontaneity, impulsiveness, and a high degree of self-disclosure. As the initiative progressed, this vice president was given more and more responsibility because she was very capable. She quickly reached the point of overload and began manifesting counterproductive behaviors such as volatility, extreme distractibility, and pure panic. Her communication patterns became dysfunctional as a result of her intense anxiety. Her erratic behavior with her followers clearly transmitted her anxiety, and she began to lose their trust. In this instance, skill, knowledge, and qualifications were not at issue. Instead, her followers feared she could not handle the heavy workload.

Congruence

The second key element of trust in this context is congruence, meaning consistency or agreement between verbal messages and the leader's behavior (Lorimer and Manion 1996). A manager/leader with a high degree of congruence between what is said and the behaviors observed by employees is perceived as more honest and trustworthy. If the leader says one thing but does another, the result is an enormous credibility gap. Most would agree that leaders must "walk the talk." The integrity and character of the manager are important. Employees need to believe that leaders act in accordance with their personal beliefs and are honest not only with themselves but also with employees. This belief is more important than agreeing with the manager's beliefs. "Effective leadership . . . is not based on being clever; it is based primarily on being consistent" (Drucker 1992, p. 122).

Lack of congruence can be thought of as a discrepancy. Discrepancies are common in any work setting. For example, one department director in the hospital maintenance department established employee work teams and assured team members that they would have input into any decisions that affected their work. After almost a year of working together as a team, they were joined one day by two new team members whom no one on the team had expected. Their manager had hired the additional members without including the team in the decision. Consequently, the team members felt betrayed by the manager, and the ensuing breach of trust was difficult to repair. They wondered what other decisions the manager had made without their knowledge or input.

One of the most serious problems with congruency is that inconsistent messages are often inadvertent. The manager/leader usually does not purposely engage in behavior contrary to previous messages sent but instead, without realizing it, acts in direct contradiction to the oral and written messages delivered. This happened in one organization where competence was a stated organizational value. When the organization needed to determine which employees would be laid off during an economic downturn, tenure was the key selection criterion, not competence. Tenure and competence are clearly not the same thing, and many employees were offended and angered by what appeared to be a decision-making criterion inconsistent with a stated, and often touted, organizational value. When this decision was questioned, the senior executive leading the initiative became defensive and angry but eventually listened to the feedback and changed the decision-making criteria. Tenure was used as a final determining factor only when the employees in question first met the criterion of competency.

A similar situation in another hospital was handled differently. When confronted with the incongruity between using the stated organizational value of competence versus tenure as a selection criterion, the administration retained tenure as the deciding factor. The senior executives reasoned that this was not the appropriate time to correct problems with employee competency issues that had not been dealt with previously by managers. Although it may sound reasonable and they felt better, their choice created a major credibility issue. They were basically admitting that they had never held true to the organization's stated value of competence by saying that managers had never dealt properly with unacceptable or poor employee performance.

We must all scrupulously examine our own behavior to avoid the appearance of incongruence, although it is virtually impossible to avoid all discrepancies. The requirement is especially important when you are serving in a leadership position. Thus, it is especially important for a manager to promote openness and honest feedback from employees. An executive team in one northeastern medical center worked diligently to establish an open environment by making certain that employees knew their leaders wanted feedback when their behaviors appeared incongruent. The leaders knew that their initial reaction to feedback would determine the amount and usefulness of future feedback, and they were very careful to listen fully when discordant messages were brought to their attention and to react nondefensively. In some instances, behavior deemed incongruent was changed to fit the message. In other cases, communication was unclear, and through sharing additional information the problem was resolved. This openness did not occur overnight. Many employees were—and some still are—hesitant to provide feedback because of fear of reprisal. This fear is a common obstacle for managers who hold a hierarchical position and have legitimate power over employees.

Giving the leader feedback on incongruent behavior is much more difficult than it may appear. Many employees simply say nothing when they feel a leader is about to make a mistake, and employees who were not well received when they did speak up in the past are unlikely to speak up again in the future. Some of this reluctance to speak freely and honestly is related to early socialization messages. According to Chaleff (1996), young people are taught from an early age to obey authority, to say, "Yes, sir" and "Yes, ma'am," and this conditioning runs very deep. It takes work to overcome these deep internal messages. "We are afraid that if we question authority we will be viewed as a nuisance, pushed out of the loop, overlooked for promotion, even fired. We fear the consequences of speaking up far more than we are afraid of the more serious consequences of not speaking up" (Chaleff 1996, p. 16).

Another way to view congruence involves congruity between what we do in our personal and public lives. People who do not live up to commitments to their family or who cheat their neighbors often hide behind the belief that what happens in their personal lives should not affect their leadership roles. Like it or not, if untrustworthy personal behavior is observed by followers, the level of trust in the leaders will be adversely affected.

Constancy

Constancy is the third and last ingredient of trust as identified by Bennis (Flower 1990). Constancy implies that the leader is reliable, dependable, and consistent. A good leader keeps commitments and follows through on promises. When it becomes clear that a promise or commitment cannot be met, the leader communicates openly and honestly with people to inform them of the changed circumstances, ideally before being confronted about it.

To many people, availability and accessibility are part of constancy. For leaders to be most effective, they must be accessible to followers at more than prescheduled, formal times. Some of the best dialogues occur in a completely spontaneous fashion. When the leader is also a manager or executive, the formal trappings of the role may serve to distance the leader from the followers. Common examples of this are isolated office locations or the presence of secretaries who see their role as protecting or buffering the leader from others. Although it would be impossible to remain available twenty-four hours a day, neither should the leader be completely inaccessible to followers. A balance must be found, because the perception that the leader is available is a potent one in creating a collegial relationship with others. The importance of this concept was underscored by the results of the research reported in chapter 5.

Visibility of the leader has long been suggested by many authors as a key way that managers create a positive work environment. Peters and Austin (1985) refer to it as management by walking around, or MBWA. It suggests that the closer a leader is physically to followers, the more a sense of connection and understanding is established. It is true that the leader who sees a situation with his or her own eyes is certainly better informed than one who hears about it from a third, potentially biased party. As time pressures increase, visibility and availability are often sacrificed. Whatever constraints may exist, they are never as serious as the threat to a leader's effectiveness from employees who do not feel a sense of connection and, as a result, do not follow.

These ideas may seem like common sense or intuitive knowledge. However, availability and accessibility are difficult to achieve in these demanding times. The rapidity and breadth of change occurring in health care today creates an environment filled with uncertainty, and people have many questions. Employees may not perceive every change as positive and may be very unhappy, even angry, about the current direction of the organization. Every manager today knows how daunting it is to face a crowd of antagonistic employees, and it is a natural tendency to avoid these situations and withdraw from contact with people during these times. This area demonstrates one major difference between the excellent leader and the not-so-effective leader: The excellent leader stays more visible and involved, more accessible and available to followers during bad times. Similar to a sporting event where a team finds inspiration from cheerleaders when it falls behind and is losing the game, the excellent leader knows the importance of being present when there is significant unrest. Such leaders understand that their mere presence is often a gift and message of support to uncertain people.

Being able to count on the presence of the leader is important to us, although some leaders feel uncomfortable when they do not have answers to the complex or difficult questions that may be raised. Many managers have been socialized to believe that the manager's job is to have answers. A good leader, however, understands and accepts that it is impossible to have all of the answers all of the time. It takes remarkable courage to stay present with others when they are being looked to for answers they do not have. Yet, we respect leaders who are not afraid to admit that they do not have the answers. People are encouraged when a leader communicates belief that the answers will be found by working together. This presence during trying times is a tremendous gift the leader gives to others.

When the three elements of trust are present (competence, congruency, and constancy), credibility in the leader and his or her actions is possible. Kouzes and Posner have studied credibility extensively. They believe credibility relates to how a leader earns the trust and confidence of his or her constituency. In their studies they have found "people want leaders who hold to an ethic of service and are genuinely respectful of the intelligence and contributions of their constituents. They want leaders who will put principles ahead of politics and other people before self-interests" (Kouzes and Posner 1993, p. xvii). Credibility is a way of maintaining or regaining people's faith in their institutions and the individuals who lead them.

Constancy of support offered by the leader is a vital issue affecting the quality of the leader–follower relationship. (This idea was identified in the research presented in chapter 5.) Support means to nurture or to provide sustenance, a two-way street within this context, going from followers to leaders and from leaders to followers. Consistency of support is critical; without it trust wavers. If support is offered only when everything is going smoothly and then withdrawn during vulnerable times, it is of virtually no value because you cannot count on it. The net result in the relationship is one of uneasiness, of being uncertain whether the support will be there this time. It is ironic that support is most needed during the times when it is most frequently withdrawn, that is, when mistakes occur and when poor decisions or errors in judgment are made. In a healthy relationship, support is consistent, offered freely, and visible to the receiver.

A manager's response to mistakes or errors is often the clue employees have to the consistency of the support extended by the leader. When punitive consequences are the norm, people do not feel supported. Punitive consequences for mistakes can occur in the form of shaming, blaming, humiliation, or reduction of future opportunities. Simply stepping in and taking over, relieving the individual of responsibility for correcting the consequences that resulted, can also be perceived as a lack of support. Interestingly, when the manager is observed behaving in a negative, punitive behavior with any employee, it is enough to damage trust even among those who were not directly involved. Of course, this is not to imply that appropriate actions should not be taken for a person making the same mistakes repeatedly.

Constancy may also refer to the stability of personal characteristics. The manager who experiences extreme fluctuations in mood, who is quick to anger, or who responds with knee-jerk reactions may have trust problems with employees. Take the individual who is excessively positive about ideas, unrealistically optimistic about the chances for success on a project, and effusive with praise one day, but the next day is exactly the opposite. Employees are left with an uncomfortable feeling of uncertainty, and trust is impaired. It is next to impossible for any of us to be completely balanced and thoroughly predictable. However, leaders who avoid such surprising changes in behavior can enhance the level of trust in their relationships. Consistency of behavior is important.

Strategy for Repairing Broken Trust

So these are the three essential ingredients of trust: competence, congruency, and constancy. Each ingredient offers challenges for healthy relationships in our workplaces. When mistrust becomes evident, examining these three areas can help the leader to sort out the probable causes. When mistrust is apparent in relationships, one possible approach to the solution is to ask, "What has happened to damage trust?" Leaders with the courage to ask this question are often rewarded with insight. Unless the question is asked sincerely, however, people may be reluctant to discuss situations in which they believe they were let down by a leader. Bennis (1989) points out that good leaders encourage respectful dissent so that they can know the truth about a situation even when it is not what they want to hear. In fact, good leaders need people around who have contrary views and serve as devil's advocates.

Rogers (1994) identifies three steps for repairing broken trust: acknowledging the problem, apologizing for the problem, and making amends.

Step 1: Acknowledge the Problem

The first step, acknowledging broken trust, is tough for many managers. Few leaders purposely set out to destroy trust, and it is difficult to admit that something has happened to damage the relationship. In fact, some people prefer to call it something else, anything else, rather than accept it as a lack of trust. Some managers and executives believe acknowledging a lack of trust implies a personal fault of some kind, and this belief makes it especially onerous for them to honestly examine these situations.

For example, Susan was a senior vice president in a community hospital in Texas. In her organization the hierarchy was very rigid, and the rules and policies were plentiful. One expectation was that all employees, including managers and executives, submitted time cards. For years employees were required to have their time cards signed by the individual to whom they reported, but this practice did not include managers and executives. Problems developed when one executive began submitting questionable entries and inaccurate records of sick and absent time. As a result, Susan began to require that all managers and executives get their time cards signed. The reaction was predictable. People felt they were no longer trusted. Susan was adamant that her requirement for the double check on the time cards was "just corporate compliance policy," but her assurances did nothing to assuage their feelings. When pushed she finally admitted that it was because there were problems with one individual. Even when confronted directly, she continued to deny that there were any trust issues. It was clearly a lack of trust (albeit well deserved) in the one individual who had been found altering and falsifying time cards.

Step 2: Apologize for the Problem

Apologizing for a breach of trust is difficult for many people. This does not mean accepting fault for something that is not the manager's responsibility. If it is your responsibility, the apology may sound like this: "I made a mistake and I am sorry" or "I am sorry that my decision has caused these difficulties for you." If you are not culpable, the apology may sound different: "I am sorry to hear that you feel this way; the decision was right for this situation," or "I am sorry that is what you heard. Let me try explaining this again." Another possibility is simply to say, "I am sorry that happened."

Apologies are very difficult for some people because they believe it diminishes their stature or damages the respect held by the other person. Many managers and executives have been socialized in a hierarchical system in which formal leaders just do not admit mistakes to employees, perhaps because they believe it may weaken their authority. The problem with this attitude is that people lose respect for individuals who cannot admit that they were wrong or made a mistake.

In one community hospital undergoing a major work-redesign initiative in the late 1990s, employees showed significant distrust of administration. Five years previously a layoff had occurred, and there were several very visible and devastating mistakes made in the way the process had been handled. Although the executives talked about these mistakes behind closed doors, employees talked about them openly. The executives closed ranks and never talked with employees about the mistakes. The result was an antagonistic workforce that did not trust the executives to manage the new challenge because employees did not believe the executives had learned anything from the previous layoff. How different the environment would have been if there had been open dialogue and a sharing of ideas about what had been learned since the layoff.

Step 3: Make Amends
The last step in repairing broken trust is to make amends. Correcting mistakes and avoiding similar behavior the future are ways to make amends. Sometimes the easiest thing to do is to ask, "How can I make this right? How can I make amends?" In many instances, an apology is enough. However, if there is behavior to be changed and a commitment is made to do so, the leader must follow through on this commitment. It may take longer to reestablish trust than expected. People will be watching closely to determine whether they can believe the leader's promises.

Making amends also implies some reciprocal behavior from the follower. When the leader changes his or her behavior and maintains it, others at some point need to let go of past wrongs. A manager in one organization found that his behavior when he was first appointed to his position resulted in a reputation that still haunted him ten years later. Such trust problems need to be addressed, and he should perhaps ask for their forgiveness in an effort to rebuild a trusting relationship.

Mutual Respect

The second essential element in forming a healthy relationship is mutual respect between the manager and the employee, which means having esteem for or valuing the other person for their skills, talents, and abilities. In a leadership relationship, respect can be offered in two ways. In the first, respect is offered unconditionally to all. Respect is not contingent on superficial attributes such as position, education, or socioeconomic status but is based on the contributions, both actual and potential, of the individual. Relating to followers as colleagues is a characteristic of a transformational leader (Burns 1978). This does not mean that you would not respect an individual's achievements in terms of education or position, but that you would not withhold respect from an individual because they do not have a particular level of education or positional authority.

In health care, because patients and families are extended unconditional respect regardless of their situation, it is often assumed that this same respect exists among and between health care workers. All too often, however, respect is offered solely on the status or authority inherent in a title. Just as a person leaving a position becomes a nonentity because they no longer have a title, certain employees are not recognized as leaders because they have no formal title. Individuals with particular educational qualifications are believed to be most capable or the only ones with the ability to solve certain problems. These are all examples of respect based on superficial attributes. A leader understands fully that in another situation positions may be reversed, placing the leader in a follower position.

Respect extended to followers is a result of a sincere belief that followers are partners and that they have ideas, abilities, solutions, and a keen interest in the situation. Max DePree says that the excellent leader begins with understanding the diversity and breadth of people's gifts, talents, and skills. "Understanding and accepting diversity enables us to see that each of us is needed. It also enables us to begin to think about being abandoned to the strengths of others, of admitting that we cannot know or do everything" (DePree 1989, p. 9). Extending respect to others includes seeking input, soliciting opinions and ideas, and using this information in making decisions. It also means providing freedom within the relationship and allowing a give-and-take to occur.

A second way respect is offered is based on performance. In other words, we observe a person's skills or abilities and see that they obtain desirable outcomes. This type of respect may be differential; in other words, the same level of respect is not guaranteed among people but is based on their individual performance. In this case, respect is withdrawn when appropriate or desirable outcomes are not achieved. In other words, the individual who makes repeated mistakes and does not learn from them may lose the respect of others and may even be removed from his or position.

Communication

The third essential element of healthy relationships is open and honest communication. No leader is effective without the ability to communicate with others. This involves excellent communication skills and a willingness to talk through issues. A leader may be highly skilled but unwilling to take the necessary time to do the time-consuming work of communicating. In chapter 5, the research found that effective communication skills were a key factor for managers in creating a positive work environment. Not only were the skills important, but the manager's philosophy about communication was key. Most of the successful managers in the research clearly said that they subscribed to a philosophy of no secrets and open sharing. They believed that employees not only have the right to extensive information about what is happening in the organization, but that the employees want to know the truth about things.

The paradox today is that leaders and managers spend more time than ever communicating with people, and yet the most common complaint of most employees is that no one tells them anything and that they never know what is going on. Communication skills have been discussed extensively elsewhere (refer to *From Management to Leadership: Interpersonal Skills for Success in Health Care* [Manion 2005] for an entire chapter on communication) and thus will not be examined closely here. Another characteristic of healthy communication is that it is predominantly positive. Too often, employees only hear from the manager when there are problems, and this habit sets up a negative relationship between the manager and the employees.

Creation of a Trust-Based Organizational Climate

The emotionally intelligent employee and manager know how to form healthy relationships with other people, they are able to assess and control their own emotions, and they can accurately assess the emotions of other people. The basic components of a healthy relationship are trust, respect, and open, positive communication. Healthy relationships among people in the workplace are more likely to lead to a culture of engagement and retention.

Healthy relationships are the foundation of a trust-based organizational climate. Effective leaders continually scan their environment and the reactions of the organization's members to assess levels of trust. We are becoming increasingly aware of the direct correlation between a positive, trust-based work environment and the competitive advantage of the organization.

> We are a society in search of trust. The less we find it, the more precious it becomes. An organization in which people earn one another's trust, and that commands trust from the public, has a competitive advantage. It can draw the best people, inspire customer loyalty, reach out successfully to new markets, and provide more innovative products and services (Ciancutti and Steding 2001, p. ix).

This message is echoed in earlier work done by Reina and Reina (1999), who examined closely the issues of trust and betrayal in today's workplaces. According to their findings, "Unmet expectations, disappointments, broken trust, and betrayals aren't restricted to big events like restructurings and downsizings. They crop up every day on the job. Leaders are beginning to realize that people's trust and commitment to the organization affect their performance" (Reina and Reina 1999, p. ix). Reina and Reina offer a model for understanding the complex and emotional issue of trust and betrayal in today's organization. They believe that it is possible to create an organizational climate in which transformative trust exists. The four core characteristics that produce transformative trust are conviction, courage, compassion, and community.

In their book, *Built on Trust*, Ciancutti and Steding (2001) talk about intentionally creating trust in the organization. They offer a model for deliberately and systematically establishing and maintaining high levels of trust. The six stages in the model include:

1. **Closure:** coming to a specific agreement with every communication about what will be done, by whom, and with a specific date of completion.

2. **Commitment:** expressing a positive intention to complete what was agreed to with no conditions. If one is unable to follow through or fulfill the commitment as agreed to for any reason, then the person speaks up immediately.

3. **Communication:** disseminating information in a direct, open, and honest way that replaces dysfunctional forms of communication such as talking behind people's backs, withholding information, engaging in hallway conversations, and so on.

4. **Speedy resolution:** clearing up unresolved issues as soon as they become apparent and as soon as possible.

5. **Respect:** using tact and respect in communications.

6. **Responsibility:** owning your own problems and helping others when needed.

In addition to these stages, they include discussion of other principles such as being responsive to each other, telling the truth, agreeing to a "no surprise practice," handling issues at the lowest possible level in the organization, and having managers who serve as daily role models in each of these aspects.

Importance of Collaboration and Partnership

Unfortunately, the healthy relationships we have been talking about here rarely exist in health care organizations. Many departments may have worked hard to create and maintain healthy relationships, but it is not the norm. Instead, relationships are characterized by conflict-aversive behavior and indirect or dishonest communication among coworkers. In such groups, some individuals are too accommodating to the needs of others and never consider their own needs, some do not behave assertively or ask for what they need and want, and some display passive-aggressive behavior. A major role of every manager and leader is clarifying the expectation that employees will develop healthy relationships and coaching them as they work to improve the quality of their relationships. Holding people accountable for the quality of their relationships is essential if behavior is to change. (This subject is addressed more fully in chapter 10.)

For leaders, establishing and cultivating healthy relationships with followers is the first essential step in developing the ability to influence others. This can be accomplished by ensuring that the three elements of a healthy relationship—trust, mutual respect, and communication—are in place. But understanding the concepts of collaboration and partnership is also important because these forms of relationship are healthier than the traditional command-and-control approach to leadership or "mama or papa" management styles characterized by unhealthy codependent relationships between employees and managers. As seen in the research findings in chapter 5, successful managers work in partnership with employees.

The terms *collaboration* and *partnership* have similar meanings. *Collaboration* refers to work or labor accomplished by two or more persons working together. The word *partnership* is derived from the verb *partake*, which means to share. The essence of a successful manager's relationship with employees, peers, and key stakeholders is a combination of collaboration and partnership. Collaboration became a buzzword in the 1990s, serving as a topic in many journal articles and workshop titles. But like most buzzwords, it is overused and misused without a true understanding of the concept. A good leader may not need to know the actual definition but certainly needs to live the concept in relation with followers and colleagues.

Collaboration

Collaboration has multiple meanings, but the most useful is working together, especially in joint intellectual efforts. In the context of the manager–employee relationship, collaboration includes interactions between manager and employees that enable the knowledge and skills of both to work synergistically to influence the decision being made or the work being accomplished (Manion 1989). *Synergy* is a biochemical term that means that the whole is greater than the sum of its parts. In the leadership context, it means that when the leader and follower work together, they are likely to generate more and better solutions and alternatives than either would by working alone. Dictionary definitions rarely bring a concept fully to life. To more completely understand collaboration, the relationship among coordination, cooperation, and mutual work is helpful to examine (Baggs and Schmitt 1988). These three ingredients comprise the whole of collaboration.

Coordination occurs when two or more people come together and share their points of view and their experiences to ensure a harmonious combination or interaction. One executive team meets regularly on Monday mornings for a short time, sharing plans for the week, discussing major issues, and briefly reviewing their members' calendars. Their intent is to coordinate efforts. Another example is a patient-care conference in a patient-care department that is often held for a similar purpose. Individuals from the different disciplines or shifts come together to compare their assessments of patients and to coordinate their efforts. Coordination is based on shared information.

Cooperation implies planning and working together in an actively helpful manner, more than being passively cooperative or simply accommodating. Cooperation as it relates to collaboration means meeting the other person's needs and yet being assertive in meeting one's own needs at the same time. Being assertive and uncooperative is being competitive.

Sharing mutual work in collaboration means sharing goals, planning, problem solving, decision making, and responsibility. Contrast this with consultation, where sharing occurs during the planning phase but the individual proceeds alone in implementation.

True collaboration requires coordination, cooperation, and mutual work in healthy amounts. Too often, a manager or administrator makes a decision and then expects others to coordinate and cooperate in its implementation. The manager may honestly feel as though he or she is being collaborative because there is a general feeling of cooperation. However, unless the decision was mutually made, it is not collaboration in the true sense of the word. The basis of any partnering relationship is collaboration.

Partnership

Successful relationships in the future will probably be characterized as partnerships at all levels in our society. Many types of partnerships are being developed today. Communities are forming partnerships with businesses and industries. Former competitors, such as Apple and IBM, are creating business partnerships. In a community in the Midwest, two hospitals from competing systems are considering building the third facility needed in their community. Strategic partnerships are appearing with more regularity in health care between health care systems as well as individual organizations (Blouin and Brent 1997). Managerial partnerships are found at the executive and managerial levels (Manion, Sieg, and Watson 1998; Heenan and Bennis 1999). Today, leaders need to work in partnership with others. It is the very essence of the leader–follower relationship. "In a world of increasing interdependence and ceaseless technological change, even the greatest of Great Men or Women simply can't get the job done alone. As a result, we need to rethink our most basic concepts of leadership" (Heenan and Bennis 1999, p. 5).

The philosophy and approach of "every man for himself" in organizational life is gradually going by the wayside. In the past, managers were often rewarded for the size of their turf. The larger their budget, the more direct reports, and the greater number of people in their departments, the greater their status. Organizational environments were competitive and predominantly unhealthy. When one manager's request was met, another's had to be denied. In today's world, the manager who is a leader understands the importance of forming alliances and partnerships with employees, colleagues, and peers with the goal of accomplishing shared outcomes. The effective leader of tomorrow will be one who is able to form collaborative associations with others to fulfill the organization's mission. The concept of partnership is much more complex than it first appears because an individual, group, or organization may at one time be a competitor, a partner, a distributor,

and/or a supplier. It takes a high level of maturity to balance such complex relationships.

Although successful leaders are willing and able to work in partnership with others, true partnership is not easy. Partnership may well
be the highest level of interpersonal development, and some people
may simply be incapable of forming effective partner relationships.

Development Continuum

S. R. Covey, author of *Seven Habits of Highly Effective People* (1989),
has identified the stages of development and their ramifications in the
professional world. (See figure 6-5.) As we develop as individuals, our
progression evolves from a state of dependence to a state of independence and finally to interdependence. Each of these stages of development represents significant and substantial progress.

In the stage of dependence, individuals rely on others. In the stage
of independence, individuals rely more heavily on themselves and take
responsibility for their own behavior, emotions, and accomplishments.
Independent individuals are capable of moving to the higher interdependence level of development to work effectively with others and
share responsibility and recognition.

Covey (1989) points out that only independent people can make
the choice to become interdependent. Highly dependent people, therefore, have little chance of moving into true interdependence. Independent people may choose not to become interdependent and, in fact,
may see it as a weakness to relinquish control to others or share decision making. Executives in health care systems across the country are
learning to balance a mixture of independence and interdependence as
they partner with employees, colleagues, and peers in a variety of ways.

This development continuum is significant in understanding
healthy relationships. Both Bennis (1989) and DePree (1989), when

Figure 6-5.   Development Continuum

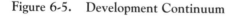

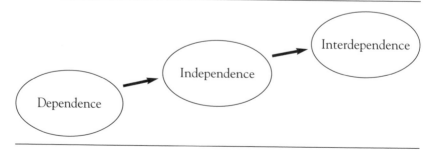

discussing leaders, describe seasoned, mature people who have recognized the need for—and have consciously chosen—interdependence with their followers. The excellent leader does not go it alone but derives energy and ideas from colleagues. Healthy leader–follower relationships are characterized by true synergy. Neither leaders nor followers exist in a vacuum but function in a reciprocal relationship that yields outcomes that exceed what either could have accomplished working alone.

Interestingly, the concept of partnership has been with us since the earliest times. In *The Chalice and the Blade*, Eisler (1987) describes the shift from a partnership societal model in earliest of human history to a dominator model. It is clear from her research that "war and the 'war of the sexes' are neither divinely nor biologically ordained" (Eisler 1987, p. xv). Based on her understanding and interpretation of historical artifacts and findings, in the earliest human societies "difference is not necessarily equated with inferiority or superiority" (Eisler 1987, p. xvii) and neither gender is subrogated to the other. The application of this concept in today's organizations is clear. Many people are involved in organizations that are "working to create more mutual relationships, democratic institutions, and equitable societies . . . [and] they want personal and social power to be used with and for others, not over or against them. They believe that conflict can be resolved collaboratively and peacefully" (Eisler and Loye 1998, p. viii).

Collective Responsibility and Accountability

In any partnership, the members must retain a sense of personal responsibility and accountability. But a new dimension is added in the leader–follower relationship: the sharing of collective responsibility and accountability. For the relationship to thrive and continue to flourish, all of the elements in a healthy relationship must exist on both sides of the partnering agreement. Both manager and employee must be trustworthy. Respect is mutual and communication is two-way. Without these attributes, the partnership withers and dies.

Conclusion

The quality of relationships in the organization is a critical element of positive work environments. Healthy working relationships consist of those characterized by high levels of trust, mutual respect, and open, positive, and honest communication. These qualities describe relationships at all levels and among all people in the organization. Especially important is the relationship between employees and their manager. A manager/leader with strong emotional intelligence and a relationship based on trust and confidence, mutual respect, and honest communication creates a vital association. The nature of the relationship is one of collaboration and partnership, neither of which is easy to attain, but a healthy relationship is worth every ounce of effort it takes to build. Relationships in today's world are "parallel and simultaneous, connected, murky, multiple, and interdependent" (Bennis 1989, p. 101). Forming healthy relationships is complex and challenging, but it is an essential component of a positive workplace.

Conversation Points

Organizational Perspective

1. Are there clearly articulated behavioral expectations of all employees that relate to responsibilities for forming healthy working relationships?
2. What are the consequences for individuals who do not build healthy working relationships with others?
3. Are issues of trust openly discussed, even when it is difficult?
4. Have there been issues of trust at the organizational level? How were they handled? How was employee pride and morale affected?

Leadership Issues

1. Use the three essential ingredients of a healthy relationship presented here (trust, respect, and communication) to assess the quality of your working relationships with employees.
2. Are there issues of trust among the people in your department? In your organization?
3. As a leader, what behavioral actions demonstrate your trust of other people?
4. Think of a time you felt betrayed by someone or something that happened in your workplace. How did you handle it? Do you carry the sense of betrayal with you, or were you able to resolve it?
5. How do you demonstrate respect for others? What behaviors do you think let people know that you respect them?

Employee Challenges

1. How much do you trust your manager? Administration? Your coworkers? If there are issues of trust, to what are they related?
2. Are employees treated with respect in your organization? What are the behaviors you see that lead you to believe you are or are not treated with respect?
3. What do you do that shows you respect others? How do you show your support of others?
4. Do people in your department feel as though they have open, flowing, positive communication with your manager and other leaders in the organization?
5. Overall, what do you think is the quality of relationships in your department or work team? What could you do to strengthen them?

7

Creating Community at Work

Jo Manion

The community exists to support its members
while they fulfill their purpose. . . .
When partnerships, management teams,
and organizations build communities,
they tap into a greater and deeper reservoir
of courage, wisdom and productivity.
—Peter Gibb (1993)

HEALTHY interpersonal relationships in the workplace are a strong measure of a positive working environment. Relationships are important in all aspects of our work lives. Chapter 6 explored the relationships among individuals such as managers, executives, and employees in the immediate work group as well as coworkers and colleagues from other departments in the organization. This chapter examines the relationships that occur in a collective entity such as a team or as a sense of community in the workplace.

The importance of effective group relationships has been the focus of many research studies on job satisfaction. The presence of healthy teams enhances affective commitment, the type of organizational commitment that develops when people feel good about their relationships with others. This chapter carries the discussion of emotional intelligence further and examines how it applies to work teams. Another way to capitalize on group relationships in the work environment relates to the creation of a sense of community among people who work closely together. A sense of community increases the sense of connection people feel with each other and builds affective commitment. Effective teams and a sense of community are factors that increase the emotional ties that bind employees to each other, to the leaders with whom they work, as well as to the team or community they form. The positive effect of community on retention has been demonstrated (Advisory Board Company 2000; Iverson and Buttigieg 1999).

Building Effective Teams

In today's work world, organizations and departments that are based on highly performing work teams have a distinct advantage over those that are undeveloped as a cohesive work group and lack a clear, concise, and collective purpose. As our work becomes increasingly complex and requires a broader range of knowledge and skills to complete, the need for well-defined, high-functioning teams is growing more apparent. Creating teams has been extensively covered in other publications (Manion, Lorimer, and Leander 1995; Manion 1997; Manion and Watson 1995), and the process for designing and developing teams is considered basic knowledge for both managers and employees alike in our contemporary health care organizations. A brief review of the process is included in this chapter because the success with which a team is created often affects the development of positive relationships within the team. A special emphasis on team emotional intelligence is included.

Teamwork Defined

Team and *teamwork* are two distinct terms that are often confused and used synonymously by people who do not understand that there is a difference between the two concepts. The word team is overused in today's world, and it is loosely applied to exhort others to perform in a particular manner, usually through teamwork. Teamwork is a way of working together, and it may mean different things to different people. For most, it implies cooperation, open communication, and pitching in to help each other out. A team, in contrast, is a structural unit, a group of people designed and drawn together to complete certain prescribed work. How they carry out the work can be described as teamwork. As adapted from Katzenbach and Smith's (1993) definition in *The Wisdom of Teams*, a team is "a small number of consistent people with a relevant, shared purpose, common performance goals, complementary and overlapping skills, and a common approach to its collective work. Team members hold themselves mutually accountable for the team's results and outcomes" (Manion 1997, p. 31).

Types of Teams

Several types of teams operate in organizations today: primary work teams, ad hoc teams, and leadership teams. Primary work teams are permanent structures organized around the primary work of a department. For example, in a business office, the teams may be organized around business functions, such as credit verification, billings, and collections. Primary work teams in a patient care department are organized around patient care. In a laboratory, teams are often designed around specialized functions, such as microbiology, hematology, and chemistry. In an emergency services department, there may be a trauma team and an urgent care team.

Ad hoc teams are temporary teams created to perform a particular piece of work, and when the work is completed, the team is dissolved. Quality or continuous process improvement and project teams are good examples of ad hoc teams, which can last for years and yet not be considered part of the permanent structure of an organization. Leadership teams are formed to provide collective leadership for a project or initiative, department, service, or organization.

Managers today may create a team for a specific purpose (such as sharing the leadership function for the department), may actually redesign their department into teams, or may share responsibility for guiding or participating in the conversion of a bureaucracy to a team-based structure. The implementation of teams in health care is discussed extensively in other publications (Manion, Lorimer, and Leander 1996; Manion 1997; Lorimer and Manion 1996; Leander, Shortridge, and Watson 1996). Exemplary leaders who understand the concepts and language of systems thinking often form diverse teams that use systems thinking to focus on critical issues. These teams are capable of outperforming individuals because systems issues require multiple approaches, a variety of experiences, and diverse thinking patterns.

Process of Team Building

Regardless of the type of team, there are six concrete steps to be followed in creating an effective team. (See figure 7-1. The key questions to be addressed in each step are summarized in figure 7-2, p. 197.)

Step 1: Define the Work

Before the team's members can be selected, the work of the team must be defined. The individual initiating the team delineates what the team is expected to do by considering several questions:

- What is the primary work to be accomplished by this team?
- Is this a problem-solving team focused on a specific issue or a project team formed to design and implement a new service or system?
- Is it providing collective leadership for the department or within the organization?

Figure 7-1.   Steps for Creating an Effective Team

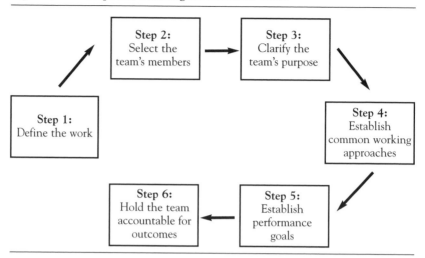

- What will be required of this team? Is systems thinking required to challenge mental models and initiate breakthrough thinking?
- What are the general goals and objectives of this group?

This step can be difficult, but it forces the leader to be very clear about his or her reasons for initiating a team.

Step 2: Select the Team's Members

Potential members are identified in step 2. The members are selected on the basis of their potential contribution to the team's work, as delineated in step 1. A team member may represent a particular part of the system or bring certain skills needed by the team. In some cases, it is impossible to obtain all of the skills needed by the team, and members may be selected for their skills potential, in which case the development of those skills is paramount. Perhaps no one in the organization has exactly the skills needed, but the team, through its work, can develop those skills.

The most effective teams are those that have a small number of consistent team members. Teams of more than twelve members run into more logistic problems than do smaller teams. In larger groups, it is easier for members to disengage and remain anonymous. Finding a common time to meet is also a problem for large groups.

Consistency of membership is critical. Frequent changes in team membership directly affect the synergy of the group and the quality of the work completed. When team members leave and are replaced, the team usually regresses in its effectiveness until the new member is brought up to speed and is fully assimilated into the group as new relationships are forged. Consistency of membership also refers to consistent attendance at team meetings. Frequent absenteeism directly affects the team's ability to produce high-quality outcomes.

Figure 7-2. Key Questions to Be Addressed during Each Step

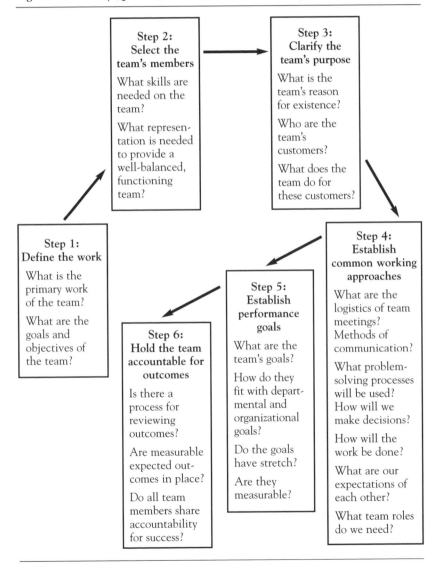

Step 1:
Define the work

What is the primary work of the team?

What are the goals and objectives of the team?

Step 2:
Select the team's members

What skills are needed on the team?

What representation is needed to provide a well-balanced, functioning team?

Step 3:
Clarify the team's purpose

What is the team's reason for existence?

Who are the team's customers?

What does the team do for these customers?

Step 4:
Establish common working approaches

What are the logistics of team meetings? Methods of communication?

What problem-solving processes will be used? How will we make decisions?

How will the work be done?

What are our expectations of each other?

What team roles do we need?

Step 5:
Establish performance goals

What are the team's goals?

How do they fit with departmental and organizational goals?

Do the goals have stretch?

Are they measurable?

Step 6:
Hold the team accountable for outcomes

Is there a process for reviewing outcomes?

Are measurable expected outcomes in place?

Do all team members share accountability for success?

Step 3: Clarify the Team's Purpose

Once team members have been identified and the team comes together for the first time, the initial work of the team is to define its purpose. Although the leader may have given some preliminary direction to the group (based on his or her thoughts from step 1), it is critical that the team actually develops its own mission or purpose statement. This statement describes what the team does and for whom it does it. In other words, the statement clarifies the reason for the team's existence. Teams that are handed a completed purpose statement or are simply told by the leader why they exist never develop the same level of ownership as those teams that actually engaged in this work. If the team is given a mission statement describing its work, one way to ensure relevancy and identification with this purpose is to have the team modify it to fit its beliefs and understandings. Even small modifications increase the team members' feeling of ownership. Team members simply do not engage with the work when they find the team's purpose irrelevant.

It is important for the leader to stay involved with the team during the development of the mission statement in order to prevent the team from heading in the wrong direction. The team's purpose must also be congruent with the organization's or department's purpose. When the two are incongruent, the team is headed for trouble. An actively participating leader does not mandate the team's purpose but is involved in guiding and setting the team's general direction.

Step 4: Establish Common Working Approaches

Once the team is clear about its mission and reason for existence, the next step is to determine and agree upon the approaches it plans to use in doing its work. "A common approach means that team members discuss, delineate, and agree on [the] ways they are going to work together to accomplish their purpose. Common refers to the collective effort that is required, not an approach that is ordinary or average. There is nothing common or ordinary about a highly effective team" (Manion, Lorimer, and Leander 1996, p. 64).

Some examples of early decisions related to working approaches include the following:

- **Logistics of team meetings:** How often will the team meet? When will it meet? Where will it meet? Will an agenda be circulated? How is the agenda developed? Who facilitates the meeting? Will minutes be needed; and if so, who will take them?

- **Methods of formal and informal communication:** Is there a need for frequent team huddles? Are team members readily accessible to each other? Do they need to be? How will they communicate between meetings? Is everyone on e-mail?
- **Methods of problem solving:** How will the team tackle problems? Is there a specific quality improvement process to be followed?
- **Steps in decision making:** What types of decisions will be made by the team? What are the boundaries in regard to the team's work? Which can be individual decisions, and which should be made by the entire team? Will majority decision making or consensus be used? When would minority decision making be appropriate?
- **Work processes:** Do certain processes and approaches need to be done in a certain way? Does there need to be consistency in practices?

Roles and responsibilities within the team also need to be discussed. The team should decide whether specific roles need to be filled by team members to ensure that work is completed. The specific responsibilities of each role need to be defined clearly. Examples of special roles include meeting coordinator or facilitator and process person. Some teams identify a celebrations role to ensure that key events and accomplishments are recognized and cheered. Some teams also identify the role of challenger. The challenger is "the team member who openly questions the goals, methods, and the ethics of the team, who is willing to disagree with the team leader, and who encourages the team to take well-considered risks" (Parker 1997, p. 8). This role is critical for most teams because the challenger is honest in reporting the team's progress and identifying problems. This individual, however, does back off when his or her views are not accepted and actively supports consensus within the team. In other words, this person does not always play an adversarial role. Another common role is the team recorder, who generates the minutes of meetings and circulates them to the rest of the team. This role is often a rotating one.

The final components of establishing common working approaches are the discussion of, and agreement on, team members' expectations of one another. Identifying and articulating behavioral expectations are key steps in early team formation for several reasons. These expectations lay the foundation for development of trust within the team. In addition, being clear about the expectations one holds of others is instrumental in preventing unnecessary conflict. Too often, people do not meet each others' expectations because they did not realize that the expectations even existed. The group discusses what they expect or need from one another in order to do a good job. Expectations for appropriate meeting participation, communication techniques, and acceptable team behavior are commonly spelled out. The following examples from real teams demonstrate expectations related to these areas.

- We expect each other to be on time and prepared for meetings and to fully participate as evidenced by an attentive attitude, clarifying questions, and open-mindedness about the contributions of other team members.
- We expect each other to communicate openly, honestly, and directly, especially when we fail to meet each other's expectations.
- We expect each other to work toward the goals of the team and support the success of the team first and individual work second.
- We expect each other to stay focused on our goals and complete tasks and projects within agreed-upon time frames (and to communicate any unavoidable delays to other team members as soon as possible).

Clear expectations constitute formalization of the team's norms, and this is one of the first steps in building and creating team emotional intelligence (Cherniss and Goleman 2001). Being willing to address another team member's failure to live up to established norms and expectations is a critical sign of the team's emotional intelligence. Fear of conflict and confrontation is a common dysfunction in ineffective teams. Seen as accountability, the willingness of team members to call their peers on performance or behaviors that might hurt the team and its performance is essential for effective functioning (Lencioni 2002). The team's emotional intelligence is discussed more fully in the next section of this chapter.

Step 5: Establish Performance Goals

The team's performance goals are closely related to the team's mission. Larson and LaFasta (1989) examined high-performing teams and found, without exception, that high-performing teams have clearly identified performance objectives and goals. The team's performance objectives and goals can also serve as a way to measure the team's outcomes; that is, they give the team a mechanism for holding itself accountable.

Team goals should be distinguished from system, organization, or department goals. "Teams take broad objectives or directives from the organization's management and shape them into specific, measurable goals for the team. Specific goals are stated in concrete terms so that it is unequivocally possible to tell whether or not they have been met" (Manion, Lorimer, and Leander 1996, p. 63). The most powerful goals provide for small wins along the way, and these intermediate victories serve to motivate and reinforce the team's progress along its chosen path.

Motivating goals are often those with stretch, that is, goals that force the team to extend itself and reach beyond its original targets. Ambitious goals produce momentum, growth, and commitment within the team. "Teams that face a significant challenge, or that develop their own ambitious goals, have a greater sense of urgency that forces them to focus their efforts in a unified direction. . . . The true strength of a team is realized when it faces and overcomes seemingly unbreachable obstacles to attain a worthy goal" (Manion, Lorimer, and Leander 1996, p. 63).

Step 6: Hold the Team Accountable for Outcomes

A final and essential step involves holding the team accountable for the outcomes of its work. This step represents a continual process of reviewing outcomes and determining whether established standards have been met and expected outcomes obtained. When its desired outcomes have not been attained, the team evaluates its process and its work to determine what went wrong, and then it takes corrective action.

The team reviews its decisions for their effectiveness and its processes for their beneficial outcomes. All team members are equally accountable for the outcomes of the team.

> Mutual accountability differentiates a real team from a working group. In both teams and working groups, individuals hold themselves accountable for the outcomes of their assignments. A team, however, takes the next step—members hold themselves mutually accountable for the team's outcomes or results. They continuously measure themselves against their established goals and objectives (Manion, Lorimer, and Leander 1996, p. 77).

Group Emotional Intelligence

The primary role of the manager in developing teams, once these steps have been achieved, is to guide the team as it builds and develops its own emotional intelligence. Group or team emotional intelligence is defined as "the ability of a group to generate a shared set of norms that manage the emotional process in a way that builds trust, group identity, and group efficacy" (Cherniss and Goleman 2001, p. 138). Team emotional intelligence emerges primarily through relationships, and it also directly affects the quality of the relationships experienced in the workplace. The relationships within the team can help the team become more emotionally intelligent, and dysfunctional relationships within the team can be destructive.

Group emotional intelligence operates in three distinct areas of interaction: interpersonal, group, and cross-boundary. As a reminder, the two dimensions of emotional intelligence include self-awareness and self-regulation. As noted earlier, the most important thing the manager or leader can do to help build group emotional intelligence is to guide the development of the norms. The norms must be consciously directed from the very beginning of the team, or their formation will be left to chance. Norms must be established for all three levels of interaction. The norms are summarized in figure 7-3.

Figure 7-3.   Group Emotional Intelligence (Cherniss and Goleman 2001)

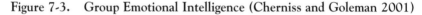

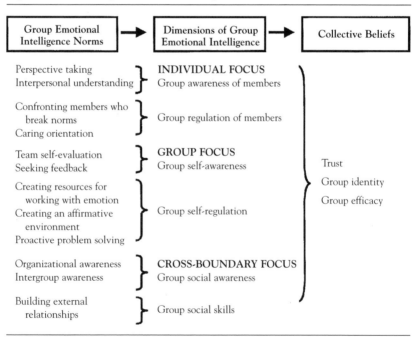

Reprinted from *The Emotionally Intelligent Workplace*, edited by Cary Cherniss and Daniel Goleman. Copyright © 2001 Jossey–Bass Publishers. This material is used by permission of John Wiley & Sons, Inc.

Interpersonal Level of Interaction

By looking at the dimensions of the group's emotional intelligence it becomes clear that norms are related to whether the interaction is at the personal, group, or cross-group level. For example, the group's awareness of individual members is an important aspect of its emotional intelligence. At the individual level of interaction, norms relate to perspective taking and interpersonal understanding. Perspective taking refers to a willingness to consider matters from another person's point of view. Perspective taking is especially important when we do not agree with that point of view. An emotionally intelligent team, then, considers all points of view, regardless of who is contributing. For example, the physical therapist assistant is not discounted because he is "only" an assistant, not a physical therapist; nor is the admissions clerk discounted because she could not possibly understand what it is like to be an emergency department nurse who is flooded with critically ill patients. People's opinions are sought, respected, and considered as the team completes its work.

The second norm emerging from the team's awareness of members is the interpersonal understanding team members have of each other. This means there is an accurate understanding of both spoken and unspoken emotions and feelings, interests and concerns, and strengths and weaknesses of the individual team members. This deep understanding exists in a close-knit work group that allows members to predict and cope with one another's day-to-day behavior. Research in this area has demonstrated that self-managing work teams show significantly higher levels of understanding of each other, they interpret each other's behavior more accurately, and they can tell whether a team member is having work-related problems or is just tired and needs a break.

The team's expectations of each other in relation to this norm are often developed when the team members are agreeing on their processes. Several examples from real teams include the following:

- We expect each other to value the diverse contributions of all members as evidenced by our willingness to hear new ideas, confront issues that arise, and consider situations from a new and different perspective.
- We expect each other to be trustworthy as evidenced by honoring and meeting commitments made, by being loyal to absent team members, and by presenting each other in the best light to others.
- We expect each other to keep sensitive information about team members private and confidential.

- We expect each other to pitch in and help when one of us is having a bad day.
- We expect each other to ask for what they need.

The second dimension of group emotional intelligence has to do with the group regulation of its members. A key task for a successful group is to create a balance between ensuring predictable team behavior and allowing members a sense of control and individuality. When the team is successful, members are more willing to put their individual needs aside for the good of the group. The norms that follow from this dimension include confronting members who break team norms and using a caring orientation. This means that when people are out of line, other team members speak up. It has been found that members of poorly performing work teams do not speak up for fear of confrontation or concern that it may make the problem worse or damage their relationships within the team. It is clear, however, that when the team member addressing the out-of-line colleague uses a caring orientation, this feedback is much better received. A caring orientation has to do with communicating positive regard, respect, and appreciation for the other person. A study of seventy-six work groups found that a caring orientation in their relationships contributed to group effectiveness by increasing each member's sense of safety, cohesion, and satisfaction, all of which increase a person's commitment or sense of engagement in their work (Wolff 1998). Caring does not require a close personal relationship, but it does require validation and respect for the other person.

Group Level of Interaction

Emotion in a group context creates a powerful force that actually overwhelms individual differences in emotion and can create a new collective group or team character. Self-awareness was identified as a crucial emotional competence in chapter 6. Group self-awareness means that members are aware of the group's emotional states, preferences, and resources for dealing with emotion. Group self-awareness requires a norm that involves team self-evaluation, the ability of the group to evaluate itself objectively and accurately, including its emotional states as well as its abilities and weaknesses in the way it interacts as a team. For example, when team decisions are repeatedly overturned and team recommendations are often not accepted as they move through the system, instead of blaming others, an emotionally intelligent team begins to ask why this is happening in an attempt to identify the team's own shortcomings. The team takes a good look at its own problem-solving and decision-making abilities. Maybe it does a poor job of analyzing various alternatives and instead relies on the same old refrain of "we need more resources" when problems occur. An emotionally intelligent team also continually seeks honest feedback about its performance.

It bears repeating that self-awareness is not enough for emotional intelligence. The second key dimension of group emotional intelligence is self-regulation. For a collective entity, it is group self-regulation. There are at least three norms in this area: creating resources for working with emotion, creating an affirmative environment, and instituting proactive problem-solving. In the case of a team, self-regulation means that the group accepts emotion as an important part of group life. It not only legitimizes the discussion of emotional issues, but develops a vocabulary for doing so. Members are comfortable talking about these issues. There is time for these discussions at meetings. Using a timed agenda has become popular in recent years, but when an agenda is enforced too rigidly, it can keep the group from addressing important issues fully. Most timed agendas take little or no account of the need to process emotions.

Creating an affirmative environment means cultivating and developing a positive self-image of the team's past, present, and future as well as comfortably using appreciative inquiry (a concept that is discussed in chapter 8) and positive expectations. As noted in chapter 4, an affirmative environment has been demonstrated to increase the team's effectiveness.

The third norm relates to proactive problem solving or taking the initiative to resolve issues that get in the way of the group doing its work at the level of quality expected. Because problem solving is such an important skill, it is discussed thoroughly in chapter 8. Examples of expectations from a real team that are related to these norms include the following:

- We expect each other to give constructive, helpful, and private feedback regarding performance.
- We expect each other to accept constructive feedback about the team with an open mind.
- We expect each other to stay focused on the goal and to complete tasks and projects within agreed-upon time frames (and to communicate immediately with all team members if there is a delay).

- We expect each other to participate proactively in solving problems faced by the team and work together until a win–win solution is developed.

Cross-Boundary Interactions

The third area of interaction for a team is the cross-boundary focus. It is self-evident that group effectiveness requires networks of relationships with individuals and groups outside of the group's typical boundary. Thus, effective groups are outwardly directed as well as inwardly directed. As a result, they are able to obtain resources outside of their boundaries. In a health care organization, for example, laboratory employees and managers are able to get what they need from materials management, nursing employees are able to obtain the support and help of human resources specialists as they deal with difficult issues, and teams in the emergency department are able to work well with employees in admissions to get what they need.

Two important norms emerge in the area of group social awareness: organizational awareness and intergroup awareness. The team recognizes and understands the social and political systems within which it works, in other words, the organization. Teams are fully aware of the other groups operating in the organization.

The second dimension of group emotional intelligence relates to group social skills, and the key norm identified is building external relationships. Research has found that the most effective teams are those that communicate frequently with the entities above them in the hierarchy, are capable of persuading others to support the team, and are willing to keep others actively informed about the team's activities and progress. Teams that are the least effective are those labeled as isolationist because they avoid engaging in boundary management and do not communicate with others to keep them informed about their activities. Examples of team expectations that are developed in this area include the following:

- We expect our team to work interdependently with other teams and departments in the organization, always seeking win–win solutions to problems.
- We expect our team to live up to the organization's mission, values, and goals when working across boundaries within the organization.
- We expect our team to stay informed of what is going on with other departments and the larger organization when it affects our work.

- We expect our team to address issues assertively and coopera-tively with teams from other departments as well as with indi-viduals outside of our team.
- We expect our team to represent itself positively throughout the organization.

Common Pitfalls in Team Development

There are many potential pitfalls in the development of teams. The most frequently observed are included here.

Often when a team is in trouble, the solution implemented includes the leader giving a pep talk or bringing in a dynamic, charismatic speaker who generates enthusiasm and excitement within the team. The results of this type of quick fix never seem to last long enough to get the team through the next crisis. Creating a sense of urgency is more effective in turning the team around. Giving the team a stiff work assignment that members see as important does more to mobilize stagnant energy and turn it into a productive force than any motivational speech could pos-sibly do.

Not recognizing the special needs and unique challenges of indi-vidual teams is another common error. Each of the three major types of teams has unique challenges, and to assume that they are all similar is to underestimate the difficulty a particular team may have. For instance, most leadership teams find defining their work and purpose difficult. This may seem contradictory because this type of team is composed of leaders who as individuals are usually self-directed and focused clearly on their work. However, most leadership teams confuse their work as a team with the work of the organization as a whole, for example, ensuring the delivery of safe, high-quality patient care to members of the community versus leading others and creating an empowering environment in which employees deliver safe, high-quality patient care.

An ad hoc team formed to lead a change initiative often has diffi-culty in handing off the project to those who will actually implement it (usually managers). The handoff is actually a basic principle of inno-vation: The people who implement a change are not as attached to the change as those who create it. The 1990s produced many examples of this in health care organizations. Quality improvement initiatives and work redesign projects in organizations were often designed by people on project teams who then handed off the implementation to man-agers who did not have the same investment or interest in the project. In many cases, full conversion and implementation failed.

Understanding the unique challenges of each type of team alerts the leader to potential problems. A more complete discussion of the three types of teams can be found in *Team-Based Health Care Organizations: Blueprint for Success* (1996) by Manion, Lorimer, and Leander.

Ignoring any one of the key elements in creating teams is another major pitfall, but one that is relatively easy to correct. For example, one team that had frequent and recurring problems finally called in an external consultant to help. During this work, the consultant discovered that the team had never established their expectations of one another nor had they agreed on common working approaches. Simply doing those two things cleared up about 90 percent of the conflicts.

Minimizing the development time required to grow a team is common. Too many managers and leaders today believe if they simply call a group a team, it will somehow become one. Not taking the time to apply the proper steps of team development often creates a situation in which the group struggles needlessly, trying their best but unable to determine why it is just not working. Unless team members come together to accomplish their work collectively, they do not become a team. Effective teams are those that are emotionally intelligent and are able to recognize and process emotion within the group and regulate themselves in response to daily organizational events. For a team to become emotionally intelligent, it is helpful, and perhaps even necessary, that at least some of the individual members have a high level of emotional intelligence (Cherniss and Goleman 2001). However, just because the team includes emotionally intelligent team members does not ensure that the team as an entity will be emotionally intelligent collectively or effective in its performance.

Being able to create high-performing teams is one of the most critical challenges facing leaders today. Virtually every future organizational structure (adhocracy, network, or clustered organization) is based on the premise that teams are to be a prevalent structure. Leaders must have the ability to tap into and release the potential of teams. Being part of a highly functioning team of people is likely to lead to strong affective organizational commitment and a positive work environment.

Development of Leadership Teams

The number of teams needed in any one organization or department depends on the size and structure of the organization and the complexity of its functions. At the very least, managers should consider forming a leadership team for their areas of responsibility. In a department, this may mean a small group of assistant managers or selected employees who work closely with the manager to perform the leadership function of the department. For example, in a hospital laboratory department, the leadership team might include the department manager, the supervisors of the different functions, the employee responsible for quality improvement processes, and/or the person who leads the employee governance council if there is one. In an inpatient nursing department, the leadership team may consist of the assistant nurse managers or charge nurses, the department educator, and the department manager.

Membership is determined by the purpose of the team. In some leadership teams, selected employees may serve on the team to provide input from a particular segment of the staff regardless of whether the employees play any specifically defined leadership role. For example, the manager may want someone from the night shift to serve on the team.

Creating a leadership team within his or her scope of responsibility is one way for the manager to broaden and deepen the leadership strength in the department. It also serves as a tremendous source of support for the manager and improves the leadership's effectiveness. Commitment to decisions made is stronger because there is group ownership and accountability. It can also free up the manager to learn additional skills and take a more strategic approach that focuses on the issues and challenges of the department or service.

Creating Community in the Workplace

A second aspect of creating a sense of connection among people at work relates to the concept of community in the workplace. Beyond the individual relationships of people, a sense of community results in a collective entity or spirit in a work group, a department, or even an organization. Because a sense of community has the power to increase people's emotional ties to each other, establishing community is also a way to strengthen retention efforts and levels of organizational commitment (Manion and Barthlomew 2004; Manion 2004a). This strategy has been found to be effective regardless of the age cohort; in other words, it is as effective for genXers as for baby boomers and may be increasingly important for nexters.

Importance of Community*

Over the past two decades, the average American worker has added an extra month to their work year (Vogl 1997). Many of us spend more of our waking hours in our workplace than with our families or loved ones. Discretionary time is at an all-time low for many Americans as we work longer hours and bring more work home. Discretionary time is further reduced by the fact that in many families all of the members who are able to work are contributing wage earners. Thus, the family's time away from work is often spent doing home maintenance, running errands, getting groceries, and completing tasks that were performed by an at-home partner in previous decades.

In today's world, a sense of community in the workplace has become increasingly important for many people because it may be the only source of community in which they participate. Decreasing involvement in family, church, and neighborhood activities; increased geographical distances from family members and childhood communities; and extremely harried and full work lives have all combined to escalate a general feeling of isolation and disconnectedness from the typical communities of the past.

Less discretionary time has led to a decline in our involvement in other communities over recent years. Our longer working hours often lead to less inclination to get to know our neighbors, and besides, we rationalize, they are just going to move on in a few years anyway! Active membership in professional associations and religious organizations is at an all-time low (Putnam 2000). "Besides the broad decline in church affiliation and attendance, so, too, there has been a falloff in membership in other organizations—trade unions, parent–teacher associations, fraternal clubs like the Elks, Shriners, and JayCees—and volunteering for groups like the Boy Scouts and Red Cross" (Putnam 2000, p. 20).

Social scientists explain the yearning for community as a reaction to decades of individualism, which peaked near the end of the last century. Americans have spent almost two centuries dismantling their roots and traditions in the pursuit of individual happiness only to find that happiness comes from community and from connection to other people. All of these factors create a longing for a feeling of community

---

*This section on the importance of community is adapted from Jo Manion, Community in the Workplace, *Journal of Nursing Administration* 34(1). Copyright © 2004. Used by permission of Lippincott Williams & Wilkins.

in some aspect of our lives, and work is where many of us spend the majority of our waking, alert time.

Many leadership scholars and experts believe creating community is an essential leadership skill. "The task for leadership in the coming century is to transform work organizations into viable, attractive communities capable of attracting workers with needed skills and talents. . . . A sense of community invigorates members' lives with a sense of purpose and a feeling of belonging to an integrated group that is doing something worthwhile" (Fairholm 1998, p. 151). Understanding the definition of community helps us to understand the ramifications of the need for community in the workplace.

Community Defined

Community has become a buzz word over the past several years and as such can be overused and misused, which reduces its influential power. According to Rousseau (1991), community is a form of human association that binds people together. It is far more than simply a group of people living or working together who share common interests and projects. It is "a psychological reality, an act of will that constructs a tie that really binds" (Rousseau 1991, p. 45). And, Rousseau believes, the tie that binds is altruistic love. Altruistic love puts the other first, expects nothing in return, and loves generously, openly, and without reservation or expectation.

Rousseau further believes that contractual relationships are incapable of producing community because they are inherently egocentric. They exist for the good of one or more of the parties and thus can only link people together in this external aspect. "Those who love contractually are seeking their own fulfillment as their end, looking to other people as the means to their own pleasure or utility, they forge no existential bonds with each other" (Rousseau 1991, p. 49).

If this is true, according to Rousseau, it would be highly unlikely that community could exist in the workplace. How much altruistic love do we experience in our business relationships? The primary nature of the relationship of employee to employer is a contractual one, as is, by extension, the relationship of employee to manager. Clearly, the organization requires certain work to be accomplished and compensates the employee in accordance with the completion of that work. Although the initial and underlying nature of the relationship is contractual, however, that contractual agreement may not be the entire essence of the relationship. In other words, the employment relationship is not merely contractual. Many employees are committed and feel quite connected to their work and can feel in community, or in unity, with the coworkers to whom they feel close. Such connections are more likely in individuals who see their work as a calling rather than as just a job. People for whom benefits or financial compensation are the primary motivators for work are, by Rousseau's indicators, less likely to feel a sense of altruistic love that leads to a feeling of community.

"Community is a psychological reality, and our motives determine whether it happens or not" (Rousseau 1991, p. 51). In other words, it is important to look beyond the initial nature of the relationship (the contract) to try to determine the motivation of the people involved. Rousseau notes that motivation, or the subjective intention of the person who decides and acts in a certain way, is the key factor for building community. It is difficult or even impossible to truly know another's motivation or in some cases even our own motivation. Rousseau suggests a way to think about this:

> It is seldom easy to achieve purity of intention, and it is never easy to know that we have. One test of our sincerity, though, is the price we are willing to pay in order to appropriate the community of being in altruistic love. If communal actions cost us significant money, time, energy, or physical pain, and we carry them out anyway, we have a reliable sign of that purity of heart (Rousseau 1991, p. 148).

A simple example in a workplace community can be evident when an individual willingly experiences the inconvenience of a scheduling change to help out a colleague who needs to change his or her schedule.

Scott Peck has studied and helped facilitate the formation of many communities. He believes that the lack of community is such a norm in our society that it is easy for us to believe that community is impossible to achieve. Community is more than simply the sum of its parts or its individual members. It is a group of individuals who have learned "to communicate honestly with each other, whose relationships go deeper than their masks of composure, and who have developed some significant commitment" to share life's deeper experiences (Peck 1987, p. 59). In this context, our work lives can be considered potentially one of life's deeper experiences.

Elements of Community

The many facets of community are interconnected and interrelated. It is helpful to understand what various scholars of community have found when they closely examined the elements within a mature com-munity. The aspects considered here are identified as essential; that is, if any of them were absent, it would be unlikely that the group could be a true community. These characteristics include inclusivity, com-mitment, consensus, realism, capacity for contemplation, safety, and a group of leaders (that is, the members all flow in and out of leadership roles). (See figure 7-4.) These characteristics are discussed briefly to stimulate self-reflection and for use as an evaluation mechanism for assessing the current state of community in your department, your work team, or your organization as a whole.

Inclusivity

Community is inclusive in nature, which means that the group is con-tinually seeking ways to extend itself and attract new members. Exclu-sivity is considered an enemy of community because it can turn the potential community into nothing more than a clique, a group orga-nized to protect against a feeling of true community. However, inclu-sivity is not an absolute (Peck 1987). There may be valid reasons a particular member should be excluded, such as when the inclusion of the individual might damage the community as a whole. Excluding a potential member is considered with great care and concern. Commu-nity requires that diversity is welcomed and celebrated. A department

Figure 7-4.   Elements of Community

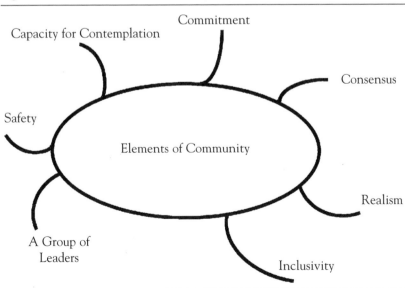

with a strong sense of community is effective at bringing in and incorporating new members into the established community. New members are welcomed, and rituals exist to help them assimilate into the group.

Commitment

Commitment is a second key aspect of community. Commitment has been defined as that which makes us continue a particular course of action even when more positive alternatives or potentially negative consequences attempt to persuade us to abandon the chosen course of action (Brickman, Wortman, and Sorrentino 1987). This means that once committed to participation in the community, a person is obligated to follow through. One of the ways this is evidenced in a community is the accommodation of individual differences and the tendency of true community to actually encourage individualism (Peck 1987). The individual's commitment is to the community as a whole; in other words, individuals bind themselves to participation in the community. Commitment requires personal sacrifice, that is, giving up something that is valued (Kanter 1972; Rousseau 1991; Peck 1987; Brickman, Wortman, and Sorrentino 1987). For example, in a patient care department, there are many occasions when individuals might prefer to do things their own way but agree to subscribe to the team's approach of handling the situation, such as staffing coverage and requested time off. In every organization there are standardized approaches and shared values and philosophies that ensure consistency in the delivery of services.

Consensus

Consensus is a way of reaching a decision about an action to be taken in which all members of the community agree to support the decision, even when they do not fully agree with it. Consensus is a process that works only in an open and trusting environment. It requires that all members have the opportunity to speak and be heard. In other words, ideas and opinions are shared openly, and even when disagreement occurs, members seek to understand each other's viewpoints. Peck (1987) shares examples of true community where consensus almost magically occurs. Consensus is not the absence of conflict, but the ability to work through the conflict. In fact, he calls true community "a group that can fight gracefully" (Peck 1987, p. 70). Many groups that suppress or deal with conflicts in a covert manner think the absence of conflict is a good sign, never realizing that they have only attained a level of pseudo community.

In pseudocommunity, a group attempts to purchase community cheaply by pretense. . . . It is an unconscious, gentle process whereby people who want to be loving attempt to be so by telling little white lies, by withholding some of the truth about themselves and their feelings in order to avoid conflict (Peck 1987, p. 88).

Pseudo community is a significant problem in health care organizations because many health care workers tend to be conflict aversive. True community is conflict resolving; pseudo community is conflict avoiding. Healthy conflict resolution skills are essential for the development of emotionally intelligent employees.

Realism

Realism refers to the fact that issues considered by a true community are addressed more realistically because of a broader treatment of issues and ideas. "Because a community includes members with many different points of view and the freedom to express them, it comes to appreciate the whole of a situation far better than an individual, couple, or ordinary group can" (Peck 1987, p. 65). This is the power of synergy or interdependent working relationships. The one-plus-one-equals-three phenomenon is at work in communities.

A classic example comes from the world of nature. The properties of hydrogen ions and oxygen ions can be studied in the laboratory, and these properties may all be described very scientifically. However, when these two elements are combined in a certain way, an entirely new characteristic called wetness is created. Neither the hydrogen nor the oxygen ions individually have this characteristic. Thus, together we are more than a simple collection of parts. All of us have experienced a day at work when staffing seemed quite inadequate, perhaps due to the sickness of colleagues or an unanticipated high work volume, and at the beginning of the day things looked quite hopeless. However, the combination of people was just right, everyone pulled together so that things just clicked, and everyone had a great work shift. This is synergy in action.

Capacity for Contemplation

True communities continually examine themselves. They are self-aware and recognize their abilities and strengths as well as their weak spots. Contemplation may start at the individual level, but it progresses to the collective level before long. No community can expect to be continually healthy and fully functioning. However, a genuine community, because of its contemplative nature, "recognizes its ill health when it occurs and quickly takes appropriate action to heal itself" (Peck 1987, p. 66).

In our work world, this characteristic is more often referred to as accountability. Accountability is the retrospective review of results to determine whether the group is working effectively. Are we achieving desired outcomes? Is our work of high quality? Why are our decisions being overturned? Why are we dealing with the same problem we had last year at this time? A true community continually reviews and self-assesses, taking corrective action when needed.

Safety

Genuine community is a place where people feel safe to express themselves and to be themselves fully without apology or explanation. The community offers acceptance. From sharing vulnerabilities a sense of connection forms, and strength grows from this support. It takes a great deal of effort and energy for a group of people to reach the safety of true community. But it is essential for the honest expression of ideas and feelings. It is also crucial in setting a climate that acknowledges mistake making as sometimes inevitable and a source of learning. This is one of the powerful benefits of community in the workplace. In times during which both the internal and external environments in health care organizations are increasingly turbulent and uncertain, the security experienced within a community can provide a haven of safety for people in the workplace.

Group of Leaders

Finally, a true community is a group of people who are all leaders. This concept is often described as a decentralization of authority (Peck 1987). Members who are accustomed to leading often feel comfortable and safe when they do not have to pick up the leadership reins. Members who are more reserved and not used to leading also feel more comfortable in picking them up, speaking out, and helping set a new direction. Peck found that "one of the most beautiful characteristics of community is what I have come to call the 'flow of leadership'" (Peck 1987, p. 72). The flow of leadership results in decisions being made more quickly and an increased likelihood that each member's individual gifts will be brought forward at just the right time.

Stages in Community Building

Communities go through several specific stages during their development. Understanding these stages helps us appreciate both the dynamic

and developmental nature of community. Instant community is an illusion. Using the concept of creating community as a retention buzz
word is inappropriate. Building a sense of community must be based on
an awareness that it is a developmental process, not the latest retention program. Although the stages in community building vary somewhat from author to author, Shaffer and Anundsen (1993) offer a
model that is applicable and easy to understand. The stages are outlined in figure 7-5.

Stage 1: Excitement

Excitement is an enjoyable phase, much like the honeymoon phase of
a marriage or relationship. The focus of the group is on its potential,
with an emphasis on positive outcomes and a minimization of the
problems that are likely to occur. The task for the group at this time is
to create a shared purpose and vision. The purpose need not be a task
to accomplish or a change to undertake. The purpose of the community may be simply to provide support to each other or to create a
workplace where we enjoy ourselves. Alignment with this purpose,
however, is important because it helps the members get over the rough
spots ahead. It often takes strong leadership and someone willing to get
the group started to move into and through this stage. This phase does
not last, and, in fact, if it continues indefinitely, the group is probably
a pseudo community, where community exists only in pretense.

Figure 7-5. **Stages of Community Development**

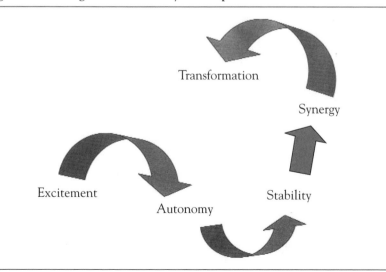

Stage 2: Autonomy

Autonomy is the focus of the second phase of community building. Often, this stage can make or break a community. During this stage, the illusion of unity is shattered, and members often become disappointed with each other, feeling angry and disillusioned. This phase passes only when members give up the fantasy of harmony without struggle. Although unpleasant, struggle is a critical part of the community's developmental process, and this phase is considered successful when the group survives and remains whole. Members assert themselves as individuals, are able to differentiate their needs from the needs of others, and yet remain committed to the needs of the whole, the community. The members consciously choose to act and work interdependently. The need for safety is paramount during this stage. When members do not feel safe within the community, its tasks are not accomplished.

Stage 3: Stability

During the third stage, community members settle into their roles and the community's structure. At this point, the fact that the community is still intact serves to reaffirm the members' caring for each other and their commitment to a shared purpose. Members know they are respected as individuals, and yet they understand the rules of the game (which they have helped establish). This understanding frees up energy to focus on the common tasks required.

A major pitfall in this stage is that members can become too settled in their roles, and the same member may continue to serve as the leader (developing agendas and leading meetings) or the resident critic (bringing up opposing viewpoints). Allowing one person or one small group to carry one role alone for too long can lead to burnout and stagnation. Our tendency when one member is especially talented (or merely willing) in one area is to let that individual carry the load, which does nothing to develop our collective abilities. This tendency can make it especially difficult for the community to embrace new leadership.

Stage 4: Synergy

Synergy is exciting and paradoxical. At this stage, members are acutely aware of their individualism and yet are more interconnected than ever before. Although aware of his or her own contributions and needs, each member is also very committed to the needs of the community. In fact, what is good for the individual is also good for the community. A characteristic of this stage is that roles reverse more comfortably, with leaders and followers flowing in and out of roles easily. Synergy, the excitement of our combined abilities, talents, and strengths, is very apparent at this stage. The illusion here is that the work is done. It is easy to believe that once you achieve synergy, it will remain and stay the same. However, all systems are continually in flux, and this community is no different.

Stage 5: Transformation

Transformation is the final stage of the cycle, when the community undergoes a death and possibly a rebirth of sorts. At this stage, the community may expand its boundaries or identity, break into smaller groups, or disband completely. Even the most successful communities reach a natural ending point, a time when members seem destined to move in new directions.

Leadership's Role in Creating Community

What can leaders do to develop a sense of community within their scope of responsibility? Unfortunately, it is not as easy as understanding the elements of community and the stages healthy communities experience as they mature. There is no guaranteed process a leader and employees can use that is certain to result in the development of a healthy community. Instead, the interventions are more general and foundational, and a sense of community develops only when the chemistry and efforts of the members determine it will be so. However, there are specific recommendations based on actual workplace experiences.

Hold a Clear Vision of the Possibility

Vision was such a buzzword of the last decade that many managers have become somewhat cynical about being told to have a vision. Yet vision is hope for the future. It is the ability to see something different than what currently exists. Vision is the ability to actively use your imagination. Using words and pictures to paint an image of community helps employees see and feel the direction in which they are heading. Few people jump onto a train unless they know where it is going. Creating and sharing a vision of community is the first and foremost task of the leader. It requires continually upholding what is possible: holding the best idea of each individual and therefore the department as a whole.

When the leader holds a vision of possibility for the department that includes a strong sense of community, this vision can actually guide day-to-day decisions and actions. Coupled with an intellectual understanding of community, interventions can be deliberate and supportive of the future vision. For example, consider the inclusive nature of community. Thomas Moore believes that one of the greatest needs of the soul is for belonging. He contends that people must be welcomed into a group (Moore 1994). Therefore, a new employee who has been hired or transferred into a department does not necessarily belong until invited. This invitation can be extended by the manager in the form of sharing his or her vision, making a strong initial connection during the interview process, and monitoring the new employee's progress closely to make sure that he or she is assimilating into the group. Invitation means looking for connections and creating opportunities for employees to connect on a personal rather than just a technical or professional level. For coworkers, this means reaching out and getting to know the new colleague and providing support as well as a gracious welcome.

Nurture Relationships

The second leadership intervention is to nurture the development of healthy relationships. Rousseau (1991) quite firmly states that community is based on altruistic love. Altruistic love means authentically caring for and about the members of the community. It extends beyond the employees in the department to include physicians, patients, and other colleagues as well.

As we saw in chapter 6, leaders can measure their effectiveness by the quality of their relationships. The strength of a community lies within these bonds. Forming strong affective relationships requires honesty, authenticity, and the capacity for intimacy. As in any relationship, it is important to realize that extending yourself to other people is taking a risk. However, the energy, support, and depth of meaning that come from working in a group of people who genuinely care for each other is profoundly rewarding. Only when we can see each individual as a gift and value their unique contributions can we develop the elements of synergy and realism that characterize community. A nonjudgmental attitude fosters feelings of safety. This is perhaps the greatest gift that a leader can give to employees because it demonstrates the tolerance for differences that is unique to community.

Genuinely caring for others is at the heart of this authenticity. Pretense does not work. Although the focus in health care has shifted toward seeing the needs of the whole person, management sometimes lags behind in seeing the whole employee. A dichotomy between work and home no longer exists because our lives are so much more complex than they were just twenty years ago, with the relationship between these two aspects of our lives interwoven and intricate. As we saw in chapter 5, ten or twenty years ago asking a personal question would have been considered intrusive, but today asking about family and being aware of your employees' personal challenges serve to enhance and build good relationships. A leader who arrives in the department (or at a meeting) and immediately begins asking rapid-fire questions about the project or tasks to be completed is often perceived by employees as caring more about work than about people.

Provide Support for Community Formation

Understanding the typical stages of community formation is essential for the effective leader. Knowing, for example, that in the early stages of community a stronger leadership presence may be required as opposed to the rotating leadership characteristic of later stages of community formation is crucial. Otherwise, a leader may inadvertently continue to exercise a strong, hands-on leadership role beyond the point at which it is healthy for the group.

Support may be needed in protecting the time community members have to spend together. The immense pressure to increase productivity in the workplace also decreases the amount of free time that employees spend together. For example, one physician remarked that ever since the hospital converted to bedside charting, he rarely talks with the nurses. The intention in this case was to streamline the documentation process, but precious time for human interactions was lost in the shuffle. In economics, this time together is called social capital, and it is considered vitally important because it produces "trust, cooperation, mutual support, bonding and . . . loyalty" (Putnam 2000). Balancing the need for productivity with the need for creating community and building social capital is a significant challenge for any health care manager today.

Seek Opportunities to Strengthen the Sense of Connection

There are endless opportunities for actions that strengthen the sense of connection people in the workplace feel toward each other. Simply being aware and looking for these opportunities is a powerful leadership strategy.

Take the example of the new nurse manager, Katie, who was faced with the need to complete seventy performance evaluations shortly after her appointment. Although she could have treated the evaluations as a tremendous burden, she chose to look at them as an opportunity to hear from each of her employees and to begin building relationships. Through this process it became clear that a major problem existed in the relationship between physicians and nurses.

Katie went to the group of physicians with this message. "I had identified my major challenge as recruitment and retention. But after listening to the staff, I understand that we have another significant problem. Nurses who have worked here for fifteen years complain that you *do not even know their names!* How do you expect me to recruit and keep nurses if you make no attempt to even know their names?"

Katie decided to remedy this situation and made a commitment to attend the physician section meeting every Friday. She highlighted a different employee each week, which required extensive research on her part. She presented three interesting things about each individual; for example, one nurse loved to garden, was a ballroom dancer, and was a Hell's Angel! Katie then proceeded to hold up a picture of the employee and announce his or her name. The physicians looked forward to these staff vignettes, and the special things that they learned about the members of the nursing staff helped to bridge the professional gap. In addition, the nurses were each given the task of learning something about each physician—hobby, children, interesting fact— and this goal was written into their performance evaluations. Relationships began to form in the spirit of community.

In her department, Katie took other actions as well. She placed the community bulletin board at the front station to increase its visibility to physicians, nurses, and auxiliary staff. The bulletin board became a space and place that community members could post items that were of interest to others such as a flyer describing a bicycle or snow tires for sale or an announcement of a staff member's special achievement. The sharing of such information increased the department's sense of camaraderie and open communication.

At a holiday gathering, physicians, respiratory therapists, physical therapists, physical therapy assistants, and nurses were asked to write their favorite vacation spot or hobby on their nametags rather than their name. This simple idea elicited many conversations that staff would have never initiated under other circumstances. It helped everyone to step outside their comfort zone. Conversations are like threads that weave a group of people together and strengthen the bonds among individuals and thereby the group as a whole. Any activity that creates personal connections or stimulates conversation encourages the formation of community. Our challenge as leaders is to constantly see and capitalize on the opportunities that exist.

When the atmosphere in the department is one of community, patients feel it. In Katie's department, even the patients began to feel as though they were members of the community. Ruth was eighty-two years old when she was admitted to the orthopedic unit with a hip fracture. Because she had no relatives and a legal guardian had not been established, her stay was extended from a week to two months. During this time, she became part of the community of the department. It was impossible not to fall in love with this pleasant and tender woman. She ate every meal at the nurses' station, and the staff eagerly devised recreational plans for her.

At the end of October, Ruth was finally discharged to an adult family home with three other residents. She was confused about the change of surroundings, but eventually she settled into her new home. Two days before Thanksgiving, the nurses received a phone call from the owner of the home. The owner said that all of the other residents were going home for Thanksgiving to their families, and Ruth wanted to come home, too. And so, on Thanksgiving Day, Ruth took her seat once again at the nurses' station so that she could eat her turkey dinner with her "family." The need for community is universal.

Benefits of Community Building

Do we need to develop a sense of community in our workplace? Arie de Geus of Royal Dutch/Shell argues that for "companies to endure they have to create a feeling of community, where workers think of themselves as members rather than employees. They belong to the organization" (Vogl 1997, p. 21). Paradoxically, although a sense of community can help create a sense of joy and connection in our work environment, community is difficult to attain in our contemporary workplaces. Reengineering, work redesign, downsizing, rightsizing, layoffs, mergers, and acquisitions have become common, almost universal experiences in our work lives. These initiatives are successful only when employees and employers work together in an atmosphere of trust and mutual collaboration. Yet, trust and collaboration are the very elements that are often destroyed.

There are other obstacles to community in the workplace as well. The increased use of per-diem and temporary employees creates continual change in the workplace. Another factor is our free enterprise system, which promotes individualism and results in subordinating the interests of community to those of the individual. Alienation, distrust, and competition are obviously major barriers to creating community. When the members' real agenda is increased personal power and fulfillment of personal needs rather than the well-being of the community, the group will not remain a community for very long (Naylor 1996).

It is precisely because of our experiences in leaner and meaner workplaces that we are seeing an increased interest in spirituality in the organization. "We humans hunger for genuine community and will work hard to maintain it precisely because it is the way to live most fully, most vibrantly" (Peck 1987, p. 137). The absence of community is keenly felt. Rather than rushing out to create community at work, it is important for managers to consider their interventions carefully and only after they have considered their own motivations. Otherwise, efforts to increase community in the workplace may backfire, leaving employees even more cynical. In his article, "The Call to Community," Zemke says that we have two options in the workplace:

> [First, community can be considered] nostalgic claptrap, a psychological retreat from what's happening in the real world. Or, as some proponents suggest, it may be an attempt to create a new, more civil code of workplace conduct, a code that accepts the realities of the modern world but holds that we can both cope with the insecurities and create openness and closeness with one another that facilitates our work and our humanity. Which assessment is correct? Will we trivialize the notion of community, or will we use it as a springboard for changing our behavior and our outlook on the world of work? (Zemke 1996, p. 30).

Conclusion

Both the formation of effective teams and the creation of a sense of community in the workplace are proven workforce retention strategies, but workforce retention alone cannot be the motivation for their creation. The motivation and commitment must be the desire to create, support, and nurture a group of people whom you genuinely value. These initiatives are ways to create a positive workplace. Creating an emotionally competent team often leads to increased effectiveness in the workplace as well as a stronger sense of connection among coworkers. When a sense of community is present, people feel connected to something larger than themselves. Both approaches build on the ties of affective commitment.

Conversation Points

Organizational Perspective

1. Are defined, developed teams an essential part of the organization's structure? Or do they exist sporadically throughout the organization?
2. Are internal resources available for the development of teams? (Resources include experienced team facilitators from human resources or the education or organizational development departments as well as time available for the developmental work of becoming a team.)
3. Does the senior executive group work as a true team and provide a clear example and role model for others in the organization?
4. Is team activity reinforced throughout the organization? (Reinforcements include but are not limited to rewards and recognition programs based on both individual and team performance and organizational leaders who understand how to communicate with and develop collective entities.)
5. Is there a sense of community in the organization as a whole? What kinds of activities and specific interventions or initiatives help the people in the organization feel a sense of community?
6. How is conflict handled organizationally? Is there a conflict-aversive culture, or is conflict handled directly and in a way that promotes the growth of people and the equitable resolution of issues?
7. How actively do employees participate in organizational community activities, such as summer picnics, holiday parties, and so on?

Leadership Issues

1. Do you have established teams within your area of responsibility? What is the purpose of these teams? How long have they been in place? Were they developed purposefully, or did they just emerge and evolve on their own?
2. If you do not have any formalized teams, are there functions or purposes that could be better met by a team? Where do you have an opportunity to improve your service by forming a team?
3. Do you have a leadership team that helps you lead in your areas of responsibility? Is it an informal work group or a true team? Could it be improved by becoming a true team?

4. Do your work groups demonstrate the essential elements of a team?
5. What is their level of maturity and effectiveness? Are they continuing to develop? Are they meeting their purpose?
6. Where in your areas of responsibility do employees experience a sense of community? Is there any place where you have deliberately tried to establish a sense of community, or has it evolved spontaneously?
7. If you see community in your areas, what stage of development is the community? Have you taken leadership action to assist in its development?
8. Are there places where you would like to see a true community form? What can you do as a leader to encourage this?
9. What are the benefits of creating a sense of community?

Employee Challenges

1. Do you function on a true team, or are you part of a work group? Would there be advantages to becoming a team? What would need to be different?
2. Do you and your coworkers understand the difference between teams, work groups, and pseudo teams? Or is the term *team* used loosely to describe any work group?
3. Are the expectations and norms within your team jointly established by team members, clearly understood by all, and lived up to by those involved? What happens when a team member does not abide by the established norms?
4. How emotionally intelligent is your team?
5. Do you and your coworkers feel a sense of community in the workplace? Where does community exist (for example, in a particular area of the department, on a certain shift, in a professional group, in the organization as a whole)? Are you certain you have a community and not a clique? (A clique is exclusive, with only certain people allowed to join, but a true community works diligently at being inclusive and including others.)
6. Have you taken any action to help the formation of community? What is your role in helping with the formation of the community?
7. What are the characteristics of community you see in your department or among people in your work area?
8. If you have a sense of community, what stage of development is it in?

8

Focusing on Results

Jo Manion and Sharon Cox

Leaders are proactive—and able to make something happen under conditions of extreme uncertainty and urgency.
—James Kouzes and Barry Posner (1993)

SAVVY LEADERS and managers intent on creating a positive workplace where people enjoy and are fully engaged in their work understand that one of their responsibilities is to focus on and obtain needed results. They understand that process for process's sake is not acceptable. How results are achieved is important, but getting results, solving problems, and making improvements are ways that effective leaders use to do their jobs and create commitment and credibility among their followers (Manion 2004b).

The ability to get needed results is tightly connected to the strategies and interpersonal skills addressed in this and other publications. For example, in *Execution: The Discipline of Getting Things Done,* Bossidy and Charan (2002) report that the first essential skill of getting things done is to know your people and to continually expand people's capabilities through coaching. When the leader's relationship with employees is healthy and positive, it is easier to communicate with each other, negotiate difficult issues, and work together to implement solutions.

This chapter explores models of shared decision-making that are in use in health care organizations today. The second section addresses several concrete process skills, such as problem solving, decision making, appreciative inquiry, and managing polarities that both managers and employees can use in getting results. An actively used continuous quality improvement process is closely linked to

Portions of this chapter are excerpted from *From Management to Leadership: Interpersonal Skills for Success in Health Care,* second edition, by Jo Manion. Copyright © 2005 by Jossey–Bass Publishers. This material is used by permission of John Wiley & Sons, Inc.

incremental improvements in our systems as well to an individual organization's success in creating an innovative culture, as discussed in the next chapter. A basic problem-solving process is offered here that is congruent with the quality improvement processes practiced in many health care organizations today. Decision making is discussed and some common pitfalls in the process are identified. Appreciative inquiry and polarity management are two additional approaches offered for tackling tough organizational issues. Polarity management is based on the recognition that not all issues are problems to be solved, but may be polarities to be managed.

Models of Shared Decision Making

Perhaps one of the most important aspects of creating a positive workplace is related to the degree to which employees are actively involved in making decisions about their work or giving valued input into decisions about their department and organization. All of the models of shared decision making that are being used have at their core the intention of transferring responsibility to employees or empowering employees. Because empowerment was a common buzzword in the 1990s, many people are tired of hearing it. It was overused and is often misused. A brief review of the concept is offered here to serve as a basis for understanding shared decision making. (For a more complete discussion of the subject, see *From Management to Leadership: Interpersonal Skills for Success in Health Care*, second edition, by Manion [2005].)

Empowerment

Transferring responsibility to others, often known as empowerment, is one of the most important processes managers and leaders need to develop. The definition of *empowerment* is "to be given the legal authority to" take a particular action. The word *power* means "the ability to act or to produce a result." These two definitions combined are "to be given the legal authority to act or produce a result." Gibson (1991, p. 351) defines empowerment as "a social process of recognizing, promoting, and enhancing people's abilities to meet their own needs, solve their own problems, and mobilize the necessary resources in order for them to feel in control of their lives."

The importance of empowering people in organizations cannot be overstated. Empowered employees are fully engaged in their work and contribute at a much higher level than their counterparts who see their work as simply a job. With the constantly shifting business climate and increasingly challenging external conditions facing health care, every organization needs the ability to respond rapidly. Quick response is virtually impossible from a workforce that has to constantly be told what to do, that is basically uninformed and unaccustomed to making decisions, and that has never participated in collaborative planning. On the other hand, organizations that have dedicated resources to the continual development of their people and treat their employees as intelligent partners in the delivery of services are much more likely to have individuals who are able to respond quickly when external and internal conditions change. These employees are not dependent on the manager or leader for direction or decisions; they can function independently and interdependently when needed.

In many organizations it is not just employees who are not developed and empowered, but also first-line managers. This creates a tremendous ripple effect in the organization. Rosabeth Moss Kanter, professor at the Harvard Business School, has been on the frontier of management and leadership for nearly thirty years. She points out the dangers of not empowering managers in the organization:

> Managers with power accomplish more because they have greater access to information, resources, and support in the company. Being busy, they pass the information and resources to subordinates. Thus, powerful leaders are more likely to delegate responsibility and reward talent.
>
> Powerless managers who can't easily get access to resources and information are frustrated and weak. The result is often petty, dictatorial managers who wield the only power they can: oppression of subordinates. It is powerlessness, not power, that corrupts (Kanter 1997, p. 6).

Empowerment does not occur simply because a leader says, "You are now empowered; go perform!" There is no Harry Potter magic wand to wave or incantation to pronounce so that people suddenly begin behaving differently. "Empowerment takes planning, patience, trust, and time. It's not something you can do overnight. If you want it to work, you have to commit to it. You must be willing to invest in it, support it with systems, and approach it in a logical, determined way" (McCarthy 1997, p. 7).

Process of Empowerment

As a process, empowerment begins with an understanding of four interrelated concepts: capability, responsibility, authority, and accountability.

The sequential application of these four concepts leads to empower-ment. (See figure 8-1.) First, the meaning of each of these terms must be clarified.

Capability

Capability refers to the ability, knowledge, and willingness of an indi-vidual to carry out the task, assignment, or responsibility. Ability is not only personal competence comprising skill and experience, but the availability of needed resources. An individual may be willing to accept a particular responsibility but simply not have the time, equip-ment, or resources necessary to do an adequate job, or vice-versa. The person may have ability in terms of both personal competence and resources but lack willingness. All elements must be present or empow-erment fails.

Responsibility

Responsibility is the clear allocation or assignment of a task or piece of work that needs to be accomplished. Responsibility also implies accep-tance of this allocation by the individual involved. The person to whom the task or assignment has been given must accept ownership before this responsibility has truly been transferred. For instance, a team accepts responsibility for carrying out its work, monitoring and controlling work flow, and making necessary decisions within its scope of responsibility and authority. It is responsible for maintaining an acceptable standard and for continually searching for ways to improve its processes and outcomes.

Figure 8-1.   Empowerment Sequence

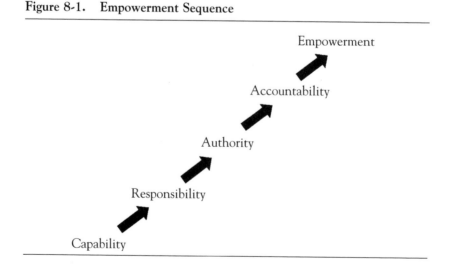

Authority

Authority is the right to act in an area for which one has accepted responsibility. For responsibility to be carried out, an individual must have a commensurate level of authority. There are four commonly accepted levels of authority, which are summarized in table 8-1.

The first level of authority is the authority to collect data or gather information. No action is taken on the data or information, and decision making is retained by the person assigning the responsibility and granting the authority.

Once the data have been collected or the information gathered, the individual involved in the gathering also reviews it and makes a recommendation based on his or her assessment and previous experience. This is level two authority. Decision making is retained by the person assigning the responsibility and granting the authority, but the gatherer's recommendation is considered in making the final decision.

At level three, the individual collects and reviews the information, makes a recommendation, and discusses it with the person assigning the responsibility. After their discussion and upon agreement, the individual proceeds to carry out the action.

Table 8-1. Levels of Authority

Level	Description
Level 1	This is the authority to collect or gather data and information. No action is taken by the person who gathered the information; the decision is made by the person who granted the authority.
Level 2	The person or persons involved in collecting the information also review it and make a recommendation based on their assessment and previous experience. The decision is made by the person who granted the authority with consideration of the recommendation.
Level 3	The individual or individuals gather and review the information or data, make a recommendation, and discuss the recommendation with the person who assigned the responsibility originally. After discussion and mutual agreement, the individual or individuals proceed to take action or implement the decision.
Level 4	This level represents independent action. The individual has the right to gather information, consider it, determine a decision or course of action, and take the necessary steps to implement the decision. In some cases, it may be a courtesy to let the person who assigned the responsibility know the outcome, but in many instances this is not necessary.

Level four is the highest level of authority because it represents independent action. It is the right to gather information, determine what needs to be done, and take necessary action. The person accepting the assignment is authorized to act in the place of the delegating individual.

In addition to these levels of authority, the individual's responsibility or authority may be limited by the constraints or parameters of a particular situation. For instance, the individual is given responsibility for making a purchasing decision with level four authority but within the constraints of an established dollar amount. Or a person may be given the responsibility to make a decision and determine necessary action but only after getting agreement from certain key stakeholders such as employees on the night shift, closely linked employees in another department, or physicians.

Accountability
Accountability is the retrospective review of decisions made or actions taken to determine whether they were appropriate. Were desired outcomes, in fact, achieved? If results were not satisfactory, what corrective action is needed to remedy the situation? This attitude of continual review is characteristic of a lifelong learner, a learning team, or a learning organization.

Application of Empowerment

When a leader applies the empowerment process sequentially, it goes something like this: Before the leader transfers a responsibility, he or she assesses the other person's ability and willingness to take over the responsibility. The leader asks the following questions:

- Does the person have the knowledge to carry out this responsibility?
- Are necessary resources, such as information and time, available?
- Has training or education been provided?

Once the leader has determined that capability is present, the leader clearly defines and communicates the responsibility. Assumptions are not enough; the assignment must be clear to both the party accepting the responsibility and the other people who may be affected by this assignment. A discussion of applicable parameters is held, and agreement on the appropriate level of authority is reached. And, last, outcome measures are determined to monitor success. The same process applies to the transfer of responsibility to a group such as a team or a department council.

The significance of empowerment as a developmental process is now clear. As an individual becomes more capable and highly skilled, he or she can accept more responsibility. The level of authority is gradually increased following successful performance of a responsibility. Parameters and constraints may be expanded as comfort with an individual's performance increases. It would be highly foolish, and even dangerous, to give a novice performer level four authority and no constraints the first time he or she takes on a responsibility.

Using this process appears simple, and yet there are many pitfalls and potential missteps in any health care organization today. When situations arise in which people feel disempowered, the process presented here can be used to assess the source of the problem and to give guidance for correcting it. Here are some of the more common examples of pitfalls with each of these elements of empowerment as they relate specifically to shared decision making.

Common Pitfalls Affecting Capability

Job requirements change as a result of new needs in the organization, and yet people stay in their positions even when they are no longer able to do the work required. This leads to an environment of entitlement. New expectations in the workplace can be communicated, education and training provided, and employees given time to adjust and meet new standards. However, at some point, these individuals can be expected to develop the abilities required or face a change in roles.

Another problematic situation occurs when individuals take on or accept responsibility for something they are not capable of doing. Perhaps they believe they have the skills, but in reality they do not. This creates frustration for both parties, the employee and the manager. It also results in lengthy and potentially costly delays in completing the task.

Some people are simply unwilling to accept more responsibility. This creates an admittedly difficult situation for a leader, manager, or coworker. With reductions in staffing levels and downsizing of organizations, everybody simply has to pull their own weight. The highest levels of performance are needed from every individual, and shortfalls from those not contributing fully can simply no longer be absorbed by others. Although you cannot force someone else to accept responsibility, acceptance of responsibility can be made a requirement of the job, which if not met means job loss.

Also, there may be insufficient resources for people to capably accept certain responsibilities. Time, equipment, money, education, training, or coaching may not be available, although individuals may be willing to accept additional responsibility. Organizations that attempted to convert to team-based structures in the last decade are a good example. Redesign of work was accomplished and team structures were determined. Employees were assigned to teams and expected to carry out their work in a new way without preparation in the form of education or training; furthermore, they reported to managers who had little or no experience in coaching teams. In addition, no extra time was incorporated into work assignments for the collective work of the team. This situation created a no-win situation for all involved.

Common Pitfalls Affecting Responsibility

The most common pitfall with responsibility is that it is not clearly communicated but is instead assumed to be understood. For instance, both managers and employees make the mistake of assuming that the job description clearly and completely defines what the employee is expected to do. Instead, they need to realize that there always are numerous other responsibilities for which an individual is held accountable, and these must be clearly articulated. For instance, as mentioned in chapter 6, employees should be told, "You are responsible for two things as an employee. The first is to do the work for which you were hired at an acceptable level of quality. The second is to form and maintain healthy working relationships with your coworkers as well as with your patients/customers." In other words, employees, not managers, are responsible for relationship issues in the workplace. Relationship issues range from resolving conflicts in a positive manner to having open, honest, and direct communication with coworkers. Managers are available for coaching in difficult situations, but it is clear that maintaining healthy relationships is everyone's responsibility. But how often is this responsibility discussed clearly among employees and managers?

Another problem with the element of responsibility occurs when there is a significant overlap of responsibility. In one organization, the chief operating officer (COO) was a cautious individual with a bad habit of asking multiple managers to do the same task. A manager asked to investigate and follow up on a problem would discover that others had been asked to assume the same responsibility. It was irritating and demoralizing to the managers to find they were duplicating one another's efforts. In some rare instances, it makes sense for several people to share a task or responsibility. But in order to avoid a disempowering and discouraging situation, the involved parties need to clearly discuss who is doing what. Few people appreciate it when their time is wasted by having to do redundant work.

In some instances, individuals have an exaggerated sense of responsibility and take ownership beyond what is intended. This can also lead to frustration and discouragement for all involved. In one organization, a team of internal trainers was created to provide the education and training for a major organizational initiative in process improvement. In the beginning, the team mistakenly believed that their role was to lead this initiative. They felt responsible for the success or failure of the effort, and it did not help matters that managers in this organization abdicated their responsibility for leading the improvement process to the team of internal trainers. Conflict and difficulties were significant until the responsibility of each was clearly defined. This particular pitfall is especially important to avoid when working with department councils and other group decision-making entities.

Common Pitfalls Affecting Authority
The concept of authority is where most confusion and problems occur for people. Many individuals believe empowerment only occurs when they have level four authority and that anything less than independent action is disempowering. Nothing could be farther from the truth. The level of authority has to be high enough to carry out the responsibility, and when the authority level is commensurate with the responsibility, empowerment results. Even a chief executive officer or system president does not hold level four authority for every aspect of his or her work. In any role, there are some responsibilities that rightfully entail a lower level of authority.

A second source of confusion around authority comes from the mistaken but commonly held belief that the lower levels of authority are not as important as the higher levels. Many mistakes and poor decisions are made in today's organizations because of this misconception. Individuals are asked for their opinion or to gather information, but because they are not making the final decision, they do a halfhearted job of collecting or giving the requested information. The individual making the final decision is disadvantaged because of poor-quality input. Each level of authority is critical, and responsibilities with each level of authority must be taken seriously.

Levels of authority may be falsely assumed by both performers and leaders unless they are specifically discussed and agreed upon. Conflict occurs when it becomes apparent that there is disagreement. Quality or problem-solving teams often run into this situation.

In one organization this occurred in the nursing department with a very visible employee team that had been asked to develop a clinical career ladder for the department. The team worked diligently for months and created an entire program based on extensive research from other hospitals.

On the verge of implementation, they were stopped by the corporate human resources department because of compensation issues and a need for equity across the entire system. Home health and long-term care had not been included, nor had any of the other professional departments. This team had unwittingly exceeded its level of authority, and as a result, a significant amount of resentment and frustration developed between the hospital nursing department, corporate human resources, and the rest of the system. The team's level of authority had been assumed but never discussed.

Changing levels of authority in the middle of a project is sometimes necessary but should be avoided if at all possible. A manager may have given an individual a responsibility and agreed upon a level of authority only to recall or decrease the level of authority when the individual or group does not carry out the work in the way the manager desired or expected. There are, however, multiple ways of achieving necessary outcomes, and a confident leader recognizes the need to relinquish control and let followers find their own way. When the project or assignment is snatched away midstream, the result leaves a bad taste for participants and an unwillingness to accept further responsibility.

New authority-related problems are appearing today with the major structural changes in the workplace. In the past, managers were clearly delegated a certain level of authority and reporting relationships were delineated and unambiguous. For many people in today's health care system, this has changed completely. Take, for example, the role of the nurse executive who is responsible for the nursing function throughout the organization in today's hospitals. The responsibility has become increasingly difficult to carry out now that it is dispersed among a variety of managers, some of whom have no professional nursing background and may report directly to a different executive. Communicating the essence of nursing issues and ensuring quality standards in the absence of line authority requires strong leadership skills.

A final problem related to authority is the reversal of authority. This occurs when a manager undermines the work of an individual or group or simply shows a lack of respect for the final decision. The most

frequent cause of this behavior is that the manager neglected to identify key parameters up front and the decision made was based on
incomplete information. Less frequently, the manager may have had
no intention of relinquishing control but wanted others to feel as
though they had participated.

In the early days of the quality movement, this lesson was frequently learned the hard way. One quality team worked for six months
on a specific problem. Their recommendation would have cost
$200,000 to implement and included the addition of several full-time-
equivalent positions to the annual personnel budget. No one thought
to tell the team that any recommendation could not exceed the current budget. Unfortunately, their experience led them to conclude that
administration was not serious about involving employees in decision
making and that quality was not a primary concern. Although members of the team were selected because of their interest and commitment, they became unwilling after this experience to participate in any
further projects. Sadly, the budget constraints might have been more
acceptable if they had been identified during the initial stages of the
project.

Sometimes group members attempt to undermine decisions. A
medical clinical affairs committee discovered this in one organization.
The director of medical affairs was given the authority to solve a problem within a certain dollar amount. Two weeks later he reported on his
actions. Two physicians who had not been present at the previous
meeting began questioning and second-guessing his decision. The
chair of the committee firmly reminded them that the director of medical affairs had been given the authority to solve the problem and that
his decision would be respected and supported.

Common Pitfalls Affecting Accountability

Although problems with authority are the most common, issues con-
cerning accountability are often the most serious. This element is potentially the weakest link in the chain. If people are not held accountable
for their behaviors and actions, whatever may be done through the first
three steps can be quickly negated. One reason so many things go right
in organizations today is because many employees and managers feel a
high level of personal accountability, continually reviewing their outcomes and learning from them. People who are continual learners
demonstrate a high level of internal accountability. Nevertheless, there
are many problems with external accountability, or the formal, traceable
lines of accountability in the organization.

Most organizations have only limited systems of accountability. It can sometimes be very difficult to ascertain what went wrong and why. Increasing numbers of part-time employees and per-diem or temporary employees have made determining who is responsible when a problem occurs rather complicated. Assignments of employees are often inconsistent, and many handoffs from caregiver to caregiver and department to department increase the difficulty of tracking.

Another issue hampering accountability is the tendency of managers and leaders to protect employees. When an individual or team makes a mistake or poor decision, the real role of the leader is to coach and support them in their efforts to correct the situation. Too often the manager steps in and takes responsibility for correcting the problem. Take, for example, a situation in which a physician has a complaint about an employee or a team and goes to the manager. If the manager takes care of the problem, the employee or team has learned little except that it is not capable of resolving its customer service or relationship problems. On the other hand, if the manager coaches the individual or team to work directly with the physician to resolve the issue, both the team and the physician benefit. The manager's behavior is sometimes motivated by his or her satisfaction in solving problems or, in some cases, by expectations within the hierarchy. Many established bureaucracies have only limited tolerance for these situations and simply want them resolved in the quickest fashion possible.

The final major pitfall for accountability is that the consequences of mistakes or poor judgment are too often punitive rather than corrective. Many organizational climates today are characterized by blame and accusation when things go wrong. These negative, punitive responses are probably the fastest way to squelch the staff's willingness to accept responsibility in the future. People are quick learners, and they watch what happens to their colleagues and coworkers. Swift retribution designed at extinguishing poor performance may end up extinguishing all performance. People are not willing to take risks in a harsh and unforgiving environment.

Shared Decision-Making Models

Having acknowledged the pitfalls with moving decision making down in the organization, most leaders in health care agree that capability, responsibility, authority, and accountability should be balanced and commensurate with each other if we are going to have effective organizations and employees with any degree of job satisfaction. Clearly, employee empowerment is a valuable concept, especially in the effort to retain top-performing staff members. It is also generally understood that the closer decisions are made to the point of service, the better those decisions will be. "Those who have to make it work should be involved in the decisions about the work" is a generally accepted management principle that goes back to the formation of quality circles for process improvement efforts in the early 1980s.

Shared Decision Making in Nursing

Shared decision making was the major underlying principle in the development of shared governance in nursing almost thirty years ago. Although the description of this concept has expanded and changed somewhat over the years to shared decision making or shared leadership, the principles hold true that professional nurses need to be making the decisions that impact their practice. As is the case with almost any major cultural change, there also needs to be a structure in place to facilitate the process, in this case, professional decision making. Dr. Timothy Porter-O'Grady makes this point emphatically as he stresses the core principle for shared decision making and employee empowerment:

> Empowerment involves recognizing the power already present in a role and allowing that power to be expressed legitimately. Empowerment does not give anything to anyone. There is no transfer of the locus of control. It is more a recognition of the legitimate location for certain decisions and structuring the system to let those decisions be made where they legitimately belong (Porter-O'Grady 2001, p. 469).

"Structuring the system to let those decisions be made where they belong" has for many hospitals involved creating unit-based councils of staff nurses around key aspects for decision making such as clinical practice, management, education, and quality. (See figure 8-2.) Typically, the elected or appointed leaders of these councils represent their patient care units on housewide nursing councils to deal with practice, management, education, or quality issues that involve all similar departments across the organization or even the system. This helps promote consistency and standards of practice and fosters a collaborative work environment. The leaders of the housewide councils form a coordinating council to act as a clearinghouse for projects or issues and to serve an oversight function of identifying and reducing any redundancy of effort or duplication among the councils. This model, or some variation of it, is in place in virtually all magnet-designated hospitals across the country and in thousands of other hospitals throughout the world (Porter-O'Grady 2001).

Figure 8-2.   Classic Model for Shared Governance

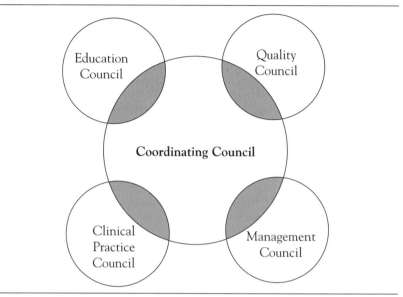

Shared Decision Making across Disciplines

Although the shared decision-making model has become a template for decentralizing decision making in nursing departments and is widely accepted as a framework for shared decision making among nurses and the management teams with whom they work, there have been only preliminary and sporadic attempts to develop similar models for employees in other disciplines. Shared decision-making models that include all disciplines across the organization have not existed until recently. Any cross-disciplinary efforts that existed previously usually developed when members of other disciplines were invited to nurse-led councils for input and collaboration on relevant issues. Nothing more formal has been used on a widespread basis in health care. Efforts to involve all disciplines in shared decision making can be categorized in one of the three following ways:

- The effort involved the formation of councils around strategic initiatives such as patient safety, customer service, or community involvement.
- The effort was modeled after process improvement techniques that have demonstrated success in the business world, for example, Lean Thinking, an approach to improve productivity pioneered by Toyota (Womack and Jones 1996), or Six Sigma, a

methodology for statistical analysis and process improvement made popular by Jack Welch as he touted the $600 million addition to the bottom line experienced by General Electric in the late 1990s (Plotkin 1999). These ideas that were so successful in business have been adapted in any number of health care organizations with significant results and a marked increase in the involvement of managers and employees in a wider range of system changes and fiscal accountability.

- The effort was apparent in other common organizational structures with goals similar to those of shared governance. For instance, organizations that implement a team-based design are accomplishing much the same end: transferring responsibility for front-line decisions about the work to the people doing the work.

For organizations that have invested in the formation of councils across disciplines or in sophisticated training efforts like those just mentioned, there is no question that they have improved employee and management decision-making skills. The result is empowered front-line employees with more ownership for process improvement and productivity that ultimately results in a positive impact on patient and service outcomes as well as financial viability. These changes represent substantial improvements over the hierarchical, top-down decision making that has characterized health care workplaces for over one hundred years.

Health care has finally begun, just in the last decade, to move toward sharing decisions with those who have to make them work. However, there is still much work to be done in fundamentally changing how decisions are made in the day-to-day operations of hospitals and other health care organizations. Too often, substantive decisions are made only at the top despite the fact that council members have been trained in the latest management techniques or that extensive time was taken to discuss issues. In the absence of a prevailing structure or infrastructure to share decision making and move decisions to the point of service, old patterns are unlikely to change (Porter-O'Grady 2001).

Two Case Studies of Shared Decision Making

Looking at two case studies of shared decision making will be helpful. The two organizations discussed here made fundamental changes in the ways that decisions are made in their facilities, and they developed an infrastructure to sustain the changes over time. Both organizations had past experience with the council model for group decision making and found that they needed to do more to substantially change their culture and move decision making deeper into the organization. Each of the organizations opted to begin by involving director-level (middle) managers in more decision making across all disciplines. They also planned to involve front-line employees more fully in the future.

Genesys Health System

Genesys Health System in Grand Blanc, Michigan, has taken the concept of shared decision making quite seriously. They began with the implementation of a design team made up of all disciplines, which over a nine-month period carefully researched and implemented a structure for shared leadership and decision making with the intent of ensuring that decisions are made with the participation of those who must execute them, ensuring a focus on continuous improvement, streamlining decision making for more timely action, and allowing leaders to think and act systemically.

Their model involves four councils: the strategy council (made up of the executive leadership team), the operations council, the patient care council, and the people and culture council. (See figure 8-3.) Each of the councils consists of ten to fourteen directors selected by the design team on the basis of specific criteria for council membership. Each council includes a member of the executive leadership team (as a sponsor) and acts as a working council that deploys teams to deal with a variety of issues. The chairs and cochairs of each council form the integration team, which coordinates the work of the four councils to avoid overlaps or redundancies and to augment collaboration among councils.

Having specific criteria for membership on the councils ensures the inclusion of members from a variety of roles and perspectives. For example, the people and culture council is made up of representatives from human resources, labor relations, organizational development, payroll, information systems, the diversity team, diagnostics direct service support (for example, case managers), and indirect service support (for example, dietary or maintenance) as well as a patient care director, a department director, a first-line supervisor, and a sponsor from the executive leadership team.

The responsibilities of each council were clearly defined by the design team prior to the implementation of the model. The level of

Figure 8-3.   Shared Decision-Making Model at Genesys Health System, Grand Blanc, Michigan

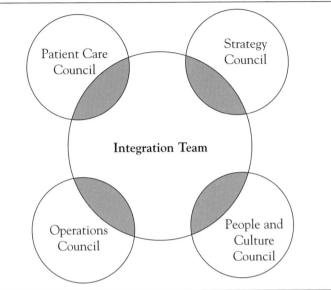

specificity in the design teams' efforts is reflected in the responsibilities of the people and culture council:

- Assisting in the development and operationalization of a cultural vision for the organization
- Facilitating the alignment of cross-functional policies and procedures with the organization's beliefs and values
- Coordinating and communicating issues related to the way we do our work and provide a forum for conflict resolution and problem solving
- Providing a think tank for operational issues and a forum for launching new projects in accordance with strategic and operational plans
- Ensuring ongoing assessment of the quality of work life at Genesys
- Fostering the growth and development of the individual
- Identifying skill and knowledge gaps between the cultural vision and where the organization is today
- Monitoring key people system indicators (for example, required training, minority representation, performance appraisals, employee surveys, and so on)

Clearly, the leadership in this organization and the depth of involvement among the council members constitute a major culture change under way in this complex organization (a unionized tertiary care medical center made up of four different organizations that merged in the late 1990s and built a new medical center to house the merged organizations). Genesys has a unique structure for shared decision making in that each council has representation from a variety of perspectives and layers in the organization that range from physicians to first-line employees such as security officers. The organization recently implemented a web site so that by employees could submit issues for consideration by the councils and keep up-to-date on the work of the councils. Any employee can access the councils' meeting agendas and minutes as well as any documents used by the councils.

The design team projects that the implementation of this model for shared decision making will occur in phases, with initial attention to core competency training such as problem-solving and process improvement skills, effective meeting behavior, and so on, as well as demonstrated success in project completion. Clearly, culture change of this magnitude requires an incremental, phased-in process and competency training, but even more important, it demands a strong, unwavering commitment from the senior leadership team and department directors. These factors are working to make shared decision making a reality in this system.

St. Alphonsus Regional Medical Center

St. Alphonsus Regional Medical Center, in Boise, Idaho, has for the last few years been undergoing a significant building program. In tandem with this project, they are moving to patient-centered care and becoming the employer of choice in their region. They developed a model to share decision making between the directors and the senior management team that has proven to be quite successful. (See figure 8-4.) While the senior leadership team focuses its efforts on strategic issues, the operations management team (made up of directors who report to vice presidents) is charged with making day-to-day operational decisions, particularly around developing and monitoring the hospital's operational budget. The operations management team has established various "affinity teams" to monitor a variety of issues, including employee vacancies, salaries, and supplies and purchasing as well as revenue management, including growth opportunities.

These wide-ranging responsibilities have created a level of cooperation and collaboration among the department directors that supports

Figure 8-4.   Shared Decision-Making Model at St. Alphonsus Regional Medical Center, Boise, Idaho

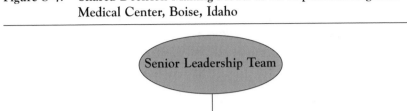

their efforts for culture change and patient-centered care. The managers who report to directors are involved with the senior leadership team and the operations management team in quarterly leadership meetings to augment their culture change efforts. During its first two years of balancing the budget and meeting financial targets, the operational management team made significant strides with managing the number of full-time-equivalent positions (FTEs). Prior to the implementation in 2001, the organization had, for example, an increase of almost 300 FTEs per year. With the work done by the affinity team for vacancy review, they reduced that number to 32 through most of 2004. This is just one of many examples of the ways in which moving decisions deeper into the organization has improved the quality of the decision making. The directors have acknowledged their growth as a team and the relationship between the senior team and the directors has markedly improved as they each assumed ownership for making shared decision making a success.

Lessons Learned from the Case Studies

These are two examples of organizations that have made a significant commitment to culture change and to shared decision making. Although the models they developed are still in their infancy, they can serve as prototypes for others who want to invest in an ongoing effort toward creating a more collaborative workplace in order to create long-overdue changes in the health care workplace.

As we struggle with ways to create positive workplaces, it becomes increasingly clear that the old hierarchical, patriarchal, bureaucratic structures increase employee dependency and have a potentially negative impact on the quality of work life for all of us, which translates into fewer positive organizational outcomes. There is no better time than the present for developing an infrastructure for shared decision making with the increased numbers of knowledge workers and genXers who want to be in the loop on decisions and recognized for their contributions. Contemporary workers know that they have a range of opportunities and that their services will be in demand for years to come as workforce shortages grow more significant. Health care organizations are under pressure to change the workplace in fundamental ways if they are to attract top-performing employees. Examining current formal approaches to shared decision making is a first step. Applying these principles throughout our organizations and systems is the second step. Building an infrastructure for shared decision making has clearly become a priority for forward-thinking organizations. While these changes will not be easy, they are necessary.

Dr. Timothy Porter-O'Grady, the respected innovator of nursing shared governance some thirty years ago, conveys a sense of urgency in making the argument for shared decision making when he writes:

> Whatever the process of changing structure, locus of control, decision processes, and team-based initiatives are called, they are essential to the future of doing health services business. From shared governance to shared leadership, shared decision making, empowerment, point of service accountability, or whatever other name might be attached to the dynamic, shared decision making is an essential element of the work of reconceptualizing and configuring health care for the future. . . . It is not possible to empower the consumer to make right choices if [the] providers who enable this empowerment are not empowered. Building a structure for empowerment is not only relevant it is essential (Porter-O'Grady 2001, p. 473).

Skills Needed for Shared Decision Making

This section of the chapter explores several key skills necessary for successfully implementing shared decision-making models. Problem solving and decision making are discussed in some detail. Two additional relatively new approaches to problem solving, appreciative inquiry and polarity management, are also discussed briefly as possible alternatives to more traditional approaches.

Problem-Solving Skills

In hierarchical, top-down organizations, problem solving is limited in terms of both who is involved and the kinds of problems around which groups meet. Group problem solving is a bottom-up process requiring a visionary leader, a manager or leader who can relinquish control sufficiently to create an environment for employee empowerment. When problem-solving groups are prevalent in an organization, it is a good sign of employee involvement. And knowledgeable leaders understand that it is difficult for individuals to feel empowered when they have no tools with which to solve pressing problems that directly affect their ability to do their work. Seeing improvement in their daily work life creates a sense of momentum and hopefulness for the future in the work group and ensures future participation in these activities. Many quality or process improvement groups are essentially problem-solving groups.

Process of Problem Solving

Most effective problem-solving processes include some variation of the following five steps, as illustrated in figure 8-5. Regardless of what

Figure 8-5. Problem-Solving Process

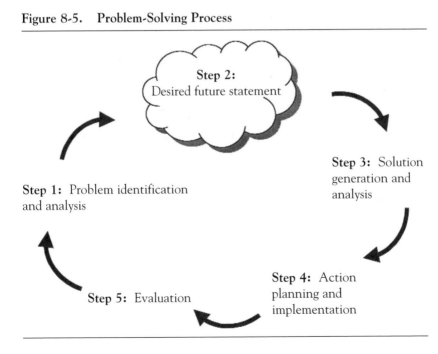

Step 2: Desired future statement

Step 1: Problem identification and analysis

Step 3: Solution generation and analysis

Step 4: Action planning and implementation

Step 5: Evaluation

these steps are called, a skilled leader understands that this process must be both sequential and methodical. All of the steps must be included and performed in the appropriate sequence in order to obtain a quality outcome. Often what passes for problem solving is some spontaneous, inconsistently applied brainstorming technique that follows no proven methodology and misses one or more important steps.

The following problem-solving process can be used effectively by either individuals or groups. Group problem solving is the format considered for purposes of this discussion.

Step 1: Identify and Analyze the Problem

In the first step of a problem-solving process, the group describes and, ultimately, defines and analyzes the problem. The discussion typically begins with descriptions of symptoms or other evidence of a problem as it affects various members of the group. In many instances, initial statements of the problem are vague and confused. Sometimes additional information is needed before a problem statement can be written.

It is important to surface as many characteristics of the problem as possible at this point and to avoid jumping to hasty conclusions. Psychologists who have experimented with thinking for over the past seventy years have discovered that once a person offers an explanation, they have difficulty revising it or dropping it even in the face of contradictory information. In experiments, subjects were shown an out-of-focus 35-millimeter slide of a fire hydrant. The psychologists found that when a person mistakenly identified the object when it was out of focus, he or she often could not identify it correctly when it was brought into greater focus so that another person (who had not seen the blurry slide) could easily recognize it. Their conclusion was significant: More evidence is required to overcome an incorrect hypothesis than to establish a correct one. Individuals who jump to a hasty conclusion are less sensitive to new ideas and information (Adams 1986).

Questions often help to define the problem more fully, for example:

- What are the signs and symptoms of this problem?
- Whom does the problem affect?
- Is its effect direct or indirect?
- What is the frequency of occurrence?
- What are all of the possible causes or factors involved?

The group may determine that more information or data are required. Many of the techniques taught through quality improvement programs, such as using histograms, fishbone diagrams, Pareto charts, and process and scatter diagrams can be helpful at this point in the decision-making process (Byers and White 2004).

During this first step, another important issue to consider is ownership. How have the group or individuals within the group contributed to or created the current problem? This factor is critical to consider because the group will have better success if it begins with alternatives over which it has control. Accepting some of the responsibility for the problem is difficult for many groups, who often begin by believing the cause and fault for the problem lie elsewhere. By pushing themselves, however, they usually begin to see how they have helped create the current situation.

Caregivers in one organization were angry because they often did not have enough clean linen in the morning to complete changing the patients' bed linens. They clearly attributed the problem to the linen services department. When forced to look at their own role in creating the problem, they were clueless. They continued to insist that it was the fault of linen services. But with persistent prodding, they gradually began to come up with ideas. "We stopped attending the liaison meeting with linen services because we didn't think they were listening to our concerns." They also recalled being told that over $200,000 in scrub clothes were replaced during the year because of employee theft. That money could have helped pay for a higher-capacity washing machine that would process linens faster. The final contributing factor that they identified was their common practice of hoarding linen and stashing it in all kinds of places so that it would be available when needed. This practice had made it impossible to get an accurate inventory count, which required linen services to plan inventory on the basis of inaccurate figures. Once these issues were identified, the group began to work more effectively on the problem.

In a radiology department, the problem was inaccurate requisitions for procedures. One way the radiology employees had contributed to the problem over the years was that they usually accepted the patients and performed the procedures in spite of being given incomplete or inaccurate requisition forms. As a result, the persons responsible for the inaccurate requisition forms never realized that they were causing problems for radiology.

The problem statement is a concise description of the problem. Novice problem-solving groups tend to put the solution into the problem statement. One group, for example, came up with "the problem is inadequate staffing." So stated, this limits problem-solving creativity because the solution automatically becomes getting more staff. When the problem statement is changed to "there is more work than the current employees can handle," multiple possibilities become apparent, including eliminating some of the work, changing the way it is being done, obtaining time-saving technology, and making temporary adjustments in staffing levels.

Once the problem is clearly identified, the group determines its level of authority in solving the problem. Determining the level of authority at this point is critical because it ensures that everyone's expectations are appropriate. Necessary communication and involvement with others in the organization can be planned. Just because a group has a low level of authority does not preclude it from working on a particular problem; clarity about authority levels prevents misunderstandings later, when it comes time to implement the decisions.

Compare the two employee groups: Both chose to work on a problem for which they had only level one authority. The issue was employee benefits. The first group was very aware of its level of authority. The members spent their time investigating the problem and gathering information, and they made recommendations for the human resources department to consider based on their findings. Their work focused on a desired future that included the successful presentation of their information and specific steps aimed at their strategies for delivering the recommendations.

The second group had not clarified its level of authority. The members proceeded with enthusiasm throughout the entire process, developing a future vision that included employee benefits offered in a cafeteria-style approach. Their action planning revolved around the implementation of the new benefits. They were excited and eager when they finished the problem-solving process only to become frustrated and angry when their work was never acted upon. The members of the group cynically observed that it was the last time they would volunteer for a problem-solving task force, never realizing that the work they had done substantially exceeded their level of authority.

Step 2: Describe the Target Outcome
A common mistake problem-solving groups make is to focus almost exclusively on the problem and its causes rather than on what they would like to build or create for the future. Russell Ackoff, the creator of interactive planning, has demonstrated clearly that solutions are more creative if the focus remains on desired outcomes rather than on details of the current problem (Ackoff, Finnel, and Gharajedaghi 1984).

This step involves asking the question: What would this look like if there were no problem, if it were solved? The group then writes a description of the ideal situation. So, for example, if the group's problem statement were "Communication between hospital and home health personnel is poor, creating problems in delivery of quality patient care," a desired future statement might be: "Communication between hospital and home health personnel is free flowing, timely, and accurate." In another system, a group was working on coordinating community services for seniors. Their desired future statement read: "Community services for seniors are coordinated and easily accessible to participants, with information flowing freely and fluidly between agencies for the benefit of our program participants."

Focusing exclusively on the problem statement leads to more limited solutions. A clear, desirable future statement creates a picture for those involved and generates more imaginative and original ideas, as well as a broader scope of possibilities.

Step 3: Generate and Analyze Potential Solutions, Part 1
Step 3 is both creative and analytical, and it is helpful to separate the two phases of this step. The group first generates all possible solutions. The first part of step 3 concentrates on identifying all of the potential solutions to be considered. These solutions are not analyzed critically until the second part of the step. Nothing impairs creative flow faster than criticism or an analysis of the ideas as they are presented. Creativity techniques are useful for noncritical idea generation. Figures 8-6 through 8-10 (pp. 252–56) outline several examples, which can be reviewed in more detail in the many books available on the subject of innovation or creativity.

Step 3: Generate and Analyze Potential Solutions, Part 2
The second part of step 3 is to analyze all the solutions generated in the first phase. Once all of the possible alternatives have been identified, the group can begin to converge regarding the most viable options. A series of helpful questions for sorting and categorizing feasible alternatives include the following:

- Are some alternatives very similar, or do they overlap?
- Can certain solutions be combined?
- Do any alternatives need to be rearranged?
- Can any be eliminated? (If the answer to this question is yes, should any worthwhile applications or characteristics of the eliminated options be considered?)
- What is good about a solution?
- How would it solve the problem or help create the desired future?
- Are there any possible unexpected consequences of this option?
- If anything goes wrong, what would be the course of action?

- What is the group's degree of control or level of authority over this option?
- Are there key stakeholders who need to be involved to make this option a success? Are stakeholders likely to support it?
- What resources would be needed to implement this solution and are obtainable?
- Are more data and information needed?

Figure 8-6.   Nominal Group Technique

Description: The nominal group technique combines quiet, individual thinking time with a structured and yet free-flowing sharing of ideas. The nominal group technique follows a specific process that often yields successful outcomes (Delbecq and VandeVen 1971). This technique is especially useful when group members possess varied levels of verbal and expressive skills. (The nominal group technique is often mistakenly confused with brainstorming, a much looser process of generating ideas.)

Process:

1. The facilitator asks a question about the problem, and then group members individually respond in a way specified by the facilitator. For instance, if the desired future is for communication between two agencies to be free flowing, timely, and accurate, the facilitator may solicit responses regarding characteristics required to achieve this state. The group members then individually write down all responses that come to mind after the leader specifies either how many ideas (say, five to ten) each participant should list or the time frame in which the list should be completed (perhaps five minutes).

2. The facilitator provides these guidelines for sharing the ideas:
   - Taking turns, every participant gives one idea at a time.
   - No one is to react in any way to the ideas as they are being presented, which means no clarification or discussion of any kind at this point.
   - If a group member runs out of ideas, they can pass until their next turn, when they may present another idea if they have one.

3. The facilitator lists each idea on a flip chart or board, with no rewording of the idea, until all ideas from the group have been written for the group to see.

4. Once the ideas are gathered, the facilitator leads a discussion of the ideas to clarify, elaborate, defend, dispute, or add to the items.

5. The list is reviewed and categories are identified. Some items may be combined or eliminated.

Figure 8-7.   Mind Mapping

Description: Mind mapping is similar to the nominal group process, but the recording of ideas is done in a circular fashion. Even totally unrelated ideas are captured because they may spark an idea for someone else. As Wycoff (1991, p. 48) explains, "Two things happen when you allow yourself to put the idea down—the first is that the mind is freed to go onto other ideas, and the second is that associations are made with this idea. This is where the best ideas come from."

Process:

1. In a box or oval drawn in the center of the chart or board, one or two words that capture the essence of the issue are printed. From the previous example it might be "communication between agencies."

2. As members contribute thoughts and ideas on the topic, the facilitator prints the key words describing those thoughts around the essence statement and then connects them to the box with lines. As ideas are generated that relate to one of those branches, the idea's key word is printed and then attached to the branch with a line.

Although this is a lengthy list of questions, each question is important. The group needs to think about the answers and get ready to move on. There is no perfect solution for the problems in organizations today, and it is better to implement something than to be caught in a never-ending spiral of data collection. When the selected solution does not work, at least the group has more knowledge and information on which to base a new decision.

At the end of this step, the group should have identified at least two or three viable solutions. Stopping at only one solution is dangerous. If it is not accepted or cannot be implemented, the group members will feel demoralized, as though they have wasted their time. Also, research has demonstrated that problem solvers are dominated by pressure to solve the problem and that adopting the first solution may reflect this pressure. Forcing the group to develop at least a second alternative results in more creative solutions because focus is on the desired future as opposed to the need to find an answer.

Deciding among the alternatives requires knowledge of decision-making approaches. There are several types of decision making, including voting and reaching consensus, which are explored later in this chapter.

Figure 8-8.   List Making

Description: List making is a conceptualization technique. It uses the construction of lists as a method of forcing alternative thinking. A simple and effective approach, it starts simply with a question or issue, and then the group members generate a list of ideas to address the subject. The value of list making lies in the fact that checklists require a person to consciously control his or her thinking in order to focus on alternatives that the unconscious mind might ignore in trying to simplify life (Adams 1986). For example, list making was used in a head injury rehabilitation center to discover ways of improving the environment for clients (Manion 1990).

Process:

1. The facilitator asks the group members to suggest items for the list. In the example above, the employees were asked to think about the things that they would miss or want if they were confined by a head injury to a rehabilitation facility for the months that recovery would require.

2. The facilitator creates a list of all of the ideas that were generated, for example:

> Pictures of family and friends
> The feel of sun or rain on my face
> The feel of sand between my toes
> The smell of coffee in the morning
> My hair and makeup done every day
> Shopping trips
> Favorite television programs
> Favorite music
> My children staying overnight with me
> Surprises
> Sleeping late in the morning
> Popcorn
> Ability to make my own decisions
> My pets

3. The list can then be used to guide changes, create solutions, or design new products or services.

Figure 8-9.   Attribute Analysis

Description: Attribute analysis involves breaking away from our common tendency to rely on generalization. When problem solvers consider the specific attributes of a situation, they come to different conclusions than they would if they applied generalized stereotyping.

Attribute analysis can be illustrated with a simple example: a standard lead pencil. The attributes of the pencil would be that it is hexagonal in shape, pointed on one end, constructed of wood with a lead center, painted yellow, and topped with a rubber eraser. Each of these attributes could then be analyzed further. For instance, the properties of wood include its ability to burn, float, insulate against electricity, and provide structural support. Then each of the properties of wood could be used to create lists of things that burn, float, or provide insulation and structure.

Process:

1.   List the attributes of the situation.

2.   Below each attribute, list as many alternatives as possible.

3.   When completed, make many random runs through the alternatives, selecting a different one from each column and assembling combinations of entirely new forms of the original subject.

Example: This approach was used by employees of a new outpatient surgical center to design a user-friendly system with correspondingly friendlier processes. They began by listing attributes of a user-friendly system: easy access to the building, convenient parking, comfortable waiting facilities for family and friends, speedy admission processes, simplified discharge procedures, a pleasant atmosphere, and procedures scheduled for the convenience of the client. They then listed the specific attributes under each of these characteristics. Below convenient parking, for example, was listed "covered, inexpensive or free, safe, and not far from the door or shuttle service." By listing these various attributes and going through the lists several times in different ways, employees generated several unique (at the time) approaches that enabled the new center to quickly capture a large segment of the market. These approaches included valet parking, procedures scheduled for the convenience of clients (hours after work were in high demand), discharge prescriptions available prior to surgery to eliminate a stop at the pharmacy on the way home, comedy videos in the waiting room, beepers for family members so they can be called back to the waiting area, and snacks or meals for waiting family members.

Figure 8-10.   Storyboards

Description: The storyboard was created by Walt Disney as a planning method for his animators (Vance 1982). It is used to develop and record the creative thinking process. It is based on the premise that it is easier to see the interconnections among ideas when they are displayed visually. This is a useful technique for stimulating and recording ideas between meetings of the problem-solving group. For example, one executive team adopted this idea for use during strategic planning. In developing a group vision, members were each given a pad of sticky notes and asked to write down one idea per note that described an element of their vision. Individuals generated as many as twenty-five items each. These were then shared and stuck on large pieces of paper around the room. As the notes were discussed, categories began emerging, and subsequent ideas were placed on appropriate pages.

Process:

1. Participants write their ideas on index cards or sticky notes and then attach them to a corkboard or wallboard accessible to everyone in the group.

2. Participants then are free to add additional cards with new ideas or expansions of other participants' ideas. They may also rearrange or remove the cards as needed.

Step 4: Develop and Implement Action Plans

Determining specific actions to be taken, the time frame within which they are to be completed, and responsibility assignments for each action must be specific and realistic. Once identified, the steps to be taken are prioritized. In many instances, they must be sequential because some are dependent on completion of others.

Once the plan is reasonably complete, costs for both current practice and recommended alternatives are estimated. Spending money or time in order to save a substantial amount of money or time can be a compelling incentive to adopt a new practice. In some instances, no more money is needed for an alternative, but quality of service is positively impacted. At this stage, a communication strategy is developed based on who needs to know about this plan and who must be included in developing additional expectations. How and when to present the results of the problem-solving group are decided.

During implementation, the plan must be monitored closely to maintain momentum. This monitoring function is assigned to an individual who can also reinstitute the group if further work is necessary.

Step 5: Establish Evaluation Criteria

The final step in the problem-solving process is to establish criteria for evaluating success and to determine who will be responsible for the evaluations. The parties involved in implementation must know up front how success will be measured. Evaluation criteria should be as precise and objective as possible, which in some instances is fairly simple. A percentage error rate, the number of completed diagnostic tests, the number of patient falls, and employee productivity figures are a few examples of easily obtained objective measures. Others are more difficult to quantify, such as improvement in relationships between teams or departments, satisfaction levels of key customers, or more subtle changes in the quality of service.

Specific review dates are established, and plans are made for celebration of the completion of this phase of the group's work. Results must be monitored and necessary corrections made. Divergence from expected outcomes means that the cause must be identified and another workable solution found. The second and third solution alternatives formulated earlier in the process are helpful in this case. At this point, the group may need to be encouraged and reminded that even if the first recommendation or solution did not work exactly as planned, the solution is now closer than it was before.

This problem-solving process was used effectively in a hospital in the U.S. sunbelt. An annually recurring problem of a lack of patient beds during the winter months with the influx of visitors from the Northern states created conflict between employees and physicians, all scraping to come up with needed resources. Finally, during the summer months, administration initiated a problem-solving team composed of employees, managers, executives, and physicians. The process took several months, but the result was a plan that increased the number of available beds during the winter months and clearly identified backup contingency plans. For the first time in years, the winter season was managed without key stakeholders coming to blows over beds for patients.

Common Pitfalls in the Problem-Solving Process

The most common pitfall occurs when the group does not distinguish when to use problem solving, appreciative inquiry, or yet another approach such as polarity management. Appreciative inquiry and polarity management are discussed later in this chapter, and both are effective ways of dealing with issues. There are simply some issues that are better tackled with an approach such as appreciative inquiry, and others that are not clear-cut problems, but instead, polarities to be managed. Determining first which approach to use can prevent a great deal of unnecessary effort.

A second pitfall occurs when the group includes a suggested solution in the problem statement. This limits the variety and creativity of alternatives the group identifies. Then it is the same old answer one more time. Not only is the solution ineffective, but everyone involved ends up disenchanted.

A third pitfall relates to the group's level of authority. Steps for action must fit the level of authority and the problem. Too often groups develop grandiose action plans that go way beyond their level of authority and any reasonable parameters. The previously mentioned quality problem-solving team that came up with a solution costing over $200,000 annually and adding another four full-time equivalents to the personnel budget is a good example.

Hidden agendas and personal platforms make up the next pitfall. Some group members may have a personal strategy they want to promote, even if it has little to do with the issue at hand. This cannot be allowed to interfere with a fully explored problem-solving process.

Yet another pitfall occurs when time frames and people responsible for each action step fail to be identified. These are critical to the implementation stage, at which point it is easy for the group to lose steam and neglect to carry out agreed-upon steps. Monitoring and follow-through are essential.

Following the process sequentially is difficult for many groups. The process is a blend of both right- and left-brain activities, and some groups have trouble with one or the other, or simply switching between the two. Identifying and analyzing problems and developing action plans and evaluation measures are all examples of logical, left-brain thinking. Establishing a desired future and generating all possible options require creativity and spontaneity and so involve right-brain thinking.

Moving from one stage to the other may be facilitated by taking a brief physical break between them or actually carrying out each step in separate meetings. This creates boundaries between the two types of thinking processes and helps members make the transition. If people in the group are characteristically logical and concrete thinkers, such as clinical laboratory professionals, the group leader may need to be very firm in keeping the group focused during the right-brain activities because there will be tremendous pressure to move to analysis and left-brain logical activities.

Not respecting the problem-solving process as a methodical, sequential process leads to several common problems. The most common is called the Band-Aid® approach, a knee-jerk reaction that occurs when the group moves straight from problem identification to action planning without taking the time to think through a desired future or develop a full range of creative options, as illustrated in figure 8-11.

Another common problem, called analysis paralysis (figure 8-12), is experienced when the group stays in the problem-identification phase so long that paralysis sets in. It seems as though there are never

Figure 8-11. The Band-Aid Approach to Problem Solving

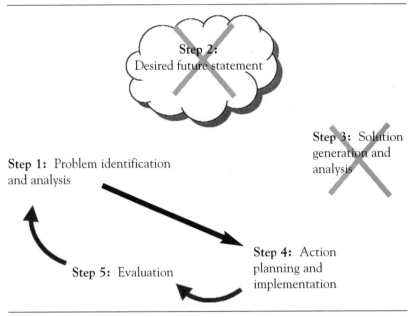

Figure 8-12. Analysis Paralysis in Problem Solving

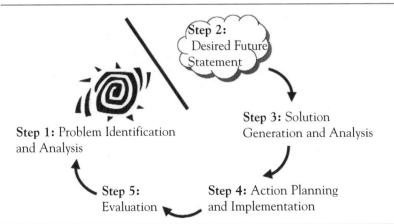

enough data to make a decision, not all the facts have been collected, or there is not enough information with which to move ahead. The goal here is to reach a happy medium between gathering the information and coming to a decision. Collect enough data to provide information for adequate analysis through a specific agreed-upon process and stick to an acceptable time frame for the problem at hand.

Some groups have an exaggerated sense of responsibility and take on too much ownership for the problems. This can often be avoided by asking the important question: What is our level of authority for solving this problem? They may discover that they do not have an adequate level of authority for implementing a solution to the problem and can therefore accept that it is not their responsibility to do so. In some instances, they may realize that they are trying to solve a problem for a key group not represented and, as a result, they must modify the membership of their group.

Reasons Groups Fail in the Problem-Solving Process

It is imperative that both individuals and groups develop effective problem-solving skills. Most groups process problems rather than solve them, continually discussing the symptoms or effects, anything but the root causes. In many instances, the problem itself escapes during the discussion without ever having been defined. There are at least three reasons groups engage in unproductive processing:

- The group uses voting to determine plans of action, which forces group members to pick sides. Once a person takes a side and another opposes it, the two opposing stances become even more adamant and continue to grow farther apart.
- Groups neglect monitoring their group process. Although members may observe unproductive process, they are too often unwilling to address it. For example, silent members are not asked to contribute, apathy is ignored, or disruptive behavior is tolerated.
- The group does not recognize or understand its patterns of behavior, which may include closing discussions prematurely or reaching decisions without fully analyzing the problem. Members may not recognize groupthink or behavior that is so polite and courteous that no one dares talk about the real issues. When the group's solutions or alternatives are not accepted, too often the group blames those with authority rather than reviewing their own process and truly evaluating the quality of their work.

Groupthink is a phenomenon "whereby team members become afraid of offering ideas that might conflict with the group's policies and actions. New ideas are often offered weakly and withdrawn quickly if opposed" (Chaleff 1997, p. 4). Groupthink can destroy creative initiative and even cause people with opposing views to be forced out. The remedy for groupthink is continual self-evaluation of the group's patterns and outcomes.

Managers and employees who understand problem solving also understand its relationship to decision making. The two are closely interwoven and highly interdependent. Good problem solvers make decisions and good decision makers use a problem-solving approach.

Decision-Making Skills

In this context, a decision is a choice among alternative courses of action that may lead to the desired result. When there are no alternatives, no decision is made. Managers and employees alike assume responsibility for the consequences of their decisions. This can be frightening at times because many decisions are made under conditions of uncertainty.

Decisions are evaluated based on their results or consequences, which are often unpredictable. An individual or group does not have to be right all the time, only most of the time. A sign in a printing shop provided this profound piece of wisdom: "Good decisions come from experience. Experience comes from wisdom. Wisdom comes from making bad decisions." If an individual or a group has difficulty dealing with uncertainty, they either postpone decisions until all of the uncertainties have been resolved or they make poor decisions because they are uncomfortable coping with the uncertainties.

"As important as sound decision-making is, many executives [and groups] neglect to use any formal decision-making process" (Clancy 2003, p. 343). Good decision makers combine a logical, systematic approach with their intuition. They sort and classify information; differentiate between the valuable, worthless, and redundant; prioritize; and integrate the whole into an accurate picture of reality. As the amount of information available increases, the complexity of decision making also increases. Managers and employees who are good decision makers evaluate and recognize what type of decision is called for from each new situation.

Types of Decisions

Five types of decisions are commonly made in health care organizations: individual, minority, majority, consensus, and unanimous. The type of decision that is appropriate depends on the specific situation.

Individual Decisions

Individual decisions are made by one person: a leader, a manager, or an individual with the responsibility and authority to decide. Others involved are expected to abide by this decision. This type of decision is most often used when the person with the decision-making authority perceives that there is no choice, the decision is not important, or the group does not want to make a decision. One example of this is called the "plop," a suggestion that gets accepted without any discussion. The plop can be offered by any member of the group.

Individual decisions are sometimes seen as an imposition or a mandated solution directed by someone with the authority or expertise to impose such a solution. Impositions are justified when the issue is truly nonnegotiable in terms of responsibility, when a group does not accept responsibility for the solution, or when the decision will have relatively little impact.

Minority Decisions

Minority decisions occur when a few people or a subgroup of the larger group involved in a situation meet to consider the matter and make a decision. When a group decides that minority decisions are appropriate, expectations must be clearly articulated between the individual or group delegating the responsibility and the minority or subset of the group accepting the responsibility. The decision of the minority group is considered binding for everyone involved.

This approach is often used by teams and large employee groups. A subset of the team examines an issue and makes a decision for the team; this can be a very effective method of decision making when it is difficult for a larger group to come together and take the time to navigate the entire process together. It requires a high level of trust within the team or group. Team members with a vested interest in the decision are expected to be part of the subset and are not allowed to sabotage the decision later. This is often the type of decision making represented by a department or employee council.

Majority Decisions

When more than half of the people involved in a situation make a decision, it is considered a majority decision and is often referred to as a majority rules vote. The resulting decision is binding on all. This type of decision is problematic because it often means that some of the members do not support the result.

A significant disadvantage to majority decision making is that it forces people to take one side or the other. Often the best solutions are found somewhere in the middle. The more firmly one argues for a cer-tain side or solution, the less likely he or she will be to support an opposing solution if it wins. This form of decision making can be use-ful when the decisions involve minor issues that do not require 100 percent support to implement or when large numbers of people are involved and there is no forum or structure for resolving minority positions.

Consensus Decisions

A consensus decision results when the entire group or team addresses a problem with all group members, who fully present their views. Con-sensus is said to exist when each group or team member can honestly make these three statements to every other member (Creative Health-care Management 1994):

- I believe I understand your point of view.
- I believe you understand my point of view.
- I believe the decision has been made in an open and fair man-ner, and I am willing to support the decision whether or not it's my first preference.

In true consensus, no majority rules voting, bargaining, or averaging of votes is allowed. The process takes more time to achieve but results in active support and prevents sabotage and undermining of decisions made. A colleague describes consensus as 90 percent agreement and 10 percent support. Consensus is especially useful when full team or group commit-ment to the decision is essential for implementation. In an organization, for example, major decisions such as whether to embark upon a major cultural change initiative or to purchase another facility should be decided by consensus of the entire executive team. If the decision is made in any other manner, support may not be present during imple-mentation, when it is required from the entire team.

Unanimous Decisions

In a unanimous decision, when each group member fully agrees on the action to be taken, there is a higher level of commitment. This may be needed when the decision significantly affects each member.

Process of Decision Making

Although group decision making generally results in a higher level of commitment to the decision than does individual decision making, the group decision-making process is also more complex, and arriving at a final decision can be more difficult. Managers and/or group leaders are usually responsible for deciding whether to use an individual or a group decision-making process. At a minimum, the following five factors should be considered:

- **The nature of the problem or task:** Some problems are more easily solved by a group and others by an individual. In creating a new alternative or doing independent tasks, individuals often surpass groups. A project such as creating a new crossword puzzle is a good example. When tasks are convergent or integrative and require that various pieces of information be brought together to produce a solution (such as solving that crossword puzzle), then a group is better. Most goal setting is also more effective in a group because it increases the variety of contributions and level of commitment.
- **The importance of acceptance of a solution:** When people participate in the process of reaching a decision, they have more commitment to the decision. They work harder and have a greater interest in making the decision successful. When an individual solves a problem or makes a decision, two things must happen: Others must be persuaded that this decision is best, and others must agree to act on the decision to carry it out. Not all decisions require commitment, and such decisions can be made by an individual.
- **The value placed on the quality of the decision:** If a manager is concerned with acceptance of a decision and with empowering others, he or she may adopt a decision of somewhat lesser quality because it has widespread acceptance. Decisions made by a group in the beginning of their skill development simply may not have the same quality as an experienced individual's decisions. If the quality of the decision is paramount, an individual expert in the field might be used. For example, if a group is having internal communication problems, it may produce and decide on the problem-solving alternatives to implement. If the outcomes are not beneficial, the group can then engage in additional problem solving. Getting it right the first time is not critical. However, if there are significant computer hardware problems with a particular application that could significantly affect the organization's information systems, a decision to bring in an external expert to solve the problem or make recommendations may be the prudent choice.

- **The characteristics of individual group members:** Effective managers consider the expertise of the various group members, the stake each has in the outcome, and the role each is likely to play in implementing the decision.
- **The operating effectiveness of the group:** It may be a better choice to ask an individual to solve a problem or make a decision than a group that is too new to make the decision or who cannot seem to work together. The skills of the group facilitator have an impact as well.

On the upside, group decision making represents greater total knowledge and information. Each group member brings a different perspective, resulting in a greater variety of approaches. Group decisions may have better acceptance and fewer communication problems. Implementation is likely to be smoother and to require less monitoring.

On the downside, there can be strong social pressure to conform in a group setting. Groups also tend to err on the side of quick convergence, perhaps settling prematurely on a decision that seems to have support. High-quality ideas introduced late in the discussion have a limited chance of serious consideration. A dominant individual can prevail because of status, verbal skills, or stubborn persistence. Hidden agendas create problems in group decision making. Unless these are surfaced, they result in skewed and sometimes unfair or poor decisions. A significant problem for group decision making is that it simply takes longer for a group to decide.

Common Pitfalls in the Decision-Making Process

One of the most significant pitfalls in the decision-making process is related to the paradox of choice. Author Barry Schwartz says that we all suffer from choice overload. Never before in human history have we had so many choices and never before have people been more dissatisfied (Schwartz 2004). Rather than exhaustively examining every alternative and every aspect of every alternative before making a decision, in order to arrive at the very best choice, Schwartz encourages people to be satisfied with a "good enough" decision. In his experience Schwartz found that there are "maximizers" and "satisficers" in terms of their decision making. Maximizers are those who expect the very best and search diligently and endlessly to find it. Satisficers, on the other hand, make a decision first about whether the issue is important enough to undertake such exhausting and endless research, and if it is not, they accept a good-enough choice and then relax and enjoy it. They save themselves a great deal of time, worry, and stress in the process of choosing. He found that maximizers often do get a little more, but they are less happy than the satisficers.

Another common decision-making pitfall is approaching decisions without due consideration of the various types of decision making. Without careful analysis of the situation or sufficient thought given to outcomes, a manager may miss opportunities for effectively engaging others in the decision. Employees can fall into the same trap. There are appropriate occasions for all types of decision making, but if employees expect to participate and reach consensus and the manager is making an individual decision, the employees' expectations will not be met.

For example, in one urgent care business, Ellen, the chief executive officer, decided to reorganize and restructure the leadership and management ranks. Several managers were furious because they were not included in any discussion but were instead simply told what the new structure would be. Ellen elected to make an individual decision, which was her right as the chief executive officer. Unfortunately, however, she had been preaching empowerment for some months, and her individual decision was seen as a slap in the face to those who were committed to building empowerment in the company. An open discussion about how decisions would be made and which were to be individual and which were to be group decisions may have prevented some of these hard feelings.

The third common pitfall is a lack of understanding of consensus. Consensus, like empowerment, has become an overused buzzword in recent years. Some people mistake participatory decision making (where the leader gets input from members, but then a small group or an individual actually makes the decision) as consensus. Consensus is first and foremost a group decision-making process. If a decision truly needs to be made by consensus, there can be no assumption that the conditions of mutual belief, understanding, and support have been met. Because reticent or disagreeing group members may not come forward or openly oppose the decision, the leader needs to ask each member of the group to openly state his or her commitment to the decision.

For example, a statewide ad hoc committee, whose task it was to recommend a new organizational structure for the state association, spent long hours debating this hot political issue. When the group finally settled on a recommendation, the leader asked for consensus.

Every group member was individually asked: "Do you believe you understood everyone else's point of view? Do you believe your point of view was fully expressed and understood by the others? Can you support this decision?" Each participant stated his or her agreement. At the annual meeting, however, one of the committee members had second thoughts when he realized that representatives from a special interest group of which he was also a member were upset about the committee's final recommendation. This member began talking with key association members, trying to engender support for an alternative and basically undermining the committee's work. During a public discussion of the issue, the committee chairman reminded association members that the recommendation had been reached by consensus, and he reviewed exactly what consensus means. When reminded that he had agreed to support the decision of the committee, the individual ceased his efforts to overturn the recommendations.

Not carefully considering the various factors in group versus individual decision making can be another major pitfall for a manager. A healthy combination of the two is important. In some instances, it is also appropriate to explain why one or the other is used.

Decision making is closely related to problem solving but involves its own special issues. Exemplary leaders and managers are good decision makers, but they also are able to relinquish control and engage others in decision making when circumstances warrant. Shared decision making can strengthen any organization as long as it follows careful consideration. Understanding and applying the four key concepts of empowerment (capability, responsibility, authority, and accountability) can help make shared decision making successful.

Appreciative Inquiry Skills

An alternative approach to traditional problem solving or process improvement methodology is a form of action research referred to as appreciative inquiry. Appreciative inquiry is based on the belief that something is already working well in the organization. Finding it and studying what is working well can lead not only to a deeper understanding, but also to insight into how to overcome the current difficulties and design a more desirable future.

It is well known in the research world that what we dwell on increases in our life. It follows then that focusing on problems is an approach that simply brings more problems or difficulties. To appreciate suggests that we hold something as positive, we see the positive traits or characteristics, and this increases its value, much as our homes appreciate in value over the years. Appreciative inquiry is based on gen-erative learning:

> An ability to see radical possibilities beyond the boundaries of problems as they present themselves in conventional terms. High-performing organizations that engage in generative, innovative learning are competent at appreciating potential and possibility. They surpass the limitations of apparently "reasonable" solutions and consider rich possibilities not foreseeable within conventional analysis (Barrett 1995, p. 37).

Traditional Problem Solving and Appreciative Inquiry

Traditional problem solving often involves looking back at our failures and trying to discover the causes. In contrast, appreciative inquiry involves inquiry into our successes so we can discover the distinctive attributes we can use to build upon performance and create new strate-gic approaches. Traditional problem solving is a more mechanized approach based on the belief that problems can be isolated, broken down into separate parts, repaired, and then restored to wholeness. As an approach it often totally misses the systems implications. And, in the same way that one can dissect the body and learn about it even at the smallest cellular level, we have yet to discover the true essence of the person, the soul or the personality, that really makes each of us who we are. In the same way, problem solving often misses the essence of a situation.

Problem solving is likely to be more effective in dealing with issues that are process improvement oriented, such as tackling the issue of inaccurate radiology requisitions or extended wait times for patients in the emergency department. Appreciative inquiry works well for issues related to less logical and methodical processes, such as changing the work culture. In some instances, a major issue might include both approaches. Improving extended patient wait times in the emergency department is an example of an issue that has both specific process improvement opportunities as well as needed cultural changes.

Proponents of appreciative inquiry point out that there are many consequences of using a problem-solving approach, including:

- **Problem solving is a limiting approach to the issue.** Often we accept the constraints of the status quo, which leads to coping with a problem rather than fixing it. Take, for example, the problem of a very high patient census and the potential need for diverting patients from the emergency department to another facility in town. Employees in one hospital were asked what they would do if the other emergency department in the city was also on divert. They were absolutely stymied and could come up with no solutions. When asked about setting a limit on elective admissions to ensure that there were beds available for emergency admissions, the employees found the idea inconceivable because they felt administration would never consider such an approach. Yet it is a solution, just not a popular one. And until something is really done to create a different scenario for these people, all of their planning is based on coping strategies for dealing with an untenable situation. At what point does it become riskier to continue to admit patients when there are not enough resources to provide for their safe care?

- **Problem solving is based on an overlearned deficiency orientation.** The assumption is that there is something wrong somewhere. Managers develop self-worth as problem solvers and so do executives. Thus, the more problems, the more important I am! This can lead to the dysfunctional behavior that occurs when we see individuals who actually seem to be "stirring the pot" or creating problems because solving crises is what they do best!
- **Problem solving is based on a fragmented view of the world.** People in the organization become more and more expert in smaller parts of the system. Along the way it is easy to lose our ability to see the system as a whole and to understand the interdependencies and the intricate connections that exist.

Ludema, Cooperrider, and Barrett (2000) sum up the consequences of an organizational focus on problem solving quite well:

> As people in organizations inquire into their weaknesses and deficiencies, they gain an expert knowledge of what is "wrong" with their organizations, and they may even become proficient problem-solvers, but they do not strengthen their collective capacity to imagine and build better futures (Ludema, Cooperrider, and Barrett 2000, p. 8).

In health care today one of the most important organizational tasks is the creation of learning cultures (Tichy and Cardwell 2002). An appreciative learning culture allows employees to explore and to extend their capabilities and experiment at the very margins of their expertise and knowledge. This serves to improve our ability to meet our mission: high-quality care for patients and clients.

Process of Appreciative Inquiry

Although there is no cookie-cutter approach to appreciative inquiry, there are several general principles and stages that have been identified. One of the most important principles is that the leader or group needs to form a positive question or statement of the topic. This is the most critical part of the entire process because it serves as an intervention in and of itself (Zemke 1999). Although it sounds easy enough to accomplish, in truth, most people when faced with a difficult issue or challenge tend to focus on the negative and to create a problem-oriented question. Take, for example, the need to improve physician and employee interpersonal relationships and communication. The tendency is to identify this issue as a "need to improve physician-employee working relationships." Inherent in this statement is the message that there is something wrong at the current time, and it carries with it complex baggage such as the unequal positional power of physicians and employees or the difference between employees and independent practitioners.

The challenge is to create questions that "inspire and encourage people to give . . . positive examples to use as models" (Zemke 1999, p. 29). So asking people in the organization a question such as, "What examples of positive working relationships between employees and physicians do you see in the organization?" and then further exploring the characteristics of these relationships, "What makes these relationships work so well?" Or another approach would be to ask people to "describe what it is like when you have a good working relationship with a physician (or with an employee)." If the topic is not affirmative, the initiative will fail.

The stages of appreciative inquiry are illustrated in figure 8-13. They include discovery, dreaming, design, and destiny.

Stage 1: Discovery
The first stage in the process is often referred to as the appreciating phase, and it involves storytelling. It is a very collaborative stage. Participants think of examples and experiences that illustrate or answer the appreciative question and share them. They focus on those moments of excellence and identify the factors and characteristics that made them possible. This stage basically answers the question, "What gives life?" From this work it is possible to build consensus around the strengths or basic principles inherent in the issue.

For example, one organization was concerned about creating a more positive work environment in order to attract and better retain

Figure 8-13. Stages of Appreciative Inquiry

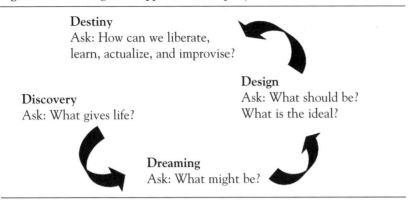

Destiny
Ask: How can we liberate,
learn, actualize, and improvise?

Design
Ask: What should be?
What is the ideal?

Discovery
Ask: What gives life?

Dreaming
Ask: What might be?

employees. They used an appreciative inquiry approach. The questions from this first stage were: "Think of a time when you felt most energized and alive at work. What was happening? Who was there? Describe the workplace environment." Some of the answers included:

- I felt valued.
- I was learning a new skill.
- My manager coached me so I could build my expertise.
- I was involved in helping make the decision.
- There was progress as a result of our actions.
- What I did made a difference.
- I liked the people I was working with.
- We had a great team.
- I was asked my opinion, and it was used in making the final decision.
- I had a high level of autonomy.

From this first step, a list of positive attributes was developed to describe these environments.

Stage 2: Dreaming
The second stage is the dreaming stage and is also known as the envisioning phase. The basic question is: "What might be?" This stage often starts off with an exercise such as: "Let's assume that tonight we fall asleep and wake up five years from now. When you wake up, the hospital has become exactly the organization you would like it to be. What do you see that is different and how do you know it is different?" (Zemke 1999, p. 30). The result of this stage is that the group comes

to some kind of coalescence around a vision for the group or the orga-nization and drafts a statement of what it will look like in the future. Based on the previous example, a vision statement might be something like: "Our workplace environment is one in which there are healthy working relationships between people, there is a high level of employee involvement in decision making, and where people are treated with respect and valued for their contributions."

This stage is similar to the visioning approach used by strong leaders (Manion 2005). It is not merely a dream, but a vision that is grounded in history, tradition, and facts. It is based on examples of what has worked.

Stage 3: Design
The third stage in appreciative inquiry is also referred to as the cocon-structing phase because the work is to design the ideal. Questions include: "What will it look like? What are the principles that will help translate this vision into action? How can we make this happen?" Many successful books in the business literature use this approach. Organizations or businesses that are successful are studied carefully to determine the principles that led to their success, and then the princi-ples are shared with others, who attempt to emulate them.

A disadvantage of trying to duplicate another organization's suc-cesses is the resistance often encountered, because no other organiza-tion or business is exactly like ours. The differences are often used as explanations for why it cannot be done. One of the advantages of using an appreciative inquiry approach within the organization is that it takes away this rationalization or excuse. For example, if this positive environment can be created in the imaging department, why can it not be done in the laboratory? After all, similar financial constraints exist, the medical staff is basically the same, community issues are shared, and so on.

Stage 4: Destiny
The fourth stage is also known as the sustaining phase, and the ques-tions focus around "How can we liberate, learn, actualize and improve?" The work of the participants focuses on how to actualize, sustain, or create these characteristics. Zemke (1999) notes that originally this stage stood for delivery and the work was focused on developing action plans, building implementation strategies, and monitoring outcomes. This concrete structured process has since been greatly deemphasized by Cooperrider and his colleagues in favor of more spontaneous, free-form sorts of activities. In other words, simply preparing people in the

organization with the process of the first three steps and then letting them apply them on their own in the organization has been successful in many different types of businesses around the world.

The end result of an appreciative inquiry process depends on the topic that started the cycle. It may be a culture change or the development of a vision and plan to be worked.

Polarity Management Skills

Still another skill set is needed to deal with challenges in getting our work accomplished. In some instances, the issue or difficulty we are dealing with is not a problem as such, but rather what Barry Johnson calls a polarity. "Polarities are sets of opposites which can't function well independently. Because the two sides of a polarity are interdependent, you cannot choose one as a solution and neglect the other" (Johnson 1996, p. xviii). Believing that everything we face is a problem results in trying to solve some problems that are simply unsolvable, even if you had all the necessary resources. By seeing polarities as problems to be solved, we greatly undermine ourselves by wasting time in futile efforts. There are many examples of polarities in our health care organizations today:

- When are leadership skills rather than management skills needed?
- When do we emphasize individual effort versus team initiative?
- When does the manager perform difficult tasks rather than coaching others on how to do them?
- When is a manager's accessibility and visibility more important than the manager's need for thinking time and privacy?
- When does the implementation of policies require rigidity and when does it require flexibility?
- When do we place a priority on the needs of employees versus the needs of patients?
- When do we need to emphasize service at any cost versus cost-effectiveness and wise use of resources?
- When do we need commitment versus when is compliance adequate?
- When is specialization of employees and physicians more appropriate than generalization?
- When is centralization of services more appropriate than decentralization?

If any of these polarities are seen as problems to be solved, we waste our efforts. There are no clear-cut solutions to these issues.

Polarity Management versus Problem Solving

Johnson's (1996) approach involves identifying when the issue is actually a polarity and managing it as such rather than treating the situation as a problem to be solved. "The objective of polarity management is to get the best of both opposites while avoiding the limits of each" (Johnson 1996, p. xviii). In other words, the manager has the judgment to reward both individual and team effort and understands that in any modern organizational system, there is not only room for both models, but a need for both. In some instances, the work is individually based while in other situations a team is much more effective. Overemphasis on either end of the polarity can result in problems.

The way to manage a polarity, Johnson suggests, is through using a grid, or polarity map, with two poles. (See figure 8-14.) The left half represents one side of the polarity, and the right half represents the other side. The upper half represents the positive outcomes that focus on the particular pole, and the lower half represents the negative outcomes that

Figure 8-14.   The Polarity Map (Johnson 1996)

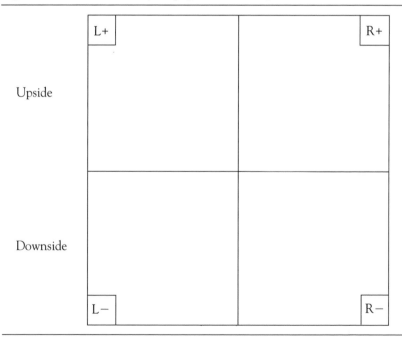

come from focusing only on that pole. Before you can effectively manage a polarity, you have to be able to see all four quadrants of the polarity grid. He suggests filling out whichever quadrants are the easiest first and then working from there.

In figures 8-15 and 8-16, polarity maps are drawn to represent the four quadrants of an issue faced by a respiratory care department in a large tertiary medical center. The pediatric respiratory therapists included those respiratory therapists assigned to general pediatrics and those who were neonatal intensive care unit respiratory therapists. Conflict arose periodically over the years about the issue of specialization versus generalization among these practitioners. The neonatologists and pediatricians were often in direct conflict with each other as well as with the manager and employees of the department about the issue. Over the years, the emphasis moved back and forth. When this issue is examined as a polarity, the underlying issue is identified as determining whether patient needs or employee needs are paramount.

Figure 8-15. Polarity Map: Patients' Needs versus Employees' Needs (Johnson 1996)

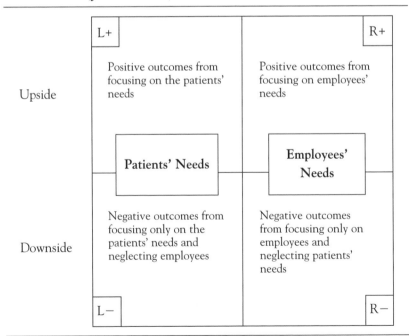

	L+ Positive outcomes from focusing on the patients' needs	R+ Positive outcomes from focusing on employees' needs
Upside		
	Patients' Needs	**Employees' Needs**
Downside	Negative outcomes from focusing only on the patients' needs and neglecting employees	Negative outcomes from focusing only on employees and neglecting patients' needs
	L−	R−

Figure 8-16.   Respiratory Therapist Example: Putting Patients' Needs First or Employees' Needs First

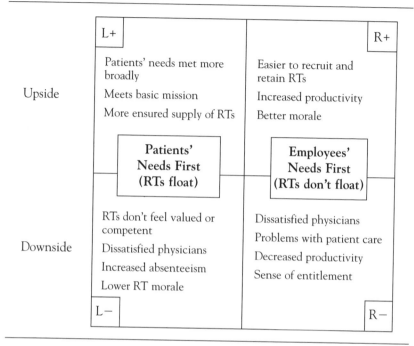

Mapping this polarity enables you to see the whole picture or structure of the dilemma. To focus exclusively on patients' needs may result in important employees' needs not being met, which may then result in lower morale and productivity, indirectly affecting whether patients' needs are met. The clearest opposites in the polarity map are the downside of one polarity and the upside of the other. Johnson calls movement through the grid the polarity two-step (Johnson 1996, p. 11). It starts in either lower quadrant and moves across, up, and down, and then it is repeated.

The difficulty in dealing with polarities occurs because the parties involved are convinced that they are right in their particular conviction and they basically see only their perception. Working the group through the polarity map helps illustrate the whole picture. Instead of disagreeing parties contradicting each other's view, the task becomes supplementing each other's view in order to see the entire picture. Parties on both sides of the polarity have key pieces to the puzzle; they just need this simple structure to help identify and share them. The opposition each side feels to the other actually becomes a key resource in dealing with the issue. No one is being challenged; instead the accuracy of each position is assumed. As a result, there is joint effort in combining two valid views of a situation in order to see a more complete picture.

Johnson (1996, p. 45) says that "in most organizations there are often very serious and costly confrontations that take place because a 'both/and' polarity is treated like an 'either/or' problem to solve." In working out the polarity map together, the possibility of each participant seeing the other quadrants and more fully understanding the issue occurs because their own view of reality has not been contradicted, but confirmed. "Successful management of polarities calls for intentional interventions that support both values (poles) simultaneously" (Wesorick 2002, p. 24).

One of the difficult challenges is knowing when there is a polarity to manage instead of a problem to solve. Johnson (1996) offers two questions to use for help in distinguishing between the two: (1) Is the difficulty ongoing, and (2) are two interdependent poles involved?

If there is a solution that is a definite end point in a process, the problem is solvable. Take, for example, the decision about where to have the holiday party. Once the decision is made, it is done. This is an either/or problem. Either we go here, or we go there. Once the decision is made, it is carried out. Problems of choice are solved the minute the choice is made. In contrast, we are continually engaged in solving polarities. Instead of reaching an end point, there is a never-ending change of emphasis or focus from one pole to another. For example, there are times to emphasize and reward individual performance, and at other times it is appropriate to focus on the team effort.

The second question is whether there are two poles that are interdependent. "The solution in problems to solve can stand alone. Unlike a polarity to be managed, the solution to a problem to solve does not have the necessary opposite that is required for the solution to work over an extended period of time" (Johnson 1996, p. 82). Polarities, instead, require both poles. The issue of manager accessibility to employees is an example. On the one hand, for the manager to be available to employees is an important aspect of the job, and yet there is also the need for the manager to have quiet, uninterrupted time in order to do work that requires concentrated thinking time.

Once the polarity map has been completed, the question is asked, "What do we need to do to stay in the upper two quadrants?" In the previous respiratory care example, how can we meet both the patients' and the employees' needs? How do we know when to shift the focus from one pole to another? The group then has identified actions to support each side of the polarity and is more likely to recognize when overemphasis on either pole occurs in the future.

Conclusion

This chapter examined the relationship between a positive work environment and the manager's focus on results. Models of shared decision making were examined as was the concept of empowerment. Several key processes that are used in obtaining results, specifically the skills of problem solving and decision making, were also presented. Two additional approaches were included to broaden the individual's results-oriented repertoire: the use of appreciative inquiry and polarity management. These skills, especially when combined with the interpersonal skills previously discussed, increase the quality of the work environment for all.

Conversation Points

Organizational Perspective

1. Is there an established continuous quality process in your organization? How widely is it used? What results does it produce?
2. Are problems actually being solved in the organization, or do you continue to recycle them (dealing with the same old problems year after year)?
3. Is there a formalized structure for shared decision making in the organization? What is it called, and how effective is it?
4. Do employees and managers feel empowered to make necessary decisions about their work? Is there an emphasis on hierarchical decision making? (that is, I take it to my boss, who takes it to his boss, who takes it to her boss?)
5. Is decision making bogged down in the organization, or is it timely and conducted at the lowest levels possible?
6. Where have you used appreciative inquiry in the organization? Have there been any change initiatives undertaken or issues resolved using the underlying principles of appreciative inquiry?
7. What are key polarities we deal with on a regular basis?

Leadership Issues

1. What are typical system or department problems you deal with currently? Do you regularly use problem-solving groups in your department? How effective are they?
2. Do employees from your department participate in organizational decision-making groups? What process do they use?
3. Think of the different types of decision making (majority vote, consensus, individual, and so on) and identify examples of each you see in your work environment.
4. How could you use appreciative inquiry to deal with issues you are facing?
5. What are common polarities you see in your workplace?
6. Have polarities been mistaken for problems? How could you use the polarity grid for achieving more effective results?

Employee Challenges

1. Are you better with right-brain (spontaneous, creative, free-flowing) thinking or left-brain (logical, analytical, and methodical) thinking? What about your work group? What is the impact on the effectiveness of your problem-solving efforts?
2. Do you serve on a department council, task force, or problem-solving group? How effective is the group? Do you follow a problem-solving process, or is it pretty loose and spontaneous?
3. Do you feel empowered in your decision making? What are examples of decisions you have a level four authority to make? How about level one?
4. How comfortable or familiar are you with the skills of appreciative inquiry and polarity management? Do you see any issues in your workplace where these approaches might be helpful?

9

Creating an Innovative Work Culture

Jo Manion

Unimpeded on a daily basis by the concern for survival,
free from the generalized assumption of scarcity,
a person stands in the great space of possibility in a posture
of openness, with an unfettered imagination for what can be.
—Rosamund S. and Benjamin Zander (2000)

A POSITIVE working environment is one in which the people who work there are able to see results as an outcome of their efforts. As discussed in chapter 8, a focus on results requires a workplace in which employees enjoy a high level of autonomy and decision-making authority. Employees are skilled decision-makers and problem-solvers. The leadership philosophy is one characterized by managers who seek to understand the problems and difficulties employees face and who continually seek improvements in work processes. The creation of a workplace environment in which innovation is not only encouraged but expected is critical to achieving results.

Health care organizations characterized by encouragement and support of innovation are certainly more likely to have a strong, viable future. Creativity and innovation are hallmarks of the most successful health care organizations in the country today. "Nothing is more risky than not innovating, with the possible exception of confusing innovation with something that fails to create value" (Hattori and Wycoff 2002, p. 25). To successfully navigate the chaos of today's business environment, the successful health care organization must be able to tap into the creative potential of its employees.

In health care today, we face a critical choice: innovate and change or expect to be replaced by organizations that do. It becomes a choice between gradual decline and eventual demise or transformation. Because health care is a mature industry, transformation is more difficult than it seems. "Although the 20th century can be remembered as the most active age for health innovation, the 21st century promises even more technical creativity and service transformation" (Porter-O'Grady 2003, p. 31). In his essay on the consequences of innovation, Ellis (2004) notes that every passing day brings innovations that seem almost more like science fiction. Examples include the regeneration of limbs and organs in human beings; the implantation of computer-assisted telepathy devices that help the disabled control their environments; the development of injectable DNA computers able to detect cancer and then produce custom drugs to treat it; and the development of gene therapies that may eliminate illnesses such as diabetes and Alzheimer's. The list goes on and on, but one conclusion is clear: Maintaining the status quo is simply not an option.

Successful innovation is not magic, and it is not something that happens spontaneously. Organizations with a track record of successful innovation understand that innovation must be managed. Innovation management requires the application of a developmental process that does not happen overnight. To succeed in innovation management, employees as well as leaders need to have a clear idea of the relationship between creativity and innovation, and they also need to be skilled implementers of ideas.

The successful organizations establish an internal climate that supports entrepreneurial activity and goes beyond paying lip service to the idea of innovation and employee intrapreneurship. They recognize that innovation must be systematic, organized, and managed for it to have a significant and widespread impact on the organization's outcomes. Innovation is expected and encouraged in the organization, and it is assumed to be a part of the work to be done rather than something that happens in addition to the real work of employees (Manion 1990). Established mechanisms for disseminating innovations are in place, and people are expected to implement new ideas.

Employee innovation and empowerment are closely related. Individuals must be empowered before innovation can occur on a systematic basis. However, some individuals who are empowered in their daily work activities may not accept the responsibility for innovation. Some people simply are not interested in being innovators. In some cases, the individual may not have the specific skills needed. For others, a traditional, bureaucratic system may place so many barriers to innovation that the individuals do not even try to be innovative.

Innovation can be undertaken by anyone in the organization. Some of the most effective innovations are developed by people who know the organization at its core. First-line employees who form the core of any health care organization are in a position to be essential innovators. On the one hand, employees who are intimately connected with the work know it better than anyone else. On the other hand, being too close to the work or having done the same work over a long period of time sometimes makes it more difficult for us to find new and different ways to carry it out. In addition, the academic backgrounds and experience of most clinicians and support workers did not emphasize innovation, and so they lack innovation skills such as creativity, business planning, intrapreneurship, and change management. Most health care workers have been socialized to their work roles in bureaucratic, hierarchical organizations whose structure alone intimidates the novice innovator. In addition, few health care organizations have had extensive experience in implementing successful and sustained innovations.

Creativity and Innovation

Innovation is the key to transformation of the health care organization and the health care system. Creativity involves thinking up new ideas or putting things together in a new way; innovation is the implementation of the new or creative idea. Innovation has been described as applied creativity, which implies that something has changed as a result of the creativity. Having a good idea is only the first step; actually converting the idea to a new reality that is useful is much more difficult. So, creativity involves thinking up new ideas, while innovation involves doing new things. If ideas are not implemented, they are useless. There is no shortage of creative ideas or creative people; there is, however, a shortage of successful innovators. Creativity does not automatically lead to innovation. It takes an individual or even several individuals with the know-how, energy, courage, and persistence to implement a creative idea. The old saying that creativity is 1 percent inspiration and 99 percent perspiration is true. Creativity is hard work more than it is genius.

Innovation is the transformation of the ideas into something of value that can be used in some way. The innovation may be a new product, service, or process. It may be as small as a simple change in the work processes of a department or team or as large as the development of a new service or the invention of a new product. Managers and executives experience more success in their roles when employees are skillful implementers of new ideas.

Many people mistakenly equate creativity with artistic talent, and so they conclude that they are not creative. Yet, creativity has been defined as a process that results in a new combination of attributes, elements, or images, as something that gives rise to new patterns, arrangements, or products that better serve a need (Raudsepp 1981). Creativity is largely the result of putting together old ideas in a new way, a technique at which any of us can increase our skill.

For those interested in learning more about creativity techniques, a wealth of resources are available through internet bookstores. Including such resources as part the organization's or department's library creates immediate accessibility to the wide variety of possibilities. Chapter 8 described several creativity techniques in the context of problem solving. In addition, some health care organizations are looking outside the industry for assistance in managing innovation and creativity, and consulting firms can bring refreshing new ways of approaching opportunities. One example is IDEO, a self-described product design and innovation strategy firm that is teaching the art of innovation to major hospital systems (Weber 2003).

In *Weird Ideas That Work: 11½ Practices for Promoting, Managing, and Sustaining Innovation*, Stanford professor Robert Sutton offers suggestions for how to generate and capitalize on new ideas. Several of his ideas may sound a bit strange, but his underlying message is clear: Innovation is not a process that is comfortable in most hierarchical, traditional bureaucracies. He says that if you want to fill your organization with good ideas, the first step is to fill it with good people. Here are some of Sutton's (2003) additional suggestions:

1. Hire slow learners of the organizational code, that is, people who ignore the way things are usually done and find their own way of doing things.
2. Hire people who make you uncomfortable, even those you dislike, and then take special care to listen to their ideas.
3. Hire people you probably do not need. Sutton's point here is to hire people with skills that the organization may not need at the moment and then ask these people how they can help you.
4. Use job interviews to get new ideas, not to just screen candidates. Give job applicants problems you have not been able to solve, and then listen as much as you can and talk as little as possible.

5. Encourage people to ignore their boss and peers. Hire defiant outsiders and encourage people to drive you crazy by doing what they think is right rather than what they are told to do.
6. Find happy people and let them fight. "If you want innovation, you need upbeat people who know the right way to battle. Avoid conflict during the earliest stages of the creative process, but encourage people to fight over ideas in the intermediate stages" (LaBarre 2002, p. 72).

These recommendations are echoed by Berwick (2003, p. 1973), who points out that "innovators will not be the easiest individuals to deal with in their organization; they may be abrasive, not invested in local networks, and demanding of latitude." All of this advice sounds straightforward enough, but when you consider what it would be like to have one or two employees with these traits in your work group, you probably start worrying. Abrasive, disruptive people (even if they are creative) are not tolerated in most organizations and are seen as trouble-makers who need to be controlled or eliminated. If health care organizations want to support innovation to any great extent, however, our organizational cultures will need to change to accommodate people who would otherwise be considered troublemakers in traditional organizations.

Innovation Management

A specific process for creating a culture of innovation in the system is useful for leaders in health care organizations who are attempting to encourage or beginning to demand more innovation from employees and colleagues. This innovation management process is helpful whether the scope includes the whole organization or just one department. Kao reports that he often hears people in health care organizations say that innovation is of great importance, and yet they admit that they are not sure where to start or how to do it.

The issue is not whether people are creative but what happens when you try to organize creativity, to weave creativity into the daily life of a system, a team, or an organization. In the traditional industrial model of efficiency and operational excellence, organizations are especially good at taking the risk and uncertainty out of people's work, so that they can perform in a predictable and quantitatively comparable way (Flower 1999, p. 15).

A process for creating a culture of innovation is also useful for giving guidance to organizational leaders who manage the process of unfolding and implementing specific innovations.

The five-stage process for managing innovation is based on an energy model adapted for organizations by Nancy Post, an organizational development consultant (Post 1989, 1993). The framework has also been used for guidance in managing energy in an organization (Manion 1993, 1994; Cox, Manion, and Miller 2005).

The five stages of innovation management are preparation, movement, synergy, the new reality, and integration. In each stage, there are specific functions that must be fulfilled and/or specific issues that must be considered. During preparation, the issues to be managed are clarity and relevancy of mission or purpose and adequacy and allocation of resources. During the second stage, structural issues such as decision making, authority levels, planning, and organizational structure are considerations. Synergy, the third stage, involves the issues of overall coordination and cooperation, priority setting, networking, climate setting, and internal communications. During the fourth stage, the new reality, productivity and the maintenance of the change are key considerations. Integration, the final phase, requires attention to quality and evaluative efforts. (See figure 9-1.)

Figure 9-1.   Five-Stage Innovation Management Model (Manion 1993)

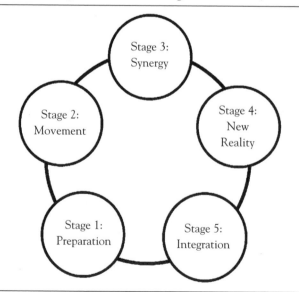

The five stages can be used as a model for balance as well as a developmental model. This means the key elements in each stage must be considered fully. When all of the issues in each stage are not addressed fully, the stage is deficient or weak, and an imbalance in the system results. Imbalances have an impact on the effectiveness of innovation management in the organization and can impair the implementation of a specific innovation. Similarly, an overemphasis on the characteristics or issues of any single stage will also result in a system imbalance. For example, in stage 1, the mission of the department as it relates to innovation and expectations for innovation from employees must match the level of resources available, or there will be dissonance and disruption. When the mission clearly states that innovation is an important organizational value, then it follows that employees and leaders will be given the resource of time in order to focus on innovation.

As noted earlier, this model is also a developmental model, and as such, it is sequential in nature. Following these stages in sequence can aid the leader in managing the process of innovation. However, the model is also interactive and dynamic. The primary issues in each stage are identified and considered sequentially, although the issues of one stage can also appear and are appropriate to consider throughout the entire cycle. For example, although evaluation is a key element of the final stage, evaluation must also occur during the entire process, not just at the end, when it is of primary importance. Figure 9-2 shows the five stages of the process with a summary of the key issues in each stage.

Stage 1: Preparation

In the first stage, preparation, purpose and allocation of resources must be considered and managed. This stage is the foundation for the rest of the process. It is primarily leader driven and the responsibility of executives and teams of internal leaders. Allocation of resources often requires management's involvement, especially when the organization is experiencing a reduction in available resources and budgets are tight.

Simply stated, innovation must be an important element of the organization's and department's mission and a part of the everyday language before it can be accepted as a value. The organization's leaders need to believe, and act on the belief, that innovation is a priority before employees will behave as though innovation is a desirable achievement. The relationship of innovation to patient care and customer service must be clearly stated and demonstrated. Not only is it important for members of the leadership team to speak the language of innovation, they must also communicate the expectation for innovation to employees. This can be further emphasized by inclusion of the

Figure 9-2.   Innovation Stages with Key Functions (Manion 1993)

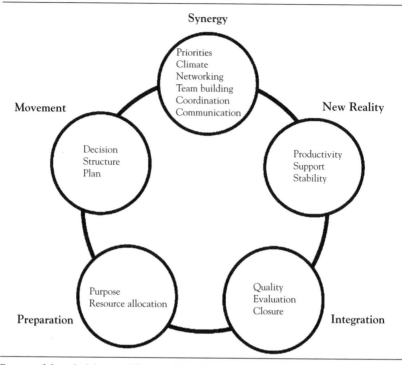

Synergy

Priorities
Climate
Networking
Team building
Coordination
Communication

Movement   New Reality

Decision   Productivity
Structure   Support
Plan   Stability

Purpose   Quality
Resource allocation   Evaluation
                                  Closure
Preparation   Integration

goal for innovation in the organization's and department's annual goals, performance appraisal process, and position descriptions. The challenge for organizational leaders, says John Kao, is "to create a context in which people understand exactly why innovation is important, and how important it is to balance the creative and the operational imperatives" (Flower 1999, p. 15).

In this first stage, the complementary issue is the adequacy and allocation of resources, including human and material resources. Adequate resources must be available when innovation is an expected part of the work of the organization. Resources include far more than mere financial resources. The first stage must consider, in addition to funding, the amount of time available, access to other stakeholders, and personal development time. It is difficult to expect people to work on innovative projects wholeheartedly in addition to carrying a full work schedule. Although enthusiastic employees are often committed enough to do so, it is an abuse of the human resources of the organization to expect this additional commitment on a long-term or continual basis. People will be used up quickly. Mentors and sponsors must be readily accessible in the organization or department as support for the innovator. Sharing resources among departments and work groups increases the environmental support for innovation.

In some instances, the organization's human resources need further development. The skills of leaders and clinical and support staff should be carefully assessed to determine the need for educational opportunities. Managers should be prepared for their roles as innovation managers. Individual innovators need educational programs or opportunities that focus on innovation and the skills needed by a successful innovator. All of the members of the organization benefit from general programs that focus on the need for innovation, essential skills, and their role in supporting coworkers who are innovators. Another important aspect of preparing people for innovation is helping them to keep up-to-date with trends and developments in the health care industry as well as other businesses.

People need to hear the innovation message repeatedly and observe actual behaviors and structural changes that support innovation before they can internalize the message that innovation is desirable and expected. The stated values and mission related to innovation and creativity, as well as the day-to-day language used by leaders, must be congruent with the behavior of leaders. In some instances, changes in the structure of the organization may be needed. It creates dissonance when executives, managers, and leaders continually espouse the need for innovation and yet employees have little to no access to funding for innovative ideas, when new ideas can only be implemented after a tedious and difficult approval process, or when the creative individual who is always searching for a new and better way is treated as a troublemaker who must be controlled. In other words, management behavior must be congruent with the message being delivered.

In terms of an actual innovation, the first stage is the time when the proposed new service, new product, or change is evaluated against the mission of the department or organization. A decision must be made on whether the innovation does indeed support the primary mission and increase our effectiveness in meeting our basic purpose. Take, for example, computerized patient record systems. Ostensibly, the main goals of implementing such a system are to increase the accuracy of clinical documentation and improve the accessibility of patient records. However, many of these systems have also been sold with the implied promise that they would reduce the amount of time clinical practitioners spend documenting the care given to their patients. Yet, first-generation versions of automated documentation systems actually increased the amount of time caregivers spent away from the patient. Only now are we getting to the point where the automated record systems may save time.

The second issue involves an assessment of needed resources against the resources available. Questions include: Are resources adequate? Do people need additional skills or time to implement or use the innovation? If additional resources are needed, how can this best be accomplished? What is the level of support for the innovation?

For example, there are many issues of resource allocation implicit in the development and implementation of computerized patient record systems. First, does the organization have the capital to invest in the extensive and expensive hardware needed to implement such a system? Is there recognition that when these systems are implemented, productivity levels often worsen for a period of time, as people learn the new approaches? Has the additional support required been assessed accurately? Do employees have the necessary computer skills to use the new system?

Examples of the application of these principles abound as a result of the wave of reengineering and work redesign projects in health care during the early to middle 1990s. For many organizations, these efforts were their initial attempt at systemwide innovation. Where the effort was successful, creativity and innovation were clearly linked to the organization's mission and its very reason for existence. Creative ideas were expected from everyone in the organization, and resources were allocated to carry out this important work. Entire teams of individuals were organized to lead the initiative, often referred to as resource or development teams. These teams included reassigned managers and employees who had the specific skills required to complete the work of redesign. Massive amounts of organizational resources were allocated to develop needed skills internally in addition to using external consultants.

Unfortunately, many organizations climbed aboard the reengineering bandwagon without paying attention to preparation issues. Their initiatives were approached as cost-cutting measures, and some organizations used reengineering to justify major changes in skill-mix ratio of caregivers, cross-training of highly skilled practitioners in all disciplines, reduction of managerial positions, and elimination of specialized and centralized departments. A number of these organizations discovered that their innovations did not make it easier to carry out their original mission of serving patients, but instead made it more difficult.

One chief executive officer summed it up by noting that when he eliminated his organization's centralized infusion therapy department, his board of directors was very impressed with the money he had saved in operating costs and gave him kudos. Within months, however, the infection rates climbed and complaints from patients increased. Two years later, when he reinstituted the centralized department, he was hailed as a hero for dealing effectively with these new problems.

If innovation is mishandled and change is not implemented effectively, the organization's resources will be depleted for several reasons. First, the process itself costs money. When the process is mishandled, employee dissatisfaction levels increase and competent employees who are able to find employment elsewhere do. The remaining employees are often left more demoralized, detached, and cynical and less willing to commit to the future initiatives of the organization.

Stage 2: Movement

Once the functions of the first stage have been addressed, an important part of the foundation is in place. People are clear about how innovation supports the purpose of the organization, and innovation is accepted as relevant by employees. The need and expectation for innovation have been consistently communicated, both verbally and through the leaders' behavior. Adequate resources are in place, and employees begin to experience actual support for innovation.

During the second stage, movement, the structural elements supporting innovation throughout the organization or department need to be established. A vision of how the innovation will be carried out and how it will result in changes is critical. When the vision is clear, the structure needed to support that vision follows.

Stage 2 includes planning and decision making. Planning for a structure that supports innovation in the organization and its many departments is critical. "Organizational structures can, in fact, be put in place that provide for a more predictable occurrence of innovation—the successful implementation of a creative idea, or an idea that is both novel and useful" (Gryskiewicz 1999, p. 18). At the organizational level, executive leaders facilitate this planning with participation and input from all levels within the departments. A process for proposing and evaluating new ideas and gaining approval and funding is established. Two separate structures may be needed, one for larger projects that involve integral changes in the organization and substantial funding and a simpler process for ideas with less impact and more modest resource needs.

One approach being used today is the establishment of a center for innovation within the organization. The center provides a structure for building a financial support base that generates revenue and receives gifts. Establishing a specific process for seeking innovative ideas from employees and guidelines for approval and the funding of decisions is part of the work of such a center and supports the work of innovation throughout the system.

Potential innovators often need skill development in the planning function. Some innovative projects are approved with very little planning because they involve a small number of people and do not require additional funding. Formal business planning, however, may be necessary for larger projects that have significant ramifications in the department and organization or require extensive resource commitment. Innovators need support and encouragement in learning how to develop a business plan. Support from other departments such as finance or marketing may be needed. Planning ways for employees to have access to these resources is important.

The complementary issue in this stage of the process is decision making, which is closely intertwined with planning. Decisions must be made as planning is completed. In some organizations, planning and decision making are clearly out of balance. Much time is spent in planning, but the plans are never carried out because actual decisions are not made. Once innovation-supporting structural changes are determined, assignment of responsibility is necessary. How will the process be initiated? Who is responsible? How will levels of authority be decided? Realistic timeframes need to be established for each element of the plan and for communicating the plan to all of the key stakeholders who are affected in any way by the plan. Clear lines of responsibility are identified, and decisions are made regarding appropriate levels of authority for those working on the project.

As the planning is completed, the need for further education and skill development for both managers and employees becomes obvious. Planning skills often need to be developed or strengthened. In addition, there must be recognition that innovation planning is a process, not an end. By its very nature, innovation does not unfold as planned, and there must be support, not just tolerance, for ambiguity, mistakes, and revisions. Visioning and strategizing are key skills for innovators in addition to the basic skills needed to lead groups, conduct effective meetings, and reach consensus-based decision making.

A potentially unexpected reaction from employees and managers sometimes surfaces during this state: anger. Although the anger may not be significant or widespread, it may be present. In establishing a structure and process that supports innovation in a department, the extremely creative individual may see it as stifling rather than liberating. Managers and leaders who have been supportive of the concept of innovation may feel irritated when they realize that successful management of innovation takes time and skill. They may need to develop new and different skills. It is important to see beyond the initial resistance and evaluate whether the established structure supports innovators or stifles their work. Too much rigid structure can inhibit creativity.

The importance of an easy-to-navigate structure that supports innovation cannot be minimized. When the decision-making structure in the organization has what is called a "tendency to no," innovation is stifled. In such structures, every decision must make its way through the decision-making channels before an answer can be rendered. At each step of the way, the proposed idea is dissected and examined for potential risks and faults until the innovator is so frustrated that he or she gives up. The likelihood of support for the idea becomes increasingly slim, and by the time the idea reaches the chief executive officer, front-line employee innovators have lost interest or are bored and demoralized.

Compare this process to how innovation is handled by an entrepreneur. If you are an entrepreneur and have a great innovative idea that requires a substantial outlay of capital, you seek out venture capitalists who are willing to invest. The first one approached may decline the opportunity, sending you on to the next, and so on. Out of seven people you approach, you may find only one who sees the same potential as you do and who is willing to invest in the idea. But all you need is one. Contrast this to the intrapreneur (an entrepreneur who is employed by someone else). You may also have a potentially solid innovation that you pitch to your manager. The manager agrees and talks with her director to obtain approval. The director thinks it is a great idea and takes it forward as does her vice president. In the end, six managers or senior leaders have given the idea their approval, but in the end the chief financial officer may refuse to approve the change because of the level of financial support it requires. The point here is that the entrepreneur deals with six negatives and one positive before the project becomes a go. The intrapreneur has six affirmatives and only one no but the project is dead in the water. This "tendency to no" is one of the true killers of organizational innovation.

This scenario is incredibly frustrating to creative employees to the point that many of them simply leave the system to strike out on

their own. When they stay, what they learn is that it is just too difficult to make significant innovation in our systems. For example, a
nurse, pseudonym Jane, contacted me for advice a few months ago.
Jane had attended a continuing education program where people
were encouraged to look for creative, innovative ways to improve
their workplace environment to help increase retention. On Jane's
return trip she had what she considered a brilliant idea that was very
simple. Instead of using expensive commercial art to line the corri-
dors and conference rooms of the hospital, why not hang pictures of
employees doing their work around the organization? Jane believed it
would be appealing to patients and visitors and it would validate
employees and communicate respect for their work. The photos
might also increase the sense of community in the organization. Jane
brought her digital camera to work one evening and took pictures of
her coworkers, which she added to a simple but attractive proposal.
To her dismay, although she has had wonderful response on the part
of many people, she has been unable to get the project approved. It
has been months since she submitted her proposal, and she is not
even certain where the idea died.

Stage 3: Synergy

After the foundation and structural issues have been dealt with in
stages 1 and 2, things begin to come together. The third stage is
described as exciting, dynamic, and seductive. It is synergy because
the innovators within the organization actually begin using the structure that has been established to support the new approaches. At this
point, it feels as though we are finally on the way. Issues of priority setting, climate, coordination, cooperation, team building, networking,
relationship building, and internal communications must be considered. Each of these issues is an important key, and lack of attention to
any one results in a system out of balance.

   Priority setting is easier when the structure for evaluating and
approving projects is effective. A formal structure facilitates the identification of the projects to be supported in the organization or department during the year. In almost every department, however, there are
many other changes and projects being implemented simultaneously.
A major concern most organizations are experiencing is the need to fix
everything yesterday. Unfortunately, when a system is engaged in too
many projects, it is less likely that any will be managed well. Determining the sequencing of major projects in the system can be difficult,
especially when other important projects are added because of external

demands. Priority setting is the difficult task of determining what is most important to accomplish with the resources available. It does not mean doing everything that needs to be done; it means making the difficult choices between those things that could be done. Priority setting requires extreme honesty by executives and the leadership team and a willingness to refuse to implement projects for which there are inadequate resources.

This process, of course, is easier to say than to do. For example, several years ago I was asked to facilitate a senior leadership team meeting in a client organization. The leaders were exhausted after trying to handle a large number of projects that all demanded their time. The first step involved creating a list of current projects. The first projects ranged from relatively small implementation projects to massive, systemwide initiatives such as merging another hospital into their system, establishing a new and extensive cardiovascular surgery service line, finishing two major construction projects, completing a housewide work redesign project, and implementing a major cultural change in the organization. To their surprise the list of current projects totaled 109! When the leaders were asked to prioritize the projects, they reported that all of the projects were critical for the organization's future viability. It was no wonder that everyone in the organization was exhausted and depleted. In order to tackle this issue in another way, we looked at possibilities for increasing resources to enable them to deal with these projects more effectively. This approach relieved the pressure somewhat as more resources were allocated to support the projects.

Establishing a climate conducive to innovation is a key managerial role. Managers must be prepared and educated about the different elements of climate and group culture and accept responsibility for the climate within their work groups. Managers must see their role as a catalyst (they release the energy of innovators within the staff). The response to mistakes is a major element related to climate. When the system or the individuals within the system have a punitive or blaming response to mistakes, the environment impedes and stifles innovation. Do employees feel comfortable about making mistakes and do they understand that mistake making is inevitable, or do employees want an environment where they don't make mistakes? When making mistakes is accepted as part of work life and as lessons to be learned, people are more likely to be risk takers and successful innovators. Companies whose very survival depends on innovation create a climate that encourages people to come forward with good ideas and to be risk takers. People are not criticized when ideas do not work out as intended or hoped; instead ideas are celebrated for what is learned from them. "Nothing will extinguish the flames of innovation more rapidly than a punitive response to ideas that don't work. Nothing is more reinforcing to creative energy than organizational tolerance for and even support of mistakes. Leaders of innovative organizations understand that the price tag of success includes the misfires" (Beglinger 2003, p. 40). This opinion is echoed by other skilled innovators, who note that successful innovation is not so much about having one good idea; instead, it is about having lots of ideas, many of which fail. And to find "a few ideas that work, you need to try a lot that don't" (LaBarre 2002, p. 70).

During this stage, attention must be paid to the coordination of efforts to prevent duplication. Roles and responsibilities must be clearly identified and boundaries established. Levels of authority and access to resources must be discussed before the innovator receives approval and begins work on a project. Too often, the limits and boundaries are not discussed until conflicts or problems occur. Cooperation must be obtained from coworkers and project team members and potentially from other departments, depending on the project or innovation. Executives and managers may need to pave the way or open the door for the innovator to obtain needed cooperation from other departments in the organization. Executives and managers who state expectations for cooperation and act as role models help innovators work interdepartmentally in finding others to cooperate with the project.

Working effectively with a group or a project team is an important skill for most innovators. Although an individual innovator may need extensive coaching to be successful in this area, it is often more productive than pulling the project from the person who had the idea and assigning it to someone in the department with these already developed skills. Innovators feel very discouraged when they lose the responsibility for implementing one their great ideas. For example, in one organization, a radiology employee had an idea for improving a process. She completed a successful trial project on the day shift. She was very committed to the success of the idea and persevered through the initial glitches of implementation. Everyone agreed that the process improved their work flow and level of service. When it was time to implement the process on the evening shift, Marjorie volunteered to work evenings to be certain that the process was successful. However, the manager was unwilling to transfer Marjorie to the evening shift because of short staffing on the day shift. Instead, the project was assigned to an evening shift employee who expressed multiple reservations about the idea. The innovation failed on the evening shift, and Marjorie was disappointed and frustrated. Because it did not work out well on the evening shift, it was no longer used on the day shift because of the need for consistency within the department. Not long after this fiasco, Marjorie left for a position in another organization.

Each situation needs to be evaluated separately. In some instances, there are overriding reasons why the creators of the idea should hand off the project to the implementers. However, in many cases, such turnovers are problematic. Innovation simply cannot be assigned. The people responsible for implementation are not successful when they are not fully engaged in and committed to the idea. This sounds like a simple concept, and yet it is violated frequently in organizations that are inexperienced in innovation. A design team works on the redesign of a department and then turns the result over to the manager and other employees to implement and make successful. When those who are responsible for implementing the idea have not had significant roles to play in the development of the design, there may be limited or half-hearted commitment to its success. Another common example seen in our organizations is when a committee takes on a problem and develops several workable solutions. Members are excited about the possibilities and then the solutions are turned over to others for what is often a lackluster implementation.

This stage also requires employees to call on their skills in leading meetings, managing group process, and using consensus-based decision making. Many project teams are more effective when they have diverse membership from various disciplines and support departments throughout the organization. Access to specialists between departments is important. Members of the project team may need training in practical creativity techniques such as games playing, brainstorming, mind mapping, story boards, and attribute analysis. (These techniques were discussed briefly in chapter 8.)

Communication is another key function of this stage. Effective innovation requires employees to have access to information about the organization and trends in health care and their particular field or discipline. Truly amazing innovations can occur when members of the department understand the big picture and the major challenges the organization is facing. Open communication among all layers of the organization is critical. Key messages often need to be repeated as many as eight to ten times through a variety of methods. Usually, the fewer layers of organizational structure, the more open the communication becomes.

Members of all departments need to learn and use direct communication skills with each other. People who manage their relationships in a healthy and productive manner are an asset in any organization. As noted in an earlier chapter, healthy relationships are not the rule in most health care organizations, and these behaviors must be continually modeled by the leaders before they are used by employees. Negotiation skills are critical human skills for innovators. Selling their ideas and concepts requires approaching the decision makers with a win–win attitude. The successful innovative idea is one that benefits the system, its customers, and the innovator.

Stage 4: The New Reality

The fourth stage in managing innovation is called the new reality. The key issues relate to stabilizing the environment, maintaining the direction that has been set, and producing results from the innovative projects and changes that have been made. A common error made in innovation management is expecting productivity improvements or gains too early in the cycle. In projects where there are expected productivity gains, it may be months before the gains are realized, and productivity measures should not be prematurely used as a measure or indicator of success. For example, one hospital halted an implementation project that involved a conversion to a team-based organization because they found teams took longer to do the work than when it was accomplished by individuals. If the organization had been patient and waited several months, teams would have settled into their work routines, other time gains would have become apparent, and a different decision may have been made.

Stabilizing the change or innovation is an important step and should be considered carefully. Ways to anchor the change must be sought. This can be done by formalizing a structure or process that was used in trial or formally communicating the improvement or new service to the entire organization. Disseminating innovation is a major challenge. The Veterans Administration Office of Special Projects has developed a systemwide, cross-functional program to diffuse innovations. Called Lessons Learned, it is basically a virtual learning center into which any one in the system can enter or review innovations. In addition, electronic communities of practice offer people the opportunity to connect with particular interest groups that may be posting innovations of interest (Charles 2000). Berwick (2003) offers several suggestions for dissemination of innovation in the overall health care system:

1. **Find sound innovations.** A formal mechanism can be established to assign responsibility to an individual for the review of key scientific or professional journals and even for attending key meetings. The responsible individual reports back to the organization on ideas that should be spread.

2. **Find and support innovators.** Because new answers to chronic, local problems tend to come from outside the current system, specific people should be assigned to scout out these solutions.

3. **Invest in early adopters.** Organizations should invest heavily in the curiosity of a few early adopters who are willing to test the innovations. Small-scale trials reduce the risk as does support in needed resources.

4. **Make early adopter activity observable.** Many people watch the early adopters, and when these people are visible, word of successful innovation spreads quickly through social channels.

5. **Trust and enable reinvention.** In innovation, new processes come from taking outside ideas and putting them to work in the system. They have to be tweaked in order to fit the unique organization.

6. **Create slack for change.** Innovators need the energy for change. Trying new things takes an enormous investment of energy. "No system trapped in the continuous throes of production, existing always at the margin of resources, innovates well, unless its survival is also imminently and vividly at stake" (Berwick 2003, p. 1974).

7. **Lead by example.** If leaders are going to be champions of the change, they must be prepared for resistance from others. Crucially important is their willingness to begin the change with themselves.

Other ways to stabilize the change are by establishing methods of rewarding and recognizing the innovator and project team. Rewards may come through increased learning and skill development, increased access to funding for future projects, educational support, and sometimes even monetary rewards. Recognition can be through sharing of successes at employee or organizational meetings, through department or organization newsletters, or through specific celebration ceremonies. External opportunities for recognition and applause are wonderfully reinforcing for project team members. Supporting publishing projects or presentations at national conferences is another way of rewarding and recognizing innovators.

For example, in one emergency department, employees were involved in several creative projects. One involved a grow-your-own graduate nurse internship program, and the second was a hospitalwide initiative to reduce admission wait times for emergency patients. Both of these innovative projects achieved outstanding levels of success. A call for a poster session at the annual meeting was received from the Emergency Nurses Association, and several of these nurses wanted to submit an abstract. The manager coached them on how to write the abstract, which was submitted and subsequently accepted. Four people from her department then requested permission to attend the national conference. Undaunted, the manager presented a proposal to the hospital foundation for funding to allow the nurses to attend. This created a high level of energy in the department, which spread elsewhere in the organization.

Productivity is highest when managers and employees are well centered with a healthy balance of energy. During periods of intense change and innovation in a department or in the organization, people often overexpend their reserves of energy, leading to overall decreases in productivity and resiliency. Encouraging self-care and paying attention to the self-care needs of managers and employees are critical in an organization that innovates successfully. Although innovation is hard work, it is energizing for many people. There is a tendency to ignore replenishment needs. Successful innovation managers recognize that change work takes a great deal of energy and that sometimes timeframes need to be modified, the frequency of meetings decreased, or extended periods away from the work encouraged. The result in the long run is increased productivity and creativity.

Stage 5: Integration

The final stage of the developmental cycle is integration or closure. The key issues in this stage relate to evaluative functions, quality, and closure. This stage is often overlooked or undervalued, and yet it is critical for future successes in the system. Although evaluation is an important process throughout this developmental cycle, at this phase it is a key issue. During the planning stage, key indicators of success were developed. At this point these indicators are used to evaluate the innovation for its beneficence and effectiveness. The process used to develop or implement the innovation is evaluated. Key questions should include: What did we learn? What would we do differently? Is there anything we can stop doing? Cultivate an attitude within the entire system that these questions are a normal part of the process. Never let the evaluation process be construed as blame placing.

The quality of the innovation and the implementation process are critical issues at this stage. How would the process be changed the next time? What are the lessons learned? In addition, the relationship between the innovation and quality of patient care should be clear and used as an indicator of success. The innovation may only be indirectly related to patient care, but the implementation of creative ideas implies that something is better as a result of the new idea. What is it that is better?

An important leadership function during this phase is to take the time to go through closure. Too often a project or innovation is completed without formal closure. Closure can occur in the form of celebrations or events that can be held even when the project or intended innovation was a failure. There are lessons to be learned and successes in the most dismal of failures. In almost every instance, innovations occur as the result of the efforts of many people in the organization. It is important to focus on the success or the process rather than the individual whose idea it was in the beginning. Recognizing and rewarding team effort communicates respect for everyone's efforts. "Innovative organizations know that celebration is an important part of completing a project" (Hattori and Wycoff 2002, p. 30).

Closure also implies letting go of things. There may be a need for grief work, the dissolution of a tightknit project team, letting go of the old way, or releasing of an old mindset. The need for grieving should not be underestimated. When grief can be expressed, the individuals involved are often ready to move on to the next project more quickly.

What's Your Innovation Quotient?

Assessing the effectiveness of innovation management processes is a helpful first step for any organization or department seeking to improve its skills. The assessment tool shown in figure 9-3 may be helpful. The items are organized in groups of ten, with each group relating to one stage of innovation management. Questions 1 through 10 relate to stage 1, questions 11 through 20 relate to stage 2, and so on. Scores of twelve or less for each cluster of ten items indicate areas that need additional work.

Figure 9-3.   What's Your IQ (Innovation Quotient)? (Manion 1993)

Directions: Answer with the same environment in mind for each question. For example, complete the questionnaire thinking of an entire organization, a department, or a specific work group. (That is, do not answer one question with a single department in mind and the next item with an entire organization in mind.) Answer by circling Y for yes, N for no, and S for sometimes.

Y   S   N   1. Does the mission statement or statement of purpose include any reference to employee creativity and innovation?

Y   S   N   2. Do job descriptions or role expectations include the expectation for individual innovation or support of innovation?

Y   S   N   3. Do the annual goals include implementation of innovative ideas or strategies that increase employee creativity or innovation?

Y   S   N   4. Are the people who are always questioning the status quo and looking for a better way encouraged and seen as "creative types"?

Y   S   N   5. Is there a lot of energy and enthusiasm for change?

Y   S   N   6. Do front-line employees have ready access to funding for innovative projects?

Y   S   N   7. Are mentors and sponsors for the novice innovator available in the organization?

Y   S   N   8. Do front-line employees and managers have time during their normal work week to work on innovations and creative projects?

Y   S   N   9. Are the boundaries and limits openly discussed with the innovator and clarified before problems occur?

Y   S   N   10. Are resources shared among departments and work groups?

Y   S   N   11. Is time taken to plan for innovation (as opposed to moving very quickly from identifying the need to actual implementation)?

Y   S   N   12. Is there an established process for managing change and innovation that internal leaders understand and are expected to utilize?

Y   S   N   13. Is a formal proposal format or business plan required before an innovative idea is considered for implementation? Do interested employees know what the expected format is?

Figure 9-3. (Continued)

Y S N 14. Is there flexibility in how the plan unfolds? (Or are people held to the specifics of the plan, that is, the timeframes, expenditures projected, process used?)

Y S N 15. Do front-line employees have easy access to the executive leadership team without having to go through multiple layers of management?

Y S N 16. Are plans developed before decisions are made?

Y S N 17. Do individual managers have control over funding so that low-cost projects can be funded without a lot of rigamarole?

Y S N 18. Are there established, agreed-upon timeframes for completion of projects?

Y S N 19. Are levels of authority clearly identified for project teams and committees?

Y S N 20. Do problems get solved in the organization so that you are not dealing with the same problems you were dealing with three to five years ago?

Y S N 21. Is there a spirit of cooperation in the organization? Can an innovator find others to cooperate in implementation?

Y S N 22. Do individual innovators retain control over their innovation as it is implemented rather than the idea being passed over to a manager or project director to implement?

Y S N 23. Does the general climate in the organization support, encourage, and seek out change and innovation?

Y S N 24. Is there a high level of trust in the organization among work groups, units, departments, managers, and employees?

Y S N 25. Are priorities established, resources assessed, and progress made on the important and major change projects under way rather than expending time and energy on an excessive number of projects at one time?

Y S N 26. Do managers and leaders act as catalysts for change and innovation?

Y S N 27. Is the majority of the management within the organization stable and effective rather than involved in crisis management, continually "putting out fires," feeling burned out?

Figure 9-3.   (Continued)

Y S N   28. Are employees and managers skilled in the application of creativity techniques such as storyboards, attribute analysis, brainstorming, and mind mapping?

Y S N   29. Can an individual innovator easily pull together a team of people from other departments and work groups to work together on a project?

Y S N   30. Are people comfortable with making mistakes rather than seeing mistakes as something to be feared and avoided?

Y S N   31. Do people in the work group, department, or organization support each other rather than engaging in a significant amount of blaming, bickering, and backbiting?

Y S N   32. Are people in the organization encouraged to take care of themselves?

Y S N   33. Do people in the organization feel like they can set limits, say no to assignments and requests, and decline involvement in particular change projects?

Y S N   34. Are managers and leaders well-centered with a healthy balance of energy rather than feeling burned out and out of balance?

Y S N   35. Is workaholic behavior and perfectionism discouraged?

Y S N   36. Is the organization basically stable and secure rather than an environment of great anxiety, high flux, and chaos?

Y S N   37. Are there mechanisms in place that give long-term support to the implementation of changes and innovations?

Y S N   38. Is there recognition and support that productivity increases occur only after the change is well-established rather than immediately?

Y S N   39. Do people talk openly about their feelings related to change? Is it okay to express negative feelings about change, or is this seen and dealt with as resistance?

Y S N   40. Are specific interventions planned and implemented to nurture people during change and major innovation?

Y S N   41. Are the values of the organization or work group clearly articulated with a clear connection between quality and innovation?

Figure 9-3. (Continued)

Y S N 42. Can employees articulate the values of the organization, and are the values articulated consistent with what is being practiced? (For example, while innovation and creativity may be articulated as important, in practice there is no allocation of resources to support it.)

Y S N 43. Are employees and leaders in the organization inspired to become involved as innovators rather than being exhausted with the day-to-day work demands?

Y S N 44. When new responsibilities and tasks are accepted, are current responsibilities and tasks modified?

Y S N 45. Are managers and leaders skilled at managing change and the emotions involved to reduce the chaos and turmoil that typically occur when something changes?

Y S N 46. Are people in the organization receptive to and excited about change rather than "fed up" with change, the "promise that things will be better after this, but they never are"?

Y S N 47. Is there a specific evaluation process to determine whether or not, or in what ways, the change has been beneficial?

Y S N 48. Are mistakes freely shared and seen as opportunities for everyone to learn?

Y S N 49. Do people feel comfortable about eliminating the unnecessary? Or is it difficult to let go of things from the past, including people or ways of doing things?

Y S N 50. Do people look forward to the future and change rather than continually lamenting over the good old days, the way things were before the change?

Scoring Directions: Each Y is 2 points, each S is 1 point, and each N is zero. Total the number of points.

Interpretation: If your total score is between 80 and 100, your environment is supportive of innovation; if the total score is between 60 and 79, your environment is somewhat supportive of innovation; if the score is 59 or below, your environment is likely to be a barrier to innovation.

Conclusion

The challenges facing health care in this millennium are perhaps some of the toughest we have ever experienced. Meeting these challenges successfully requires all of the strength the organization and its people have to offer. Having innovative, empowered employees is not merely desirable; it is absolutely essential for survival.

Creating a climate and structure within a system that empower employees and managers alike takes a strong commitment and consistent effort by the executive and leadership team. To make the leap from creative ideas to a new reality requires a process for managing innovation. It requires the establishment of a supportive climate and individuals who have advanced skills in creativity, new ideas and plan development, and change management. Transformation of the organization is the potential result.

Conversation Points

Organizational Perspective

1. Is innovation a highly held value in the organization?
2. Is the need for innovation emphasized anywhere in the organization's or department's mission statement? Do leaders talk about the need for innovation?
3. Is there a structure in place that supports innovators and makes it easy for them to be successful?
4. How innovative is the organization? How successful is it at creating and handling change?
5. When major changes or innovations are made, how well are they assimilated into the organization?
6. Is there a "tendency to yes" or a "tendency to no" in the organization?
7. How are individuals with new ideas and the enthusiasm to push them treated in your organization?

Leadership Issues

1. Do you have any innovators within your work group? How do you support them?
2. Do employees frequently bring forth new ideas? Do they offer implementation suggestions or just expect others to do the work of making them happen?

3. Do you have adequate autonomy and leeway to make decisions about ideas employees bring that relate to your areas of responsibility? Or do you have to seek permission from others in the hierarchy?
4. How skilled are you at leading creativity groups and coaching employees in innovation?
5. What new ideas have been implemented in your department or area of responsibility in the past year? How did the implementation go?

Employee Challenges

1. If you have a great new idea that will help solve problems or create new processes, is it easy to get heard?
2. Do you know how to get a new idea implemented?
3. How comfortable are you with creativity techniques such as attribute analysis, nominal group technique, or storyboarding?
4. If you yourself are not intrapreneurial, how do you support peers and colleagues who are?
5. Who do you think is responsible for innovation in your department?
6. Is there time to create new approaches and implement improvements?
7. What new ideas have been implemented in your department in the past year? What role did you play in the implementation? How did you support the implementation?
8. What is your department's IQ (innovation quotient)? What can you do to help improve it?

10

Influencing Performance

Jo Manion, Sharon Cox, and Mary Jenkins

*In today's organizational environment, there is little prospect
that any one will be "taken care of." Believing that
is another illusion that yields resistance to owning one's work.
We will each have to manage our own work and cherish
the responsibility of creating the organization where we work.*
—Dick Richards (1995a)

A KEY ASPECT of a positive work environment is an organizational culture in which problems are solved, systems are improved, and innovation is encouraged. In addition, there is a need to influence people's performance in a positive direction by encouraging and coaching colleagues and employees to continually grow and develop their skills. In some instances, this may require us to respond to, and deal with, inadequate or unacceptable performance or behaviors on the part of others. Although the majority of effort in managing and influencing performance, likely around 95 percent, focuses on encouraging and recognizing good performance, it is often the remaining 5 percent that causes us the most difficulty. It was clear from the findings of the research presented in chapter 5 that successful managers do not let the presence of workforce shortages frighten them away from dealing with unacceptable or inadequate performance. They deal with problems head on by actively coaching employees, and they are not afraid to take appropriate action even when it means ending the employment relationship with an individual.

This chapter discusses two of the most common approaches to influencing performance: formal performance appraisal systems and coaching. This chapter also discusses job fit and job sculpting to improve job alignment, feedback, and positive discipline. Finally, the chapter offers suggestions for dealing with negativity in the workplace and extreme behavioral disruptions.

Performance Appraisals and Performance Management Systems

Conversations about managing performance often bring to mind the annual performance appraisal, which, for many of us, causes us to groan inwardly and immediately tune out. Health care organizations have invested massive amounts of resources, both human and financial, to develop, implement, and maintain systems of formal performance appraisal because they believe they are beneficial for employees and the system. But do they really improve performance? Do they improve communication between employee and manager? Do they increase the alignment of the employee's goals with the department's or organization's goals? Do they motivate employees and help them with their career planning and progression? Are they an effective method of distributing pay increases and determining job promotions?

These questions are raised in a provocative book by Coens and Jenkins, *Abolishing Performance Appraisals: Why They Backfire and What to Do Instead* (2000). When the title of the Coens and Jenkins book is shared with managers, most of them perk up immediately and their interest becomes obvious. Some of them actually cheer! Perhaps it is because they know, if only on an intuitive level, that formal performance appraisal systems are not delivering on the promises made. As Coens and Jenkins suggest, it is time to acknowledge that improving the level of performance in our organizations, including health care organizations, is not about building bigger, better, or different appraisal systems. It is time for us to question the underlying assumption that such an approach can actually accomplish the positive results we are looking for.

Even more disturbing is the realization that the appraisal systems in which organizations have invested so heavily not only have failed to bring the positive outcomes anticipated; they can actually result in quite serious consequences for the organization. We all know how disappointing it is to leave that annual appraisal session realizing that our manager or supervisor does not really recognize all of our accomplishments or even understand everything that we do. Even worse, because the process is usually tied directly to the determination of pay increases, the process may actually impede deeply felt conversation and honest feedback. Ask most employees (as many research studies have), and they will tell you that these systems are ineffective.

Furthermore, the annual appraisal approach to performance management is solidly ingrained in unhealthy organizational assumptions such as:

- Employees need to be told what to do.
- The manager is better able to judge and evaluate the employee's performance than the employee is.
- Employees are not smart enough or insightful enough to evaluate their own performance.
- If given the opportunity, employees would inflate their ratings because they only see their positive traits.
- Employees are not capable of holding themselves accountable for their performance without the guidance of their managers.

It is past time that these assumptions were challenged. Noted author Peter Block uses the formal performance appraisal system as a key example for pointing out just how "patriarchal and demeaning institutional life can become" (Coens and Jenkins 2000, p. xiv).

Chapters 1 through 9 of *Create a Positive Health Care Workplace!* emphasize the need to apply affirming principles and approaches to the workplace. The chapters present new ways for both managers and employees to approach the issue of healthy work environments. The contention here is that formal performance appraisal systems are not the best approach for managing employee performance. And perhaps even more significantly, the entire concept of performance management ought to be approached in a different way. Paramount to the idea of abolishing performance appraisals is the idea that *"employees want to be and are fully capable of being responsible for themselves.* With a supportive work culture and access to helpful resources and training, employees will take responsibility to get timely and useful feedback, grow their skills, and improve their performance in alignment with organizational needs" (Coens and Jenkins 2000, p. 9).

Rather than exploring the issue of performance appraisal systems more fully in this chapter, the reader is referred directly to Coens and Jenkins's book and encouraged to use it as a resource and a thought-provoking guide to considering the issue. This chapter concentrates on several other ways of influencing employee performance, including coaching, giving feedback, using positive discipline when needed, and dealing with specific challenges such as negativity in the workplace and disruptive employee behavior.

Coaching for Performance

When most people in health care organizations think about managing the performance of employees, the annual performance appraisal comes to mind. Coaching, however, takes a different approach. Coaching others for optimal performance is an ongoing process embedded in the everyday work of the manager or expert colleague. Coaching is a process engaged in by anyone in the workplace who has some responsibility or interest in helping other workers to develop and improve their skills. Although the coach is often the individual's manager, educators and trusted colleagues with special expertise may assume the role of coach at various times. Many health care providers also serve as coaches for the patients and clients they serve. For purposes of discussion, we will confine our discussion to the coaching role involved in influencing or improving the performance of employees. The concept is presented briefly here, and the reader is referred to *From Management to Leadership* (Manion 2005) for a more complete exploration.

Coaching can be defined as "a process of facilitating an individual's or team's development through giving advice and instruction; encouraging discovery through guided discussions and hands-on experiences; observing performance; and giving honest, direct, and immediate feedback" (Manion 2005, p. 276). To be effective, the coaching relationship between two individuals must be based on a relationship characterized by trust, openness, mutual respect, positive and ongoing communication, and support. The effective coach is also familiar with the principles of both intrinsic and extrinsic motivation.

Briefly, a coaching process begins with some idea of what is to be accomplished. The desired outcome is identified as a goal that can be used to measure progress and achievement. Once the goal of the coaching has been identified and agreed upon, an assessment of the performer's current abilities is conducted. This assessment of the employee's previous experience and opportunities results in a conclusion about the person's current standing in relation to the goal. For example, perhaps you are coaching an employee who has just assumed responsibility for leading a key task force. It is helpful to know that the employee has had similar experiences with leading committee work before but that the previous work did not include committees with systemwide membership with physicians and community members a part of the process. As a coach, you can use this knowledge to key into the specific processes and concerns that the employee needs to understand in order to be successful.

Once the assessment is complete, the coach and performer work to develop a clear understanding of the task force members' roles and responsibilities. The coach and employee can also look for additional training opportunities when they are needed. In order to determine the effectiveness of the coaching, the next step is for the coach to observe the employee's performance. This can be achieved through direct observation, progress reports, and/or outcomes analysis. Finally, the coach provides feedback to the individual on how well he or she performed, and the process is complete. The rest of this section examines several specific aspects of coaching for performance.

Giving Feedback

Feedback is a critical element of coaching. Feedback validates or expands the performers' assessment of their achievement. Whether we realize it or not, we are giving other people feedback all of the time. Whenever we respond to a person's behavior, we are letting that person know whether we are pleased, excited, disappointed, dismayed, angry, or whatever. We give feedback through simple nonverbal cues and facial expressions such as a frown, a look of confusion, or a smile. Our body language lets other people know our reaction to what they have done or said. We also give feedback to others by what we pay attention to and notice. For example, a group of managers in an organization was responsible for organizing and providing leadership development programs for their peers. They not only arranged for the speaker, they obtained the necessary facilities and notified everyone in advance of the program. To add a special touch, they also arrived early and expended a great deal of effort on decorating the conference room with a seasonal touch. When the chief executive officer walked into the room, he took one look at the tables and asked in a critical tone of voice, "Where's the water pitchers for the tables?" The team felt let down and demoralized that he never noticed the hard work and effort they had gone to in preparation for the day.

Interpersonal feedback is a crucial aspect of helping people improve their performance. Seashore, Seashore, and Weinberg (1999, p. 3) define feedback as "information about past behavior, delivered in the present, which may influence future behavior." They note that feedback gives us the ability to test our perceptions, reactions, and observations. It is a primary method for influencing someone to start, stop, or change their behavior in some way. "Feedback in the workplace is fundamental for helping those who wish to improve their performance reach an objective, or avoid unpleasant reactions to their efforts" (Seashore, Seashore, and Weinberg 1999, p. 7). Feedback is the final step in coaching. It closes the loop for the performer and lets him or her know the degree to which a goal has been successfully attained.

Those of us who share feedback with others need to be reminded that it is always the receiver of the feedback who, in reality, determines whether he or she internalizes the message and acts on the feedback given. Although we each can learn ways to improve our skill in giving feedback, delivering the message effectively does not necessarily mean the receiver is going to change his or her behavior. When the person delivering the feedback is a credible source of information and has your best interests at heart, your willingness to accept the feedback increases. However, additional factors play into whether you act on the feedback. For example, perhaps the potential consequences of not changing your behavior are significant enough that you make the necessary alterations. Or perhaps you have heard the same message on previous occasions, and it is starting to make more of an impression on you. Sometimes the behavioral change requested is just too hard to make, or the suggested change is related to behavior that is an inherent and permanent part of your personality.

Although giving feedback is an important step in the coaching process, many people find the process difficult. When the feedback is positive and consists of observations that the recipient is likely to want to hear, the process is usually less difficult. But it can be a different story when the information to be shared may be perceived by the receiver as negative criticism. Negative feedback often feels confrontational and uncomfortable to give. In some instances, we may feel uneasy about our right to deliver the message. When you observe someone who needs feedback and you find yourself reluctant to give it, Clarke-Epstein (2002) suggests that you ask yourself three questions:

1. If I were the person in this situation, would I want to be given this feedback? Would I want to be told about my behavior?
2. Can the person change their behavior, given the feedback?
3. Will I be embarrassed to give the feedback, or will it embarrass the other person to hear it? If the answer to either of these questions is yes, take the time to organize your thoughts and carefully craft your message rather than delivering a spontaneous remark.

As Clarke-Epstein suggests, when giving feedback is difficult because of the negative content or potentially uncomfortable nature of the feedback, it is helpful to write a script for yourself. It forces you to think carefully about what it is you need to give feedback about and allows you time to allow strong emotions such as anger or disappointment to fade. When we deliver feedback at times when we are feeling a strong emotion such as anger, the emotion often drives our response and aggression is the result. Similarly, when you are feeling fearful, you may come across as passive and unassertive. The challenge is to share your information with the other person clearly and assertively but in a manner that does not result in the individual feeling angry or demeaned.

Writing a script also allows us to practice giving feedback when the situation promises to be especially difficult, as may be the case when you need to give the person to whom you report feedback about their annoying or destructive behavior. Scripting helps prepare us for what may be highly charged interpersonal interchanges. The basic elements and structure found in most feedback scripts include the following four elements:

When you _____,

I felt _____.

This causes a problem because _____.

I would like you _____.

This basic model provides a structure you can use to complete the sentences and form your script. Thus, giving an employee feedback about behavior may look like this:

When you responded to Susan's request for help negatively and with complaints about your own workload,

I felt angry because I have seen this pattern in your relationships with coworkers before.

This causes a problem because we have to help each other in this department so that our patients receive the kind of care they need.

In the future I expect you to help others and to be more positive about it.

There are several common difficulties with using this model. Some people feel that beginning with the phrase *when you* is too confrontational and that a softer approach would be more effective. However, the feedback giver's tone of voice and body language have more to do with expressing a confrontational, aggressive style than do the actual words used. If you start with *when you*, it cues the person that you are giving specific feedback, and it says "this is about you." Most of us are so inundated with massive amounts of information that we do not fully listen to messages unless it is clear that the message is about us or is about something of value to us.

The second issue arises with the *I felt* portion of the structure. In initial efforts to develop a script, we have a tendency to describe observations rather than true emotions. For instance, a person might write, "I felt like you did not take the other person's needs into account." This statement does not describe an emotion; it is a factual statement. Writing this part of the message in a way that shares the emotion you are feeling would be something like, "I felt angry that you did not take your team member's needs into account." Being willing to share how you are feeling, although not appropriate in every instance, is a clear, positive sign of confidence and assertiveness.

Developing the *this causes a problem because* part of the script is probably the trickiest but most important part of the message. In this part of the message you are giving the receiver a reason to change his or her behavior. The most common mistake we make is giving the receiver a reason that is important to us but may not be important to the receiver. To make it more likely that the feedback will result in a desirable action, you should think about what the receiver values. For instance, people and relationships are highly important to some of us though less important to others.

In addition to people and relationships, there are at least three other common value categories: image, goals and achievements, and facts and information. People who highly value image tend to be more concerned about things such as reputation and how the world sees them. Other people are more concerned with their ability to accomplish goals and reach achievements, and others are more likely to be swayed by factual information such as data.

When you can give people a reason to change their behavior that is important to them, you are more likely to influence their behavior. For example, suppose you were that manager giving an employee feedback on the effects of her response to teammates who asked her for help. In the first example, the reason given was based on a value related to goals and accomplishments:

> *When you* responded to Susan's request for help negatively and with complaints about your own workload,
>
> *I felt* angry because I have seen this pattern in your relationships with coworkers before.

This causes a problem because we have to help each other in this department so that our patients receive the kind of care they need.

In the future I expect you to help others and to be more positive about it.

Examples of ways to change the third portion of the script on the basis of different values include:

People and relationships: This creates a problem for you because others will be less willing to help you the next time you need it.

Image: This creates a problem for you because your coworkers will see you as a whiner, complainer, and nonteam player.

Facts and information: This has created a problem because I've had to step in and deal with one of your irate coworkers four times in just the past week.

Finding the right approach to motivate different individuals may take some experimentation. If you do not see improvement after your first attempt at giving feedback on a problem, try another reason for the person to change when the behavior comes up the next time. Sometimes it is difficult to determine from cues in a person's language which of the four values is most important for that individual, especially when you do not know the person well. In such cases, start with what you think the person values but be willing to change your message when a behavioral change is not apparent. When the feedback does not work, be careful not to fool yourself into thinking that the responsibility is all yours and that the problem must be in the way you gave the feedback or in the words you chose to use. Be sure to remember that it is up to the receiver to decide whether to make use of the feedback you offered or ignore it.

Receiving Feedback

Receiving feedback and being comfortable with the process is probably as important as being able to give feedback well. Coens and Jenkins (2000, p. 144) suggest that the receiver of feedback has "at least as much responsibility, and probably more, than the giver of feedback." All of us are privileged to receive feedback from others at various times. How we respond in the immediate situation as well as how well we incorporate the feedback into future behavior choices often determines whether the person who offered the feedback will do so again in the future. Obviously, our reactions certainly influence the comfort with which your coworkers will approach future feedback opportunities.

Negative feedback is frequently uncomfortable for both the giver and the receiver. Clarke-Epstein (2002) suggests specific responses that we can use in such situations. Sometimes our initial response to negative or critical feedback is shock or surprise. When you have no idea of how to respond, simply do nothing. You can say something like: "I am completely surprised. I need some time to think about this. When can we talk about it again?" An angry response to feedback someone has given us demands a similar reaction. Clarke-Epstein recommends that when we feel anger in response to feedback we should do nothing and realize that you will get past the feeling. Then, once you have calmed down, you can offer a reasonable response instead of a biting, angry, or sarcastic retort.

A second typical response we experience when confronted with negative feedback is rationalization. Before we know it, we have lined up our excuses and defenses. However, before sharing such responses with anyone else, it is helpful to listen carefully to yourself and try to separate your purely defensive responses from your legitimate ones. When we sound defensive, much of what we offer may be disregarded when in fact there may be a worthy explanation. Our tone of voice may also reduce the effectiveness of our message.

Finally, in some instances, our reaction to negative feedback may simply be acceptance. We know that the feedback is true and that the giver has shared this information with us in order to help us improve in some way. Occasionally, negative feedback may concern behavior that we have already recognized in ourselves but we were not certain that others had noticed. In this case, you should respond assertively and ask questions about what is unclear, for example: "Can you give me another example to help me understand?" or "I want to be sure I understand what you are saying." Although we need not accept all of the feedback, we do need to think it through and take what is helpful and put it to use.

Recognizing Problem Performers

Managing problem performers ranks right up at the top of the most difficult challenges a manager or leader must address. In fact, few issues trigger more angst or cause managers to feel more helpless than the daunting task of confronting poor performers. Why? The answer is often all too predictable and follows themes such as the following:

- Confronting the problem is not worth the effort because the organization's performance appraisal system is so cumbersome that it is easier to work around the employee.
- The human resources department does not support managers in their efforts to remedy poor performance and instead works as the employees' advocate.
- The performance problem has existed for years, and no one has ever attempted to address it.
- The employee has a volatile personality, and the manager is afraid of the employee's reaction.

Although confronting employees with performance problems is never going to be easy, demystifying the process of identifying and addressing the root causes of good and poor performance may help. The case studies described in figures 10-1 and 10-2 shed light on the process and should help you to understand how to coach people for improved outcomes.

Each of the individuals described in the two case studies elected to take on a new position. Although both employees held demanding positions that required hard work, one was struggling and had lost the sense of joy she felt in her previous position, while the other was thriving.

To understand why one employee performs better and experiences less stress than another, we need to understand exactly what factors drive performance. The most important factor in performance is the alignment of an individual's values, interests, and skills with those required by the position and the organization. How well matched the person is to the requirements of the job and the organization is the key to performance and certainly is related to the ability to experience joy at work. When any of the three elements of values, interests, or skills is out of alignment, the level of stress increases and generally the level of performance decreases. Although Mary's performance was acceptable, she was putting tremendous stress on herself. This situation is not unlike driving an old Ford that is out of alignment. You may be able to get to your destination, but the attention and physical effort required to drive it there tires you out and you may do permanent damage to the car if you keep driving it in that condition for too long. In contrast, Sharon fulfilled her goals with ease and enjoyed herself doing it. Her situation is like driving a new Lexus with automatic steering and cruise control and your favorite music playing.

The importance of alignment was profoundly illuminated in the 1980s, a period marked by extensive downsizing in many organizations. Outplacement firms were flourishing as major companies reduced staff by 10 to 20 percent. In many cases, organizations targeted individuals they believed they could most afford to lose: poor or marginal employees. In droves, these individuals were informed of their separation and quickly sent off to the care of outplacement counselors, whose first job was to help them deal with the pain and shock of losing their

Figure 10-1.   Case Study: Struggling to Perform

Mary was an exceptional obstetrics nurse and was often asked to help with complicated cases. She loved her position and the opportunity to touch the lives of so many people. There were some drawbacks, however, including salary and shift changes. So, when offered the opportunity to become a nurse manager, she quickly accepted the new position with only a passing thought about the supervisory skills that would be required in the new assignment. Mary knew she was a good learner and had always adapted well in the past; besides, she could really use the salary increase and was excited about spending more weekends and holidays with her family.

After a few months on the job, Mary felt frustrated with her position and began feeling guilty about not effectively addressing the people problems in her department. She understood that her work would be easier if she could learn how to deal with difficult people without internalizing the conflict. She considered reading a book or attending a class to help her learn the new skills she needed.

Mary's boss was also concerned. Mary was not getting her schedules completed on time, and she seemed to be on edge most of the time. Her nursing staff was growing increasingly disgruntled with how Mary barked orders and spent most of her time in the office. It was clear that she was trying very hard and putting in unusually long hours to stay on top of the demands placed on her. Her coworkers reached out to try and support her, but she did not respond to their offers of help.

After a year as a manager, Mary felt burned out. Although her administrative skills had grown, the effort was leaving her exhausted. She felt distant from the patients, and rather than having more time with her family, she was spending even less time at home than before. When she was home, she felt distracted or tired. Mary knew the quality of her work had improved; however, she frequently felt that her work was no longer meaningful. Although Mary's boss was satisfied with her performance, she avoided involving Mary in any special assignments for fear that Mary would not be able to handle the additional workload.

---

jobs. Once stabilized, individuals were taken through a series of self-assessment instruments designed to increase their self-awareness. Armed with a greater knowledge of themselves, individuals then began the search for new positions that were deemed a better *fit;* that is, positions that were in better alignment with each individual's values, interests, and skills.

The outplacement counseling had an interesting result. The majority of individuals were perceived as strong performers in their new position. Most of them received significant increases in pay and reported greater satisfaction on the job (Brightman 2002). These employees

Figure 10-2. Case Study: Working in Alignment

Sharon's job as a marketing specialist for a health system foundation seemed to be an odd match to many of her friends. They had known her as a physical therapist, and her love of the field was evident in her interactions with others. In fact, when anyone in her family or circle of friends had health care questions, Sharon was called for advice before anyone else.

When Sharon first took the marketing position, she had strong reservations about her ability to handle the responsibilities. Her predecessor had a degree in marketing and had worked in several nonprofit organizations before joining the foundation. Sharon had neither a relevant degree nor the appropriate experience, but somehow Sharon's manager was confident in her passion and knowledge of health care along with her excellent interpersonal skills.

Sharon often felt up to her eyeballs with work and sometimes found it difficult to leave the office on time, but she rarely felt overwhelmed. At first, Sharon thought the contacts with potential donors would be awkward and uncomfortable. However, she quickly found that it was easy to enroll others with her vision of what was possible, and she thrived on the opportunity to talk with people about what she loved. Sharon also received positive feedback from community members for doing what came naturally to her: engaging people in dialogue about current health care issues and opportunities.

Sharon's manager was extremely pleased with Sharon's work and was confident that the department was going to overachieve its financial goals for the year. Sharon attended a couple of marketing courses to learn the technical side of the field, but it was her knowledge of health care and interpersonal skills that made her a real standout. She found it hard to believe a year had passed since she started her marketing position, and she was confident that she would soon secure enough donations to fund the opening of an adjacent building for the new residency program.

were the same individuals who had been perceived as poor performers in their prior positions and organizations, but with better job alignment they seemed like different employees.

The lack of alignment, or fit problem, can be related to the skills or interests of the employee or to the fit between the employee's values or behaviors and the culture of the organization. In Mary's case, for example, the problem was a lack of alignment between the skills needed to perform the job effectively and the skills Mary possessed. As a result of trying to compensate for her skill shortcomings, Mary found that the effort required to stay afloat in her new position left her feeling exhausted at the end of the workday. In other situations, the employee may be able to apply the necessary skills but have no interest in the work to be done, or the employee may have the necessary skills, find the work interesting, but disagree with the predominant values underlying the organization's culture.

In other words, individuals thrive when they are placed in circumstances where the values of the organization feel right, the skills needed to perform are available, and the work itself is interesting. For the individuals studied after being downsized in the 1980s (Brightman 2002), finding the right fit in their new jobs made all the difference. Many of them said that they wished they had found self-understanding earlier in their careers. Since that time, some organizations have even begun to offer self-assessment courses to their employees.

Chris Oster, director of organizational development for General Motors Powertrain, believes that self-understanding, once identified, can become a source of stability in an unstable world. "Identifying your enduring values, interests, and skills gives you a strong sense of control. You are able to more effectively direct your career rather than being at the mercy of someone else's view of what's right for you" (Oster 2004).

Too often, the attraction to making more money or having more prestige or some other external motivator clouds self-awareness and pulls us out of alignment. In some situations, we may assume that there are no employment options available that would better suit our unique needs. Without pausing and taking personal stock in who we are and what lights us up, it is easy to go off track. There are lots of Marys out there who, without self-knowledge, keep their heads down, continue to work hard, and continue to feel miserable. Whether at the initiative of the employee or through the coaching and support of a supervisor, exploring issues of alignment or fit may very well be the key to engaging people more fully and facilitating higher levels of productivity. It is also one of the first areas to explore when performance is less than satisfactory, and exploring fit issues offers employees the opportunity to *participate* in identifying the root cause of their own poor performance. Imagine Mary: If she had recognized that her interests and skills were not well matched to her position, she might have been able to take the steps necessary to get her career and personal life back on track.

All too often, early opportunities to assess the roots of poor performance are missed. Even though a manager may be aware that an employee is performing at a level below what is required, the manager may choose a wait-and-see attitude rather than addressing the problem immediately. So, just how can we determine whether a performance problem is serious enough to warrant significant action?

Defining Problem Performance

One of the hurdles to improving problem performance is deciding whether an individual's performance is unacceptable enough to warrant action beyond regular coaching. In other words, is the performance really that bad, or is it just marginal? Making this determination is a judgment call. Most managers have a gut sense of when a problem warrants significant action. However, having a working definition can be a useful tool. To identify exceptional performers (both at the top and the bottom of the performance spectrum), Coens and Jenkins offer the following definition:

> An exceptional (or problem) employee has inarguably stood out from the rest of the work team for a sustained period of time in contribution as evidenced by the results achieved and/or the behaviors exhibited. [A problem employee] is easily declared by those that know him or her. . . . Exceptional, given its most elementary definition, is rare. To identify more than a few individuals as such negates the exceptional label and makes it [an] intolerable contradiction. It is more likely a given work team will have NONE rather than ONE exceptional team member (Coens and Jenkins 2000, p. 175).

By definition, problem performers are readily identifiable. But notice that the definition includes an element of time, varying circumstances, and a consistent conclusion by multiple people who know and interact with the individual. Although judgment is required, in the case of performance it is a conclusion arrived at after carefully sorting out all possible factors that influence performance but are outside the control of the employee. Reacting too quickly may cause a manager to attribute the cause of problems to an individual simply because he or she was nearby when the problem occurred. ("Because of recent flash floods, we have fired our weatherman!") Of course, the opposite is also true.

Credit may also be given to individuals for making improvements and performing well when they had no control over the situation. They were just lucky. ("Congratulations, Ms. Tucker, on your award for most outstanding school nurse. During the past year, there were no reported cases of measles in your district!") These examples are extreme, but they point to common mistakes in judgment with regard to performance problems. Individual performance is highly interdependent with numerous complex variables in the work environment. As a result, variation in performance may occur but have nothing to do with individual effort and skill. A healthy dose of skepticism about using data and observation over time is the best way to determine whether special attention is warranted.

Assessing Individual Problem Performance

After ruling out various system- or environment-related causes of poor individual performance, managers may conclude that the problem is rooted in the individual's behavior and/or capabilities. At this point, the options fall into three categories:

- Helping the individual improve to an acceptable level
- Altering the job or finding a position that is better aligned with the individual's skills and potential
- Taking measures to remove the employee from the organization in a manner that is respectful and caring

Choosing the correct course depends on the facts of the case as well as good judgment. The first option, helping the employee to address the performance problem, should always be the beginning point unless it is absolutely clear that any such efforts would be futile. The second option affirms the belief that performance is a function of fit and holds on to the possibility that the employee would be productive if he or she were placed in another more appropriate position. (Cases such as Mary's fit this description.) Organizations that readily dismiss poor performers create a cloud of fear for the remaining employees and damage overall morale. (Although it is demoralizing to keep a nonproductive person in a job, coworkers still expect the organization and manager to treat that the person fairly.) In cases where finding a better fit would not be wise, justifiable, or possible, then the third option, dismissing the employee, must be pursued.

As a guide for determining the best course of action, Coens and Jenkins (2000) offer several questions for managers to ask when facing a serious performance problem. The questions are listed in figure 10-3.

Figure 10-3. Questions to Ask When Facing a Serious Performance Problem (Coens and Jenkins 2000)

Checking for fit

- Is the performance a pattern or a recent development?
- Does the person have the necessary skills, knowledge, abilities, and temperament to do the job?
- Does the person like the work? Do they like the organization?

Checking for bias or inconsistent expectations

- Is this the first incident of this type, or have variations happened in the past?
- Can the observations of the supervisor be confirmed by others?
- Is there a personal, chemistry, or political issue that may have triggered the problem?
- Has the person received adequate training, guidance, and feedback?
- Has the job undergone significant change recently?
- Have management or performance expectations changed? Does the individual understand these changes?

Assessing the influence of systemic issues on individual performance

- Has the same performance deficiency/problem been observed with other people in the same job?
- How long has the person been in the job? Could subpar performance be explained by insufficient time on the learning curve, stagnation, or burnout?
- Has there been a change in the workload, volume, increase in stressors, staffing shortages, or other changes that may be be triggering the performance issue?
- Are there barriers or issues that are causing the performance problems that are not the fault of the individual? (e.g., proper tools, equipment, training, support, etc.)

When these questions do not lead to a solution and involuntary separation seems to be the only logical course, there is still another option: voluntary separation.

Sometimes open and honest dialogue about performance issues can lead individual employees to resign voluntarily. For legal reasons, certain safeguards must be taken in such cases. In such cases, working in partnership with your human resources department can be helpful and is required by many organizations. Human resources staff can also provide guidance on the process of dealing with unacceptable performance, should it be necessary.

Although taking steps that eventually lead to either voluntary separation or involuntary termination can be emotionally difficult, not taking them often leaves managers in a state of paralysis while the situation continues to deteriorate. It is all too common to observe two polarized approaches, neither of which is helpful to the individual employee, manager, department, or organization:

- **Waiting until the situation becomes intolerable before making the decision to terminate the employee immediately:** Human resources professionals report that it is more common than not for them to be contacted only at the point of termination, which makes it difficult at best to go through the necessary legal steps of intensive coaching and documentation.
- **Deciding to do nothing:** At this point, facing the discomfort and conflict entailed in confronting the employee seems too difficult. Managers resort to a default strategy: They hope that the situation will go away, that the employee will leave or transfer, or that they will find ways to work around the problem individual.

Waiting too long to move into an intensive process makes a difficult situation almost impossible to deal with. Although doing nothing feels like the easier path to take, it exacts a heavy toll. Most obvious is the disillusioning effect on the immediate work group, who often need to take on extra work to make up for the problem employee's poor performance. Less obvious but even more destructive is the tendency of managers and organizations to create policies based on the actions of a few poor performers rather than addressing performance issues on an individual basis. For example, a manager may find that tardiness is an issue for a handful of employees. To address the problem, he may establish a policy that stipulates how many times each individual employee is allowed be late during a specific time period, say, three times per year.

The policy stipulates that the employees' pay will be docked and disciplinary action will be taken when they are late a fourth time, and so on. The policy seems objective and fair to everyone, but the problem is that it eliminates the element of judgment. Eventually, policy manuals become filled with policies meant to address the behavior of a few but affecting everyone in the organization. Employees get the message: This organization does not trust its employees. Consider the following example from the "I-am-not-making-this-up" department:

> The human resources vice-president for a large healthcare system shared an example that demonstrates this tendency. Over the years, his organization had created many policies for all employees that were really designed to make it easier to correct the behaviors of a few. One of these policies dictated the number of times someone could be tardy in a year. When an employee was late more than the number of times allowed according to the policy, the employee was subject to disciplinary action. To emphasize the importance of coming to work on time, the organization also issued quarterly perfect attendance awards in the amount of $500 for those employees who were neither late nor absent during the preceding three months.
>
> During one unusually harsh winter, snowstorms left several inches of accumulation on the ground, and road conditions were sometimes treacherous. One day when snow had decreased the level of visibility on the roads, a multiple-car accident closed the main expressway for several hours. As might be expected, several employees on their way to work were delayed by the traffic jam and they were late for work. The tardiness of employees on this day was recorded, and disciplinary action was instituted for those who had exceeded the allowable level of tardiness.
>
> As might be expected with so much at stake, those who were stuck on the expressway because of the accident asked to have the tardiness for the day removed from their records because they were late due to circumstances beyond their control. The organization's decision? The tardiness on that day was not removed from the record because "others who were not stuck in the accident arrived at work on time." Fairness, it was determined, had nothing to do with the circumstances! The policy was black and white, and so it was applied without exception.

When managers are confronted with inappropriate behavior or a pattern of unacceptable performance, the tendency is to create a solution and impose that solution on all employees. The cumulative effect of these actions unintentionally erodes motivation and the health of the work environment. The message to people: "You are inferior and untrustworthy, even when the official rhetoric speaks of respect for people" (Scholtes 1998, p. 297).

With this broader view of what often results from avoiding the per-formance problem or waiting too long to seek assistance, the best course of action is to contact the human resources department to ask for support when you suspect that a performance problem may be lead to a separation or termination.

Taking Action to Address Problem Performance

Once it has been decided that a performance problem must be addressed, the next challenge is to determine the best course of action. Generally speaking, there are two distinct approaches:

- **Performance improvement:** The performance improvement approach is a rigorous feedback and documentation process that generally spans sixty to ninety days, depending on the nature of the problem. It is designed to clearly specify the performance expectations, identify the gap, document what is expected in the future, and articulate how management will support the individual. This intensive process serves the dual purpose of providing rigorous support in the hope that the individual can improve their level of performance and documentation in the event the outcome results in involuntary termination.
- **Corrective action:** The corrective action approach follows a path of progressive discipline. In some organizations, this approach takes the form of positive discipline, which will be discussed later in this chapter.

Broadly speaking, health care organizations tend to rely heavily on the use of the corrective action method, although a few organizations have implemented a positive discipline approach. However, exercising a corrective approach misses the mark when the root cause of the prob-lem is rooted in capability or skill deficiencies. The decision on the path to take should be based on an accurate assessment of the under-lying cause of the problem and matching it to the process that is most likely to facilitate improvement.

Consider a similar situation in another context. The Harper fam-ily has two children, Bill and Sarah. Ironically, both brought home report cards one quarter with a class grade of a D; Bill's was in math and Sarah's was in French. Bill is an active child, plays sports, and has a very full social life. He rarely studies for math and often misses his homework assignments. Sarah, on the other hand, studies, asks for assistance from her teacher after school, and even sought out help from a tutor. Despite this effort, something does not click with Sarah, and she continues to do poorly on her French tests.

Both children are performing at an unacceptable level. Should the action taken by Mr. and Mrs. Harper be the same for both? Should both Sarah and Bill be grounded? The action of grounding is the family equivalent of the corrective action path. Bill neglected his studies even though he knew that the consequences would be an unsatisfactory grade and trouble with his parents. Grounding may be an appropriate way to convey to Bill the need to make better decisions and choices about how he spends his time. It helps clarify his parents' expectations and demonstrates the consequences attached to the willful or intentional act of ignoring his homework. The result may very well be an improvement in his performance in math as he learns to rebalance his time.

But would grounding Sarah have the same result? Clearly, her performance was not the result of neglect, but rather a more fundamental comprehension or skill problem. Grounding Sarah would have no effect on her French grades, and it might actually make them worse. Sarah is likely to benefit more from targeted support. Perhaps putting together a study plan designed by her teacher and supported at home would be of greater value. This path would be akin to performance improvement planning. The plan may result in improvement, and that is certainly the hope. It may also help confirm that French is not the best language for Sarah to master, and other decisions might be considered. Perhaps learning Spanish, for example, would be easier for Sarah.

Performance Improvement Approach

The performance improvement planning (PIP) process is directed more toward the correction of unacceptable performance than toward unacceptable behavior. PIP is typically exercised when regular feedback and coaching have not sufficiently raised the individual's level of performance. The purpose of performance improvement planning is to give the individual every possible chance to correct the deficiencies while at the same time creating a documented record of the actions taken by the manager. It is considered a serious process, and it may end in termination when performance does not meet improvement goals. Performance improvement plans vary considerably in format according to the type of work and the type of problems to be addressed, but every PIP should be designed to fulfill the following goals:

- Point out the difference between present performance and agreed-upon expectations

- Describe the specific changes to be made
- Document the actions that will be taken to support the employee, including periodic reviews of progress
- Document the duration of the plan (usually thirty to ninety days, depending on the circumstances and results expected)
- Clarify the actions (that is, transfer, demotion, or termination) that may result if performance does not improve to an acceptable level by the end of the designated period of improvement

The performance improvement planning process protects the employee from unfair treatment as well as the organization from potential litigation. In a performance-related discharge, a paper trail describing the performance problems and the remedial efforts to counsel and assist the employee before discharging should be continuous. Too often, managers think of compiling a paper trail only after they have decided that termination is the best course. They rush the improvement program and try to fire an employee who has years of tenure with only three months of documentation, because they did not document their actions during the long period of time they earnestly spent trying to help the employee through informal coaching. The deficient paper trail leaves the impression of a very unfair or biased discharge and becomes the basic ingredient for a potential lawsuit.

Whenever serious performance problems arise, formal meetings must be held with the employee to provide the necessary guidance and counseling and to accumulate the needed documentation. Documentation of the performance improvement process can include appraisal forms, e-mails, memos, and formal notices of deficiency. After remedial measures have failed to lead to improved performance, involuntary termination may become necessary. The following facts need to be confirmed before the actual termination meeting can take place (Coens and Jenkins 2000, pp. 239–40):

- The employee clearly knew what was expected of him or her.
- The employee was given all of the information, training, and resources needed to perform adequately.
- The deficiencies were serious enough to warrant action and specific examples of the deficiencies have been documented (for example, if the employee repeatedly failed to complete major projects on time, documentation needs to show exactly which projects were left incomplete or submitted late, how the employee know that the projects were a priority, what the consequences of the employee's poor performance were, and so on).

- The details of how and when the employee was advised of the deficiencies have been documented (for example, the content and times of counseling and meetings with the employee, forewarning that the employee would be terminated for continued poor performance, and so on).
- The particulars on any special help, counseling, assistance, retraining, or other measures offered to help the employee have been documented.

Obviously, this description of how to handle and document performance deficiencies of a serious nature is a bare-bones overview of the process. For more details, you should consult a more complete treatment of the subject, such as the *Supervisor's Guide to Documenting Employee Discipline* by Lee Patterson and Michael Deblieux (1993).

Corrective Action Approach

The choice of corrective action or positive discipline is pursued in cases where the incident or the performance issue is willful or intentional on the part of the employee. Making this distinction is important. Corrective action is appropriate only in cases of gross misconduct, improper behavior, insubordination, or violation of a clearly defined work rule. Although many organizations pursue a progressive path (increasing the duration of the time without pay with each additional infraction), the process can be stepped up when the seriousness of the infraction warrants immediate termination. Theft, harassment, abuse, and immoral or indecent conduct are all examples of acts that can result in immediate termination. The actions to be taken in response to such infractions depend on the circumstances surrounding the case, the nature and severity of the offense, the employee's past record, and the past practices of the organization. With all of these variables at play, it is advisable to seek counsel from the human resources department so a more systemic view of the circumstances can be considered.

Conventional wisdom in health care has been that when employees fail to meet performance standards or guidelines for attendance or personal conduct, managers should put them through a disciplinary process, or as one manager bluntly stated, "Get their name and write them up!" Traditionally, health care managers have seen discipline as something they have to do to the employee in order to bring them back in line. Inextricably woven in this punitive mind-set are the concepts of discipline and punishment. Paradoxically, this line of thinking leads managers to treat employees worse and worse while hoping that their behavior becomes better and better. Seldom, however, does any employee come back from a suspension with a good attitude.

Despite the lack of evidence that this system for dealing with behavior problems engenders good outcomes, most health care facilities adhere to this 1930s human resources philosophy and euphemistically call their system progressive discipline. In reality, there is very little about this approach that is progressive. It is based on the belief that the failure to comply with standards or meet expectations should be met with punishment. Often, the only question asked by managers is, "Did the punishment fit the crime?"

Discipline and punishment are so intertwined in the culture of most health care organizations that the two terms are synonymous for many of us. Managers are expected to enforce compliance, which they often refer to as their law enforcement or policeman role, and most admit privately that they regret and dislike this role, especially when experienced and knowledgeable employees are involved. Regret and dislike are not the only side effects of this outdated approach. Managers also report that they are averse to taking on what feels like a controlling, parental role when they are trying to foster adult professional behaviors. Sometimes managers put off dealing with issues because they feel that there are so many stifling requirements placed on them by the human resources department. Employees often complain that managers allow some individuals more leeway than others. Savvy employees learn how to play the game, and after a while punishment loses power and being written up is no longer of significance. Employees simply accept their warnings and there is little discussion of taking ownership or committing to a personal plan for change in the future. They know there are no real consequences for their actions.

The entire concept of escalating punishments (verbal then written warnings followed by suspension and finally termination) as a means of bringing about behavioral change totally undermines the goal of progressive managers who want to work in partnership with their employees. It is increasingly obvious that "little of value comes out of the common belief that discipline and punishment go hand in hand" (Harvey 1986, p. 2). Clearly we need to revisit this age-old mind-set if we hope to create a culture of engagement and retention.

Positive Discipline Approach

In many areas of business and industry, the outdated punitive approach has already been replaced by a genuinely progressive system. Beginning in the mid-1980s, large corporations such as General Electric, Proctor and Gamble, Penzoil, and others opted to reorient their approach to discipline by moving away from punishment and toward building commitment. In his now classic article, "Discipline versus Punishment," Harvey states that:

> Successful organizations no longer look upon "discipline" as something that a manager *does* to a poor performer when he or she misbehaves. Instead these companies now approach discipline as something that must be *created*. They have abandoned traditional punitive measures, and in their place have developed systems that require acceptance of personal responsibility, individual decision making and true self discipline. They have made the transition from the concept of "doing discipline" to the more constructive perspective of "being disciplined" (Harvey 1986, p. 2).

Ironically, developing a system with the intent of encouraging commitment rather than executing punishment is not a difficult process. The process looks similar to the more traditional approach, but the premise on which this system rests is substantially different. (See figure 10-4.) The positive discipline approach is based on the basic belief that managers in an organization are responsible for leading the establishment of standards and expectations for performance. They are also responsible for letting individual employees know when those expectations and standards are not being met. The employee is the only one who can decide whether to adhere to the organization's standards and meet its expectations. In other words, the employee owns the choices regarding his or her behavior, not the manager.

Changing how we deal with disciplinary issues can create a more engaged and committed workforce, and it speaks volumes to employees about the organization's desire to help them be the best that they can be. The positive discipline process is not a panacea for every problem related to discipline, nor does it fit every situation that requires intervention on the part of the manager. It fits well, however, when managers are dealing with one of the following situations:

- The misconduct warrants a response other than formal discipline or termination.
- The problem is not a skill deficiency, but a behavioral issue.
- Using this approach will most likely prevent further problem behavior.
- The employee takes ownership for the misconduct and expresses a willingness to change and sustain the needed changes (Murray 2003).

Figure 10-4.   Model of the Positive Discipline Process

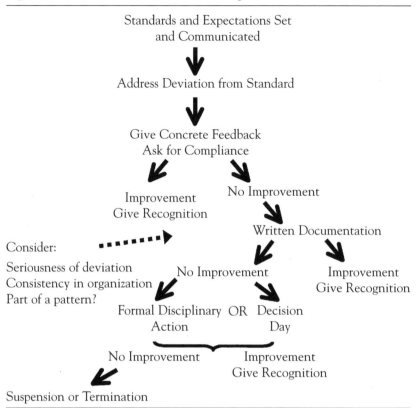

Standards and Expectations Set
and Communicated

Address Deviation from Standard

Give Concrete Feedback
Ask for Compliance

Improvement   No Improvement
Give Recognition

Written Documentation

Consider:

Seriousness of deviation   No Improvement   Improvement
Consistency in organization   Give Recognition
Part of a pattern?

Formal Disciplinary   OR   Decision
Action   Day

No Improvement   Improvement
Give Recognition

Suspension or Termination

Managers in health care organizations must deal with such situations on a regular basis, and most managers would probably welcome a more workable solution that focuses on ownership and accountability for personal behavior instead of a system of escalated punishments. For example, one manager in Arizona said, "Since we adopted this approach it has made my life easier by putting the onus for change back where it belongs and getting me out of the policeman role."

The underlying shift in basic beliefs is from punishment, "get their names and write them up," to encouraging self-discipline and making employees responsible for maintaining reasonable standards of conduct. This is a crucial difference and cannot be underestimated. This is a fundamental change in the underlying assumptions and beliefs that are the underpinnings for a system of discipline and cannot be taken lightly or covered quickly or superficially in one management meeting. If managers simply use new language as they continue to behave in the same old parent–child manner, employees do not feel supported in recommitting to anything but a job search. Employees are smart enough to recognize the change de jour or "flavor of the month" bandwagon and simply assume that the managers have been to another workshop and are now using different words to "bring them back in line." Harvey is adamant about this as he writes, "the impact of the change on the organization will be no more than that of putting a Mercedes emblem on the hood of a rusty Pinto. What is required is a total organizational commitment to an entirely different approach to the issue of managing people, performance and professionalism" (Harvey 1986, p. 3).

Treating employees as responsible adults (since we are expecting responsible behavior) may well require intentional work with managers about how to give feedback and what to do when the conversation does not go well and employees decline to take ownership for their behavior. When employees take on a victim role and blame everyone else or when they give lip service to expected behavior change, managers need coaching on how to respond in ways that are adultlike rather than the "critical parent role" that comes naturally with frustration. The manager must continue to uphold appropriate standards. There are always some employees who do not want to accept ownership for their behavior, but the vast majority of employees appreciate being treated as adults and supported in efforts to change. These people recommit to the organizational standards when the situation is dealt with in a fair and professional manner. By pointing out the gap between expected behavior and actual behavior and offering to support the employee in closing that gap as they move forward, the focus shifts to the future and supports commitment to that future rather than punishing for past behavior. This emphasis on moving forward rather than rehashing old patterns tends to promote a mutual respect and partnership between employees and managers. Obviously, this is a welcome change for managers who become more likely to confront gaps in behavior when the process they use feels more professional and affirming rather than punitive.

When managers feel more comfortable confronting marginal behavior and pointing out the gap between what is observed and what is expected, they are more likely to deal with these issues as they occur and not put them off. The majority of employees who are meeting or exceeding standards are reassured in knowing that when colleagues are not measuring up, they will be confronted. When behavior does not measure up to agreed-upon standards, most employees prefer that this be dealt with early on rather than waiting until some event necessitates a meeting of those involved.

Experience with this approach in business for the past twenty years has also demonstrated positive outcomes with respect to labor relations. Because positive discipline relies on the employee committing to behavioral expectations and developing their own action plan, there is less likelihood of wrongful termination suits. Labor unions report fewer grievances since the emphasis in on problem solving and supporting the employees' efforts to change rather than "making the punishment fit the crime" (Harvey 1986).

It goes without saying that if this approach is preferred in unionized environments, if managers are more likely to deal with a performance issue instead of putting it off, and if employees are simply following their own identified plan for moving forward, then managers have more time to recognize and support those who are doing a good job of meeting expectations. Finally, we can move away from having "problem employees" consume so much of the managers' time and emotional energy. Most important, employees take ownership for their own behavior and feel more committed to an organization in which they are treated as adults and are supported in their efforts to improve (Murray 2003).

Increasing numbers of health care organizations have undertaken the philosophical shift to positive or nonpunitive discipline. Their experience has provided further evidence of the many benefits of this approach. The numbers of grievances and suspensions have been reduced, and managers have more time for recognizing high-performing employees and promoting healthy interpersonal relationships, which result in a sense of partnership among employees and managers.

For example, a employee relations manager in a tertiary care center told a story about a long-term employee whose behavior had deteriorated to the point that it was no longer meeting the organization's customer service standards. To address the customer service problem, the employee's manager initiated the positive discipline process. When the employee returned to work after a one-day leave during which she completed a self-assessment and performance improvement plan, the employee called the employee relations manager to let him know where she was in the process and that she was optimistic about her ability to get back on track. She explained that the day away had given her some time for personal reflection about how much she really wanted to keep her job. She told him, "You know, I think it is really good of my supervisor to give me this time to sort things out. . . . She could have just fired me, but instead she is working with me on this and that makes me want to hold up my part of the deal."

Similarly, a director of nursing operations in Idaho was so impressed with the positive changes he has seen in the two years since the implementation of a positive discipline approach that he wrote about their experience in salvaging good employees. In his article, "Positive Discipline Reaps Retention," he explains that "prior to implementing this approach there were 30 suspensions or disciplinary actions in process. That number dropped to 12 in the first year of implementation and was again cut in half in the next quarter" (Murray 2003, p. 20). He also reports that the implementation of this approach has been transformational for the organization because communications among employees and managers are now on a more mature level, and employees are behaving in a more empowered manner as they take responsibility for their own behavior. Managers in the organization have found this system to be much easier to use than past disciplinary programs, and much of the animosity that existed between operational managers and human resources staff has dissipated because the process is so clear and workable. Managers using this approach follow an agreed-upon policy that has also been communicated to employees and includes the following directions for managers (Murray 2003):

- Informally communicate to employees that you value their role and expertise.
- Build the confidence level of your employees by reminding them that they have the ability to change.
- Provide direction and guidelines with communication of expectations for change and continued success.
- Draft a standard of expectations memo when formal communications are needed.
- Determine whether the employee will accept responsibility for his or her actions or continue to deny ownership.
- Continue with positive reinforcement for behavior change, and if the behavior does not change, provide the employee with a day off with pay as a time for reflection.

It should be noted that the policies on positive discipline typically stipulate that the one-day self-assessment/decision-making leaves that are granted to employees are offered only once per employee. The employee typically returns from this day of leave having reflected on their willingness and responsibility to change their own behavior and having developed a plan for sustaining the needed changes. This plan is reviewed with the manager and signed by both the employee and the manager (Murray 2003).

Another major medical center implemented a system for positive discipline in the nonunion parts of the organization and found that, in addition to the benefits mentioned earlier, they also noticed that immature and acting-out behavior diminished when managers addressed employees' unacceptable behavior or performance issues in an adult manner. The director of employee and labor relations for the system commented on how impressed she had been with the quality of the performance improvement plans that employees developed. In reflecting on their progress after one year using this system for discipline, she stated, "It has become clear to me that when we treat our employees as adults and support their efforts to change, then they respond as adults and often exceed our expectations" (Searcy 2003).

The insight into culture change reflected in this comment points to a key aspect of how we handle discipline in health care organizations. The approach we use with employees when the need for discipline arises says a great deal to them about the fundamental values of the organization. Authoritarian and punitive responses from managers negate whatever sentiments may be posted in the lobby about how the organization values each of its employees. "It is through the discipline system that the organization's culture is revealed most directly to the individual" (Harvey 1986, p. 5).

Slowly but surely health care organizations are revisiting some of their basic beliefs and assumptions. According to Harvey (1986), the success of so many organizations that have implemented positive discipline systems is encouraging:

> They recognize that whatever the "real world" may be, it was created by management behaviors and beliefs, and therefore can be changed through different behaviors and beliefs. They realize that commitment cannot be mandated—it must be built. By eliminating punishment, by recognizing good performance, by creating effective administrative systems that emphasize individual responsibility and decision making, commitment to high performance and achieving organizational goals is for them a workplace reality (Harvey 1986, p. 5).

Asking for Assistance from the Human Resources Department

Addressing performance problems is difficult no matter what system we use. Perhaps it is because we have so much at stake that we look for inflexible policies to guide us through the process. Unfortunately, the most effective actions often require the application of judgment and the consideration of each case's unique circumstances at various points along the way. In the initial stages of the process, we need to ask ourselves:

- Is the problem rooted in a system-based cause? (This is the same question posed by most nonpunitive risk management policies in an attempt to promote a safe environment.)
- Is the problem a fit issue that can be better addressed in partnership with the employee?
- Has everything been done to support the employee's ability to succeed?

At the point of taking action, we need to ask:

- Is this a behavioral problem or a competency/skill problem?
- How serious is the problem?

Finally, we need to assess the outcome of the process:

- Has the performance improved to an acceptable level? If not, is a job transfer, demotion, or separation appropriate?
- Has the case been sufficiently documented in the event of litigation?

Each of these decision points is tough to face alone, and the process usually can be effectively addressed when the manager works in partnership with the human resources department. The support that human resources professionals can provide spans a number of areas, the most important of which are the development and application of clear policies and guidelines, consultation and support, and education and training.

Clear Policies and Guidelines

Clear policies and guidelines help ensure the staff's awareness of the organization's policies as well as the consistency of policy application across the organization. New employee orientation programs usually include a review of the organization's human resources policies. Orientation gives employees who are new to the organization an opportunity to ask questions and gain an understanding of the organization's expectations of employees, given that human resources policies vary among organizations, depending on each organization's values and services.

Consultation and Support

By design, human resources brings an objective perspective to the processes of performance improvement and discipline and can readily assist the manager in determining appropriate actions. Human resources professionals deal with cases across the organization on a daily basis, and so they are able to guide managers in a way that ensures consistency but accommodates any circumstances unique to individual cases. They are the repository of information on past precedents, another important checkpoint. Finally, they are professionally trained in how to conduct these sometimes difficult conversations and can serve as a much-needed support for managers faced with employee performance issues.

Education and Training

It is critical that managers receive training so that they can thoroughly understand their organization's human resources policies and definitions of specific performance problems. Human resources professionals can also help managers build their counseling skills and apply performance management tools effectively. Although these steps cannot eliminate every problem associated with confronting a performance problem, they can certainly help managers stay on track and avoid predictable pitfalls.

Taking action to address performance problems is an important leadership function, and one that is best approached with adequate knowledge, skill, and support. Adequate preparation helps us to overcome our natural tendency to avoid unpleasant situations. Working in partnership with human resources during the early stages of the performance improvement process also helps managers avoid the missteps that can make the process longer or more difficult than it needs to be.

Extreme Performance Challenges

In this final section of the chapter, several difficult challenges are addressed. These include managing negativity in the workplace and dealing with especially difficult employee behaviors.

Managing Negativity in the Workplace

In some workplaces, the culture is characterized by negativity. Complaints predominate, uncooperative behavior is the norm, and coming to work just seems to become more burdensome every day. This kind of climate is demoralizing and depressing for all who work in it. Sometimes it has been a long-term characteristic that simply worsens over time, especially when it was left unchecked for years, while in other instances it may be a more recent development, perhaps in response to a specific situation such as employee layoffs or severe financial difficulties.

Most of us become frustrated with constant negativity and complaining. And worse, the impact on productivity is significant. As noted in chapter 4, there is a strong business case for a workplace where people are happy, and the reverse can be extrapolated from the research. When people are unhappy, creativity is lower, satisfaction is less common, absenteeism is higher, attention spans are shorter, problem-solving abilities are decreased, and cooperation is nil. This entire book has been about creating a positive work environment. And, although there were specific suggestions made in chapter 4 for finding happiness in the workplace, this section briefly summarizes steps we can take to deal with a negative work environment.

Five-Step Process for Addressing Negativity

There are five specific steps that can be taken to address negativity in the workplace. They are:

1. Examine your own behavior and make necessary adjustments.
2. Establish clear expectations for behavioral norms.
3. Address deviations in acceptable behavior in others.
4. Give each other direct and honest feedback.
5. Use deliberate approaches for helping people substitute the positive for the negative.

Step 1: Examine Your Own Behavior
One of the first questions to ask is: Am I part of the problem? The research on emotional intelligence has clearly revealed that the emotions of the leader have a significant impact on those of the people with whom the leader works. And in any workplace, we are usually closely involved, at least geographically, with the people around us. Increasingly complex, difficult challenges in our organizations help create a work environment where emotions are running high and difficulties require a lot of energy to surmount. You can perform a quick self-assessment by answering the following questions:

- How do I respond to problems and issues?
- Do I still have faith and optimism that most problems can be worked out?
- Do I have the ability to rise above the difficulties of the day and hold fast to a new vision for the future? Or am I so tired and bogged down with the everyday details of my work that I am as demoralized and downtrodden as anyone in the department?

- How do I respond to the good news that people bring? Do I reinforce it, or am I cynical and pessimistic?

Doing a quick self-assessment can reveal opportunities for immediate change and improvement. Of course, if you are a paragon of positivity, there may be no room for improvement and you can proceed directly to step 2!

Steps 2 and 3: Establish Clear Expectations and Address Deviations
Steps 2 and 3 are inextricably linked. Establishing clear expectations was discussed briefly in an earlier chapter. This is an intervention that works most effectively when establishing the expectations is done with the active involvement of employees. The basic approach would be to facilitate a discussion with staff members about what the mutual expectations should be in order to create a more positive working environment. In some instances, however, when there is a great deal of negativity in the department, you may encounter significant resistance from people as you try to facilitate the development of expectations. You may bring the group together, but members sit back, do not contribute, and basically just refuse to participate. In this situation, the manager can say something along these lines of:

> Okay, I've asked for your help in establishing our expectations of each other. You don't seem to be willing or interested in doing so. That means you are granting me the authority to set these for us. The trade-off here is that when I develop these expectations, you will be responsible for living up to them.

If you need to resort to this tactic, do not hesitate to do so. You do not have to let resistant or obstructionist behavior on the part of employees keep you from establishing expectations for a more positive workplace. You will find there are members of your work group who are secretly glad you are tackling this issue because they may be facing tremendous pressure from their peers to be negative.

This is an instance, however, of where you need to work closely with a colleague from human resources as well as with the person to whom you report. They can review your expectations to determine whether they believe they are realistic and clear. You are also going to need their support as you hold people accountable for meeting these new expectations.

As you address people's deviations from the newly established norms, working closely with specialists in human resources helps you go as far as you need to in order to deal with any deviant behavior. If you have particularly toxic employees who are influencing the rest of the staff, simply dealing with one or two very firmly sends the message to the others that you are not going to tolerate destructive or inappropriate behavior.

Once you have established the expectations, an important next step is to share them with employees. You can begin by saying something like:

> It feels like we have gotten very negative here in our department. This makes it harder for all of us to come to work and I believe it is beginning to impact the quality of service we are providing. This is a good time to start fresh with clear expectations. Let's look at what I have developed. I would be happy to hear your feedback and additional suggestions.

Pointing out to people that this is a new start puts everyone on an equal footing, and it does not hurt to let bygones be bygones.

Developing concrete expectations for a positive workplace is not easy to do. We are often so afraid that we cannot be concrete enough around attitude issues that we fail to address these problems. As a leader you can expect certain things from the people with whom you work. For example, it is possible and even desirable to say that the organization needs employees who:

- Speak positively of others
- Encourage others around them
- Have a can-do attitude
- Find the positive about an idea or situation before complaining about the negative
- Treat each other courteously and kindly
- Work interdependently with others
- Have a positive and upbeat approach to things

Step 4: Give Direct and Honest Feedback
The process of giving feedback was explored more fully earlier in the chapter. This step can be difficult to do if you are in a very negative workplace. However, you simply must be committed to delivering feedback, or people do not understand how they have deviated from the expectations. Admittedly, this takes a significant amount of energy in the beginning when people test your intentions and fortitude. It is human nature to challenge limits that have been placed on us. We want to see whether the person plans to live up to their statements and

expectations. Each of us needs to be willing to hear feedback on our own behavior without becoming defensive or angry.

Step 5: Help People Substitute the Positive for the Negative

Chapter 4 explained specific interventions from the field of positive psychology that can help increase happiness levels in individuals and in the workplace. These include approaches such as the gratitude letter, the blessings activity, letting go of grudges, and so on. All of these exercises can substantially improve the atmosphere at work. For example, using appreciative inquiry as an approach to issues is more positive than focusing on problems.

Additional Interventions

In addition to the approaches discussed in earlier chapters, leaders can use myriad other interventions. Three additional approaches are helpful for addressing common issues.

Balancing Exercise

During times of great change, there are often occasions when staff members can only grumble and see the negative side of the situation. This exercise can be performed quickly during a department meeting or as an individual intervention. It is simple and consists of making a list on a piece of paper. On one side you list the things that may be gained as a consequence of the change, and on the other side you list the things that you are likely to lose because of the change. You think of as many ideas as possible. Then, working with a partner, you review the list, and the partner adds two to three new items to each column.

People who focus predominantly on the losses change brings have a harder time dealing with change. Those who can see only the positive also have difficulty coping with change because they fail to anticipate their losses and often experience them as unpleasant surprises. This simple activity helps us balance our perspective and find a much healthier approach to change.

Reframing

Reframing is another powerful technique for focusing on the positive. Reframing means simply that we change the frame in which we perceive an event in order to change the meaning of the event. When the meaning changes, so do our responses and behaviors. This approach was developed years ago in Bandler and Grinder's (1982) work on neurolinguistic programming. It is best illustrated by a very old Chinese Taoist story about a farmer in a poor country village:

> [The farmer] was considered very well-to-do, because he owned a horse, which he used for plowing and transportation. One day his horse ran away. All his neighbors exclaimed how terrible this was, but the farmer simply said, "Maybe."
>
> A few days later the horse returned and brought two wild horses with it. The neighbors all rejoiced at his good fortune, but the farmer just said, "Maybe."
>
> The next day the farmer's son tried to ride one of the wild horses; the horse threw him and broke his leg. The neighbors all offered their sympathy for his misfortune, but the farmer again said, "Maybe."
>
> The next week conscription officers came to the village to take young men for the army. They rejected the farmer's son because of his broken leg. When the neighbors told him how lucky he was, the farmer replied, "Maybe."

This approach can be used in the workplace to change the context of the complaint or issue that people feel negatively toward. For example, one emergency department charge nurse reacted in this way when employees were complaining that they had held a patient in the department for almost three hours and an inpatient bed still was not available. The charge nurse said, "Look at it this way, we're now three hours closer to getting that patient upstairs." Using reframing is a way to identify the positive aspects of a situation. In this way, a difficult customer service situation gives us an opportunity to hone our skills in conflict resolution and to make a needed improvement in our system. A difficult day in the department reveals more information about the skill levels and working relationships of employees. It is not just putting a superficially positive spin on things; it is truly finding what is positive about the situation.

Years ago I became ill with appendicitis the day before we were planning to leave for a long-anticipated vacation, and I ended up hospitalized after the surgery. Although we were disappointed initially, overall we were relieved that the attack came the day before our vacation rather than while we were on vacation because my being hospitalized away from home would have been much worse. We were able to reschedule the vacation after I recuperated. It was one of the few times I had a clear desk and could take the unanticipated recovery time with ease. People who cope well with adversity usually use reframing as a technique.

Forward-Focused Meetings

Forward-focused meetings are meetings during which the manager or leader deliberately ensures that the process does not deteriorate into a gripe session. When a meeting starts, the leader can take one of several different steps. The first is to remind people of the parameters of the discussion. For instance, if the discussion has gotten off track and become a very negative discussion of an unrelated issue, reminding the group that they have only a certain amount of time left in the meeting can bring them back onto the subject they need to deal with. Another key question to ask the group to think about is whether the issue that has come up is one that they can do something about. In other words, if we have no control or influence over this issue, we should not waste our time talking about it. Bringing the focus back to what is working and why it is working is another way to convert negative to positive energy in a group.

Converting a negative department climate to one that is positive is time-consuming and challenging. However, a chronically negative workplace is a tough place in which to exist. Even small improvements can make a big difference to the people there. When the organization's climate is pervasively negative, the challenge is even greater.

Dealing with Extreme Behavior

One of the most difficult challenges faced by managers, leaders, and employees alike is dealing and coping with extreme behavior. Toxic, caustic, and destructive behavior on the part of people in the workplace leads to the development of a toxic workplace. "The operational definition of a toxic workplace: it's a place where people come to work so they can make enough money so they can leave" (Webber 1998, p. 156). When destructive, negative behavior is tolerated, no one feels safe.

Extremes in behavior are often the result of mental illness, and like the general population, employees in health care organizations are vulnerable to psychiatric disorders such as clinical depression and substance abuse. Although managers usually are not expected to handle these issues directly, mental illness among employees and managers can have a drastic effect on individual job performance as well as a negative impact on coworkers and patients. In its most extreme forms, mental illness, especially substance abuse disorders, among health care providers can actually place patients and coworkers at serious risk for physical harm.

Most managers in health care organizations are not equipped to recognize specific psychiatric problems manifested among their colleagues and employees. However, personality disorders, depressive disorders, and anxiety disorders, as well as substance abuse disorders, are as common among health care providers as among the general population. Managers are not expected to be mental health experts, but they should be able to recognize the warning signs of the most common psychiatric disorders as well as the symptoms of alcohol- or drug-related impairment so that they can refer troubled individuals to a source of professional mental health services as soon as possible. It may be useful to ask the director of the organization's employee assistance program to provide an in-service for the management team on the subject of recognizing and managing employees with personality disorders, substance abuse disorders, and other mental health problems.

Some mental health problems are the result of acute illness (for example, a treatable episode of clinical depression), some are chronic but treatable (such as posttraumatic stress disorder), while others (particularly personality disorders) are relatively permanent features of behavior. Working with or managing employees with psychiatric disorders can be a challenge, as can managing employees whose behavior is affected by substance abuse or addiction and other forms of impairment.

The first step in dealing with a troubled employee should always be referring the employee to the organization's employee assistance program. Managers should also document their efforts to intervene with troubled employees and discuss any related problems with the employee relations manager in human resources as early as possible. It is important that managers maintain complete records of the conversations and coaching and counseling efforts they provide for use in any possible litigation in the future (Cavaiola and Lavender 2000).

It is also essential for the manager to maintain the confidentiality of employees with mental health problems. Employees with mental health problems deserve the same level of respect as employees with medical problems. Tossing around diagnostic labels when referring to employees is inappropriate.

A detailed discussion of the impact of severe mental illness and substance abuse on health care workers and organizations is beyond the scope of this book. Instead, we have chosen to focus on the kinds of extreme behavior that lead to a negative workplace: bullying and disruptive personalities. In no way is this brief discussion intended to provide a manager with enough information to diagnose or treat a psychiatric disorder.

Bullying Behavior in the Workplace

One of the most challenging situations in the arena of workplace interpersonal relationships involves the presence of individuals who use bullying behavior to get what they want. "Bullying is not something confined to schoolchildren. It is a widespread form of abuse to be found in all forms of employment, cultures, and religious congregations" (Arbuckle 2000, p. 25). Obviously, bullying is extremely costly in both human and financial terms. "In the United States, businesses are losing an annual five to six billion dollars in decreased productivity alone, due to real or perceived abuse of employees" (Arbuckle 2000, p. 25).

Arbuckle (2000, p. 25) defines bullying as "persistent, unwelcome action or verbal, psychological, or physical aggression that is knowingly or unknowingly directed by an individual or group against people who normally are not in a position to defend themselves. It is irrational behavior, evoking strong emotions in both the bully and victim." Bullies try to force other people to do what they want them to do and are willing to try any kind of intimidation to achieve their goal. One form of bullying has recently received increasing attention in health care workplaces and is referred to as horizontal violence. This represents damaging behaviors that occur between two employees. It must be noted, however, that bullying behavior is not limited to employee–employee relationships. Managers and supervisors also use bullying behavior and intimidation tactics to coerce others in ways that are self-serving rather than beneficial to the organization as a whole and the people within it.

Abrasive and abusive behaviors used by managers and supervisors include both engaging in the toxic behavior themselves and ignoring the behavior in others. In one hospital, a director of perioperative services was being bullied by physicians who did not want to make changes that needed to be made. Several physicians threatened the manager and her family with bodily harm during a meeting attended by the organization's chief executive officer, who did nothing to stop the attacks. In a self-protective effort, the director began parking in a variety of different places from day to day because of threats to her person and property. The manager was actually pushed down a stairwell in the hospital, and still no action was ever taken against the bullies. Most of us find it hard to believe that this kind of behavior can occur, but naïveté is no excuse for refusing to see or deal with bullying behavior.

Bullying behaviors on the part of managers include (Ryan and Oestreich 1991, p. 74):

- Chilling silence
- Glaring eye contact
- Abruptness, shortness
- Snubbing or ignoring people

- Insults and put-downs
- Blaming, discrediting, or discounting others
- Aggressive, controlling mannerisms
- Threats about the job
- Yelling and shouting
- Angry outbursts or losses of emotional control
- Physical threats
- Sexual harassment

Bullying behavior among employees can range from mild forms such as making sarcastic comments, refusing to help others, or just not including individuals in normal kinds of department activities to more serious and dangerous behaviors such as threats and actual physical assaults. Farrell (1997) offers a "professional terrorism" list that sorts the various kinds of bullying behaviors on the basis of whether they are active or passive, verbal or physical, and direct or indirect. Figure 10-5 includes some of Farrell's examples as well as others reported in the literature.

Figure 10-5.   Examples of Bullying Behavior

	Direct	Indirect
Active	**Verbal** Expressing disdain Making snide remarks Constant criticism Screaming at each other Racial slurs **Physical** Assault Property damage Sexual harassment	**Verbal** Talking behind your back Sabotaging behaviors Reporting false information Malicious gossip Persistent nitpicking **Physical** Whipping others into action
Passive	**Verbal** Cattiness Chilly silence **Physical** Refusing to help Refusing to speak to a colleague Turning away Humiliating behaviors	**Verbal** Withholding information from a colleague **Physical** Refusing to move out of the way Ignoring a colleague Blocking opportunities

Thomas (2004) has done extensive research on how nurses handle their anger and reports that one of the most disturbing aspects revealed is the vehemence of nurses' anger directed at each other. The anger described in the research interviews is not a healthy kind of anger that can occur in any workplace, but destructive anger. Thomas writes about the faultfinding, bickering, backbiting, needling, snapping, and cutting remarks that are common in the work environment. Furthermore, she reports that nurses "were constantly writing each other up," which included nasty notes on locker rooms doors as well as reporting each other to supervisors. "Today, hostile messages from coworkers can be transmitted even faster in workplaces with networked computers—in those snippy e-mails with a little zinger at the end" (Thomas 2004, p. 116).

Sometimes the bullying results in performance that can actually threaten patient care. In one department in a large tertiary center in the Midwest, one employee in the department was a vicious bully who embarrassed and humiliated other employees and then employed the threat of physical harm to keep her victims from complaining to management. When the behaviors came to the attention of the assistant manager, he addressed the issue and involved the department manager. As a result, the individual was terminated. However, the bully had quite a following in the department, and the assistant manager soon found himself the target of retaliation in the form of employees calling in sick on his shift and refusing to come in and work when they were needed. The situation actually became quite dangerous before it was addressed. In the end, the assistant manager transferred to another department.

There is no doubt that bullying and other disrespectful behavior can result in negative outcomes in our workplaces. In one study of rudeness, insensitivity, and disrespect in the workplace, the investigator found that most people who were the targets of bullying behavior at work retaliated against their employers rather than the bully. Twenty-eight percent lost work time to avoid the bully; 22 percent decreased their efforts at work; 10 percent decreased the amount of time they spent at work; and 12 percent changed jobs to avoid the bully (Lee 1999). Jeffrey Pfeffer, the Thomas D. Dee Professor of Organizational Behavior at the Stanford Graduate School of Business, insists that organizational loyalty is not dead; instead, toxic companies are driving people away. He says that "there isn't a scarcity of talent—but there is a growing unwillingness to work for toxic organizations" (Webber 1998, p. 154).

So how can we deal with this dysfunctional and destructive behavior? The first step is to be aware of the possibility of bullying and to recognize it for what it is. Dealing with the behavior directly prevents it from escalating out of control. Here are some specific suggestions for dealing with a bully or bullying behavior in the workplace:

- Develop a zero tolerance policy for bullies and bullying behavior. Be very clear that it will not be tolerated, regardless of where it is found. Work with your human resources department to develop appropriate policies and protocols.
- Keep accurate information about the times and places of the bullying behavior. Documentation is critical. Work with human resources specialists to ensure that documentation is complete and adequate.
- Bullies love to dominate. When you are the victim of abuse, do not meet with the bully alone. Request support from the manager or a peer. As a manager, do not expect employees to handle these behaviors alone. Often managerial authority is necessary to deal with this dysfunctional behavior. As a manager, this is not a time to tell employees to "just work it out." That approach amounts to throwing your support on the side of the bully.
- Logical and rational arguments usually do not work with bullies. When such people are confronted with factual information or their deviant behavior is addressed, they often become more enraged and vindictive. Do not expect a reasonable response, and avoid letting your temper flare. It only escalates the emotion in the situation.
- A true bully wants the victim to feel guilty, humiliated, and powerless. Victims of the bully are encouraged to respond with nonviolence but to avoid appearing humiliated. In other words, they should not remain passive but instead should find some nonviolent way to reassert their dignity, perhaps by taking actions or responding in a way that embarrasses the bully (Arbuckle 2000).
- Deal with the unacceptable behavior and do not blame the victim. The victim must feel safe and that someone understands what is happening to him or her. "To overlook what is happening is to collude in the intimidation" (Arbuckle 2000, p. 32). And while whistle-blowing increases your chance of becoming the target of the bully, it is the only ethical course of action under the circumstances.
- Recognize that in some instances the victim of a bully may need the support of a counselor to deal with the aftermath of

emotion. In one study, the researcher discovered that health care workers who experienced bullying behavior often showed symptoms of posttraumatic stress syndrome (Doherty 2002). A referral to your organization's employee assistance program or to another source of professional help may be appropriate.

- Develop an action plan to enlist the help of other employees and managers. If possible, get agreement and commitment from others to help make the work environment a safe and positive place.

Personality Disorders in the Workplace

Without realizing it, we encounter people with personality disorders every day. In fact, most individuals with personality disorders do not even realize that they have a problem. To them and often to their families, friends, and coworkers, their behavior seems perfectly normal. Still, some of the most common personality disorders can result in a significant amount of disruptive behavior inside and outside the workplace. They can also be at the root of individual performance problems, and when that is the case, significant change becomes much more unlikely.

We have all had a coworker who was extremely difficult to work with. Managers often say, "We have this one employee who just keeps things stirred up, and I'm at my wits end as far as how I can deal with her!" This exasperation should be a clue for managers that they may well be dealing with an issue that is more significant than the usual interpersonal differences we encounter every day in our stressful work environments. It is relatively easy for managers to address everyday interpersonal problems by providing feedback or coaching, and most employees eventually recognize their part in a conflict and are able to change their behavior and maintain those changes over time.

When the call for change goes unheeded, however, or when employees refuse to recognize how their own behavior contributes to a problem, you need to consider the possibility that the employees involved may be suffering from a common mental health problem called a personality disorder.

Dr. Vicki Lachman, a well-known nurse consultant who also has a private practice in psychotherapy, defines personality disorders as:

> Enduring patterns of perception or behavior that are inflexible and maladaptive and cause significant stress. Personality-disordered individuals often see themselves as victimized by the "system" and have little insight into how they contribute to their own problems or how to change. The individuals' personality problems often appear to be acceptable and natural for them. . . . They typically are not compliant

with agreed upon standards, goals or counseling agreements and may discount their need to change by claiming they have "always been this way." They manage their anxiety by acting out rather than [by] talking out their issues . . . (Lachman 2001).

The American Psychiatric Association's *Diagnostic and Statistical Manual* estimates that about 10 percent of the general population in the United States meet the diagnostic criteria for a having a personality disorder. In addition, an individual can be diagnosed as having more than one personality disorder at the same time. Another complicating factor is that people with personality disorders are prone to developing additional mental health problems, especially clinical depression and substance abuse disorders.

Some individuals with personality disorders display behavioral patterns that are relatively mild and manageable (for example, perfectionistic or overly dramatic behaviors), while other individuals with more severe personality disorders may behave in more maladaptive ways that have a damaging impact on interpersonal behavior and vocational functioning. For example, individuals with borderline personality disorder can be very volatile and they often engage in intense and stormy interpersonal conflicts that disrupt an entire department.

In their classic book on this issue, *Toxic Coworkers: How to Deal with Dysfunctional People on the Job*, Cavaiola and Lavender (2000, p. 6) make note of the fact that all too often "personality disorders go unrecognized and yet they create a substantial amount of stress in the workplace." They offer a list of the personality disorders that are most commonly found among employees in the workplace (Cavaiola and Lavender 2000, pp. 4–5):

- Paranoid personality disorder, which is characterized by highly suspicious and distrustful behavior
- Schizoid personality disorder, which is characterized by behavior indicating no desire for affiliation or friendship
- Antisocial personality disorder, which is characterized by an apparent disregard for social morals and the rights of others
- Narcissistic personality disorder, which is characterized by self-centered and grandiose behavior that indicates a lack of empathy for others
- Histrionic personality disorder, which is characterized by dramatic, overly emotional behavior
- Borderline personality disorder, which is characterized by moody, intense, and angry behavior and stormy interpersonal relationships

- Obsessive-compulsive personality disorder, which is character-ized by extremely perfectionistic and inflexible behavior and overconcern for details

In the healthcare workplace, as in any other work setting, we can see evidence of many of the personality traits mentioned in this list. At one time or another, we all have found ourselves feeling a little suspi-cious or moody. The difference between a personality trait and a per-sonality disorder is the maladaptive and inflexible nature of personality disorders, which can adversely affect occupational functioning and interpersonal relationships. Without medication and psychotherapy to help them control their emotions and gain insight into their behavior and perceptions, people with personality disorders are usually unable to change their inappropriate behavior. It is obvious that employees with personality disorders have the potential of disrupting teams and undermining employee morale.

In her coaching seminars for nurse managers, Lachman (2001) identified narcissistic personality disorder and borderline personality disorder as the personality disorders that have the most impact on a typical work environment. The narcissistic personality characteristi-cally manifests as grandiose, flamboyant behavior. Narcissistic individ-uals are also hypersensitive to criticism. At the same time, they lack empathy for others, although they are sometimes able to take advan-tage of the feelings or needs of others for their own personal gain. They require excessive admiration and often have fantasies of brilliance (Lachman 2001). They are very manipulative in getting their own needs met, and for these reasons they create problems for work groups. A common phrase "it's all about me!" might well be the motto of indi-viduals with a narcissistic personality disorder.

For the manager or leader dealing with someone with a narcissis-tic personality disorder, it is important for the manager to:

- Be aware of ways you can be manipulated. When the employee gives you effusive praise or extensive accolades, you should be pre-pared for the demands for special treatment that may soon follow.
- When employees complain about the ways in which the indi-vidual with a narcissistic personality has taken advantage of them, be prepared to coach the staff on ways they can negotiate for better outcomes next time.
- Be honest in giving feedback to this individual but begin with the things they are doing well before coaching them on the areas in which they need to make changes (Lachman 2001).

- Help them to set realistic goals and to have more realistic understanding of their skills and abilities. Coach them in specific ways to be a team player (Cavaiola and Lavender 2000).
- Provide positive feedback and recognition when there is evidence that they are empathetic to others or are making an effort to work as a member of a team.
- Build bridges with a narcissistic individual rather than engaging in confrontation.
- Stick to your agenda, not theirs (you may want to correct his or her errors in logic but it is best not to) (Cavaiola and Lavender 2000).

Equally challenging is the person with a borderline personality disorder. Just as a "the world revolves around me" attitude is often a sign of narcissistic personality disorder, people with borderline personality disorder can often be recognized by the intensity and changeability of their moods and the comments people make about the person ("she runs hot and cold and you never know what to expect" or "we are all walking on eggshells wondering what will trigger her outbursts this time"). A person with a borderline personality has no real sense of self-identity, and so even slight changes in the environment can trigger an overreaction. Their impulsive behavior and intense anger are particularly problematic in a work setting (Lachman 2001). Coworkers quickly learn that they may be viewed as friends one day and enemies the next. Needless to say, this makes team building difficult. The turmoil created by their overreactions or intensity often makes the workplace feel like a soap opera. Perhaps the movie *Fatal Attraction* provides the most memorable example of the havoc that can be created by an individual with borderline personality disorder. In a work setting, such employees can often be recognized as the ones who "keeps things stirred up" and "act out" rather than processing an issue and choosing a more mature response (Lachman 2001).

A manager who steps in to manage a daytime soap opera starring an employee with this disorder should consider the following pointers:

- Help the employee see the gray in an issue rather than the black-and-white thinking that often leads to an intense emotional response.
- Set limits but expect the limits to be tested repeatedly. The broken record technique may be helpful.

- Seldom if ever make special arrangements for the employee because this will likely lead to additional requests for special treatment.
- Deal promptly with strong, emotional responses and role-play what the employee should do the next time a similar situation comes up.
- Notice nonverbal behavior (for example, rolling of the eyes, turning away, and so on) and ask about employee's feelings so that the employee is less likely to have an explosive emotional reaction (Chambers 1998, p. 138).
- Let the employee know about an upcoming change ahead of time so he or she is not caught off guard (Lachman 2001).
- Expect some moodiness but avoid overreacting to the employee's mood state (a simple "I hear you" is usually sufficient).
- When possible, limit the employee's contact with others (the less stimulation in their environment, the better).
- Provide positive feedback when good decision making or effective coping is observed (Cavaiola and Lavender 2000).
- Help the employee transfer effective behavior to new situations, but do not be surprised when the employee is unable to apply the same skills in a similar situation.

Conclusion

Influencing the performance of others is an important aspect of creating a positive work environment. For leaders and managers this means working in partnership with employees on performance improvement and skill development. Important aspects include being actively engaged in coaching and giving helpful feedback even when it is difficult. In some instances, sculpting the job to better take advantage of an employee's signature strengths may be the intervention required. In cases where performance or behaviors are not acceptable, the manager needs to apply appropriate processes that are implemented fairly and in full partnership with the employee. And finally, dealing effectively with toxic behavior prevents deterioration of morale.

Influencing and managing performance and problem behavior is probably one of the toughest challenges faced by organizational leaders. Yet it is directly linked to quality of work life for people in the organization and must be undertaken without fail. The payoff is worth it in the end. Finding allies and support in human resources is a strategy that helps lighten the burden and ensures that there is support for both managers and employees in the system.

Conversation Points

Organizational Perspective

1. How effectively does the organization's current formal performance appraisal system work? Is it motivating to employees? Are employees treated as partners in the process, or is it a manager-driven approach?
2. How do managers feel about the performance appraisal system? Is it connected to pay increases?
3. Are organizational managers expected to be actively engaged in coaching employees? Or are work schedules so full of meetings and other commitments that proactive, consistent coaching from the manager is rarely possible?
4. Is there ongoing dialogue and feedback among people throughout the various levels of the organization? Are employees taught how to receive feedback? Is there an openness about sharing feedback even between levels in the hierarchy?
5. Is corrective discipline or positive discipline the approach used in the organization?
6. What are the underlying assumptions about employees and the employee–manager relationship that are driving the development of policies and practices in the system? Are they positive or based on negative perceptions about employees?
7. Is there a zero-tolerance policy on bullying behavior in the workplace? Is it applied equitably and fairly at all levels of the organization? For example, how is physician bullying behavior dealt with? What recourse does an employee have who is being bullied by a manager?
8. Are there any pockets of negativity in departments? What is the level of support available for manager and staff dealing with this problem?

Leadership Issues

1. How actively are you involved in coaching and developing your employees and colleagues? Is your coaching proactive and consistent or sporadic and related only to performance problems?
2. How comfortable are you giving difficult feedback to others? Do you use a model for scripting difficult feedback? Have you taught the model to employees? How comfortable are you with receiving

feedback from those around you? Are you able to listen without becoming resentful or defensive? What could you do to improve your skills in giving and receiving feedback?

3. What is your working relationship with the specialists in human resources? Do you engage human resources early when you suspect that you are facing a potential problem situation?

4. How thorough is your documentation of performance issues? Is it complete and appropriate or sketchy and inadequate? How might you strengthen your approach to documentation of performance issues?

5. Is chronic negativity a problem in your department? If it is, what have you tried in dealing with this issue? Do you have specific techniques or approaches for keeping things focused on the positive?

6. Do you see or suspect any bullying behavior in your area? If you do, who is it? Does this person have a following? What have you tried in dealing with this behavior? How has it worked? What resources do you have to help you? If you do not see any evidence of bullying behavior, have you ever had to deal with this issue?

7. Do you see any of the personality disorder behaviors in people with whom you work? Are the behaviors you see just personality traits, or are they more persistent? What is the effect on the work group?

Employee Challenges

1. How do you prepare for your annual performance appraisal? Do you refer to the goals established at different points throughout the year, or does the form go in your file, only to be reviewed when next year's date rolls around? Do you provide any sort of self-assessment in preparation for the appraisal?

2. Do you find the performance appraisal system helpful and motivating? How would you change it if you could?

3. Is there someone who actively serves as a coach for you in the workplace? How helpful is your coach? What kinds of things does this coach work on with you?

4. How open are you to receiving feedback? Do you actively seek out opportunities in your daily work life to ensure you are taking advantage of the feedback around you?

5. Do you feel comfortable giving your coworkers or manager feedback on behavior that you would like to see them change?

6. What is your knowledge of the corrective action or positive discipline process in your organization? Have you ever experienced it firsthand? Did you feel like you were supported in the process and encouraged to improve?
7. What is the climate like in your department? Is it predominantly positive or mostly negative? Why? What are the behaviors you see that make it so?
8. Are there any bullies in your workplace? Who are they? What bullying behavior do you see? Does management know about it? How is bullying behavior dealt with in your organization? Do you feel supported and safe in your workplace? Why?

Postscript:
Going Forward

Jo Manion

If it is to be, it is up to me.
—Anonymous

A POSITIVE work environment is a key competitive strategy for both today's and future healthcare organizations. Without it, recruitment and retention of high-quality, fully engaged employees are much more difficult, if not downright impossible. And achievement of the organization's mission as well as its strategies and goals is impossible without a skilled and talented workforce. The people who comprise your workforce are the ones who attain results for the organization and your patients or clients. Even with automation poised to take over some of the more routine work in our organizations, as good as machines may become, they will never be able to care nor to innovate, both of which are necessary components of a successful healthcare organization. Many people in our organizations today are struggling, trying to do a good job with decreasing resources, escalating regulatory constraints, and a multitude of other intensifying pressures. In spite of difficulties, however, they are finding ways to create a positive work environment that makes theirs a better place to work.

This book has explored many of the various components connected with a positive work environment. What we know about the intrinsic motivators has been reviewed. If these key factors can be incorporated in the workplace, it is more likely that members of our workforce are motivated and enthusiastic about their work. If their working relationships with others are healthy and positive and if individuals can see how their work makes a positive difference for others and is meaningful, intrinsic motivation is more likely. If the system supports and demands personal and professional competence and offers choice and autonomy in the work, intrinsic motivation grows. And finally, hope of progress and a sense of achievement taps into people's internal sense of motivation.

The concept of organizational commitment was explored because we want people who not only come to work on a consistent basis, but are engaged and committed while they are there. Commitment is emotional, it engages the heart, and it provides sticking power for us when the going gets tough. Affective and normative commitment, considered to be the two stronger forms of organizational commitment, were explored in some detail. Specific steps for building these forms of organizational commitment were examined.

The new field of positive psychology offers much hope to us in increasing our understanding of what brings happiness, both at a personal as well as a professional level. Although the field is still in its infancy, the research findings offer us guidance and evidence-based interventions for creating a better, healthier workplace. Happiness has been too narrowly defined in the past, and when it is examined in its fuller context, it offers us direction for ways to increase both our own levels of happiness as well as in those with whom we work. The three components of happiness include the amount of pleasure in your life, the degree to which you are engaged in your work or activities, and finally, the depth of meaning with which you imbue your work or activities. All three aspects suggest concrete, specific ways we can increase our own happiness as well as positively influence the happiness levels in our workplace as well.

In the second part of this book we began by reviewing a research study through which experienced, successful health care managers shared what they do to create a positive workplace. All of the study participants acknowledged that they alone could not create a positive workplace, but that they worked in partnership with their employee–colleagues to do so. There were four additional key managerial strategies that emerged from this research and these included: putting the employee first, forging strong connections with people, coaching employees for their development, and focusing on results. Based on these findings, the rest of the book presented detail on strategies for achieving these goals.

Focusing on relationships, both at the individual and group levels, was the theme for two chapters. Emotional intelligence, both for the manager as well as the team or work group, was explored. Concepts for developing teams and a sense of community in the workplace were reviewed. Another two chapters were aimed at strategies for getting results and understanding organizational innovation. The final chapter presented the issue of influencing the performance of others, detailing coaching approaches a manager can take to deal with ineffective performance or inappropriate conduct.

Returning to a question asked in the early pages of this book, "Why is a healthy, positive workplace so important? After all, when all is said and done, it's a paycheck and that's what really matters." But the truth is that money is not all that matters, nor is it even the most important element in our work world, and we are only fooling ourselves if we believe that. Of course, if none of the intrinsic motivators nor the elements of positive organizational commitment present, it may be only money that is keeping people there. And you cannot count on them staying, because all it takes is for another organization to match or increase what they can make financially and most of them leave.

Most of us spend the majority of our awake, alert time at work, employed by others. Our work is capable of bringing great meaning and joy to our lives, if we would but expect it and let it. It is an avenue where we can share our strengths and talents with others. Our work is an integral part of our life's journey. It shapes and informs our personal world. It is one way we leave a mark, a legacy for others. Life is simply too precious to squander in a job or an organization where we are miserable, where the negative energy drains us of all enthusiasm and joy, and leaves us feeling depleted.

A positive work environment is possible. But don't wait for someone else to create this positive workplace that you envision. It is up to each and every one of us to take action, to be part of creating a healthier environment. If you are not actively working to make things better, you may be part of the problem. What have you done this week to make your workplace a great place to work? How many times have you laughed with colleagues or stopped to reflect on what a wonderful contribution you make? How many times this week have you encouraged someone around you or helped them without first being asked? When was the last time you showed your gratitude to others who may not hear many thank-yous? Not just your peers, but the chief executive officer or your department manager? Or the person who cleans your department and empties the trash, or the security guard who is in the background making certain that the environment is safe? What can you do to create the kind of workplace where you are excited about going to work? Where you find support and fellowship and the confidence of knowing you are doing good things? The power of ten small words sums it up best, "If it is to be, it is up to me."

References

AbuAlRub, R. F. 2004. Job stress, job performance, and social support among hospital nurses. *Journal of Nursing Scholarship* 36(1):73–78.

Ackoff, R., Finnel, E., and Gharajedaghi, J. 1984. *A Guide to Controlling Your Corporation's Future*. New York City: John Wiley & Sons.

Adams, J. L. 1986. *The Care and Feeding of Ideas: A Guide to Encouraging Creativity*. Reading, Mass.: Addison–Wesley.

Advisory Board Company, T. 2000. *Reversing the Flight of Talent: Nursing Retention in an Era of Gathering Shortage*. Washington, D.C.: Advisory Board Company.

American Hospital Association. 2001. *Patients or Paperwork?* Chicago: AHA.

American Hospital Association. 2003. Staffing Watch. *Hospitals & Healthcare Networks* 7(9):22.

American Nurses Association. 2001. *Nursing World Health and Safety Survey*. Washington, D.C.: Nursing World.

Amott, T. L., and Matthaei, J. A. 1991. *Race, Gender and Work: A Multicultural Economic History of Women in the United States*. Boston: South End Press.

Anderson, P. 1990. *Great Quotes from Great Leaders*. Lombard, Ill.: Celebrating Excellence Publishing.

Anonymous. 2002. Attitudes. *Training and Development* 56(2):27.

Applebaum, H. 1992. *The Concept of Work: Ancient, Medieval, and Modern*. Albany, N.Y.: State University of New York Press.

Aptheker, B. 1989. *Tapestries of Life: Women's Work, Women's Consciousness, and the Meaning of Daily Experience*. Amherst, Mass.: University of Massachusetts Press.

Arbuckle, G. A. 2000. Cultures of bullying. *Human Development* 21(1):25–33.

Aronson, E. 1995. *The Social Animal*. Seventh edition. New York City: W. H. Freeman and Company.

Atchison, T. A. 2003. Exposing the myths of employee satisfaction. *Healthcare Executive* May–June, pp. 20–25.

Baggs, J. G., and Schmitt, M. H. 1988. Collaboration between nurses and physicians. *Image: Journal of Nursing Scholarship* 20(3):145–49.

Bandler, R., and Grinder, J. 1982. *Frogs into Princes: Neuro Linguistic Programming*. Moab, Utah: Real People Press.

Barker, J. 1990. *The Power of Vision*. Burnsville, Minn.: Charthouse Learning Corporation.

Barney, S. M. 2002. Radical change: one solution to the nursing shortage. *Journal of Healthcare Management* 47(4):220–24.

Barrett, F. J. 1995. Creating appreciative learning cultures. *Organizational Dynamics* 24:36–49.

Barsade, S. G., and Gibson, D. E. 1998. Group emotion: a view from top and bottom. In D. H. Gruenfeld (ed.), *Research on Managing Groups and Teams*, volume 1, pp. 81–102. Stamford, Conn.: JAI Press.

Bartel, C. A., and Saavedra, R. 2000. The collective construction of work group moods. *Administrative Science Quarterly* 45:197–231.

Bateson, M. C. 1990. *Composing a Life*. New York City: Plume Publishing.

Becker, H. S. 1960. Notes on the concept of commitment. *American Journal of Sociology* 66:32–40.

Beckhard, R., and Pritchard, W. 1992. *Changing the Essence: The Art of Creating and Leading Fundamental Change in Organizations*. San Francisco: Jossey–Bass Publishers.

Beglinger, J. 2003. The innovative organization for the 21st century. *Nurse Leader* 1(1):39–41.

Bennis, W. 1966. *Changing Organizations: Essays on the Development and Evolution of Human Organization*. New York City: McGraw–Hill.

Bennis, W. (ed.). 1970. *American Bureaucracy*. Boston: Aldine Publishing.

Bennis, W. 1989. *On Becoming a Leader*. Reading, Mass.: Addison–Wesley Publishing.

Berry, L. L. 1992. Qualities of leadership. *Retailing Issues Letter* 4(1):1–4.

Berwick, D. M. 2003. Disseminating innovations in health care. *Journal of the American Medical Association* 289(15):1969–75.

Blouin, A., and Brent, N. 1997. Strategic partnering: clinical and risk management concerns. *Journal of Nursing Administration* 27(6):10–13.

Bookman, A., and Morgen, S. (eds.). 1988. *Women and the Politics of Empowerment*. Philadelphia: Temple University Press.

Bossidy, L., and Charan, R. 2002. *Execution: The Discipline of Getting Things Done*. New York City: Crown Business.

Bowles, M. 1991. The organization shadow. *Organization Studies* 12(3): 387–404.

Bowles, M. 1997. The myth of management: direction and failure in contemporary organizations. *Human Relations* 50(7):779–803.

Brickman, P., with C. B. Wortman and R. Sorrentino (eds.) 1987. *Commitment, Conflict, and Caring*. Englewood Cliffs, N.J.: Prentice-Hall.

Brightman, S. 2002. Former consultant with Drake Beam Morin. Personal conversation. New York City, February.

Buckingham, M., and Coffman, C. 1999. *First, Break All the Rules: What the World's Greatest Managers Do Differently*. New York City: Simon & Schuster.

Burns, B. M. 1978. *Leadership*. New York City: Harper–Collins.

Byers, J. F., and White, S. V. 2004. *Patient Safety: Principles and Practice*. New York City: Springer Verlag.

Byrne, J. A. 2003. How to lead now: getting extraordinary performance when you can't pay for it. *Fast Company* 73:62–70.

Caudron, S. 1997. The search for meaning at work. *Training and Development* 51(9):24–27.

Cavaiola, A., and Lavender, N. 2000. *Toxic Coworkers: How to Deal with Dysfunctional People on the Job*. Oakland, Calif.: New Harbinger Publications.

Chaleff, I. 1996. Effective leadership. *Executive Excellence* 4:16–17.

Chaleff, I. 1997. The groupthink challenge. *Team Management Briefings* June, p. 4.

Chambers, H. E. 1998. *The Bad Attitude Survival Guide*. Reading, Mass.: Addison–Wesley.

Champy, J. 2003. The hidden qualities of great leaders. *Fast Company* 76:135.

Charles, R. 2000. The challenge of disseminating innovations to direct care providers in health care organizations. *Nursing Clinics of North America* 35(2):461–70.

Chawla, S., and Renesch, J. (eds.). 1995. *Learning Organizations: Developing Cultures for Tomorrow's Workplace*. Portland, Ore.: Productivity Press.

Cherniss, C., and Goleman, D. 2001. *The Emotionally Intelligent Workplace: How to Select for, Measure, and Improve Emotional Intelligence in Individuals, Groups, and Organizations*. San Francisco: Jossey–Bass Publishers.

Ciancutti, A., and Steding, T. 2001. *Built on Trust: Gaining Competitive Advantage in Any Organization*. Lincolnwood, Ill.: Contemporary Books.

Clancy, T. 2003. The art of decision-making. *Journal of Nursing Administration* 33(6):343–49.

Clarke, J. 1999. *Connections: The Threads That Strengthen Families*. Center City, Minn.: Hazelden Publishing.

Clarke-Epstein, C. 2002. Truth in feedback. *Training and Development* 56(11): 78–80.

Clegg, S. R. 1990. *Modern Organizations: Organization Studies in the Post-modern World*. London: Sage Publications.

Cline, D., Reilly, C., and Moore, J. 2003. What's behind RN turnover? *Nursing Management* 34(10):50–53.

Coens, T., and Jenkins, M. 2000. *Abolishing Performance Appraisals: Why They Backfire and What to Do Instead*. San Francisco: Berrett–Koehler Publishers.

Collins, J. 2001. *Good to Great: Why Some Companies Make the Leap . . . and Others Don't*. New York City: HarperCollins.

Cordeniz, J. A. 2002. Recruitment, retention, and management of generation X: a focus on nursing professionals. *Journal of Healthcare Management* 47(4):237–49.

368   References

Covey, S. R. 1989. *The Seven Habits of Highly Effective People: Powerful Lessons in Personal Change*. New York City: Simon & Schuster.

Covey, S. R. 1992. *Principle-Centered Leadership*. New York City: Simon & Schuster.

Covey, S. R., Merrill, A. R., and Merrill, R. R. 1994. *First Things First*. New York City: Simon & Schuster.

Cox, S., Manion, J., and Miller, D. 2005. *Nature's Wisdom in the Workplace: Managing Energy in Health Care Organizations*. Bloomington, Minn.: Synergy Press.

Creative Healthcare Management. 1994. *Leaders Empower Staff*. Minneapolis, Minn: Creative Healthcare Management.

Csikszentmihalyi, M. 1990. *Flow: The Psychology of Optimal Experience*. New York City: Harper & Row Publishers.

Csikszentmihalyi, M. 1997. *Finding Flow: The Psychology of Engagement with Everyday Life*. New York City: Basic Books.

Csikszentmihalyi, M. 2003. *Good Business: Leadership, Flow, and the Making of Meaning*. New York City: Penguin Putnam.

de Man, H. 1929. *Joy in Work* (E. C. Paul, trans.). London: George Allen & Unwin.

DeChick, J. 1988. Most mothers want a job, too. *USA Today* (July 19):D1.

Delbecq, A. L., and VandeVen, A. H. 1971. A group process model for problem identification and program planning. *Journal of Applied Behavioral Science* 7:466–94.

Denhardt, R. B. 1981. *In the Shadow of Organization*. Lawrence, Kans.: University Press of Kansas.

DePree, M. 1989. *Leadership Is an Art*. New York City: Doubleday Publishers.

Diener, E. 2000. Subjective well-being. *American Psychologist* 55(1): 34–43.

Diener, E., and Diener, C. 1996. Most people are happy. *Psychological Science* 7(3):181–85.

Diener, E., Sandvik, E., and Pavot, W. 1991. Happiness is the frequency, not the intensity, of positive versus negative affect. In F. Strack, M. Argyle, and N. Schwarz (eds.), *Subjective Well-Being: An Interdisciplinary Perspective*, pp. 119–39. New York City: Pergamon.

DiSciullo, M. J. 1997. Remembering Joy in the Therapist and the Psychotherapeutic Process. Unpublished doctoral dissertation, Pacifica Graduate Institute, Carpinteria, Calif.

Dobbs, K. 1999. Winning the retention game. *Training* 36(9):50–56.

Doherty, K. 2002. Work Related Posttraumatic Stress in Nurses. Presented at the American Organization of Nurse Executives annual meeting, April 8, 2002, in Orlando, Fla.

Drucker, P. 1992. *Managing for the Future: The 1990s and Beyond*. New York City: Penguin Books.

Dumaine, B. 1994. Why do we work? *Fortune* 130(13):196–204.

Durning, A. T. 1993. Are we happy yet? How the pursuit of happiness is failing. *Futurist* 27(1):20–24.

Easterbrook, G. 2003. *The Progress Paradox: How Life Gets Better while People Feel Worse.* New York City: Random House.

Eisler, R. 1987. *The Chalice and the Blade: Our History, Our Future.* San Francisco: HarperSanFrancisco.

Eisler, R., and Loye, D. 1998. *The Partnership Way: New Tools for Living and Learning,* second edition. Brandon, Vt.: Holistic Education Press.

Ellis, D. 2004. What if … the consequences of innovation. *Hospitals & Healthcare Networks* 78(8):39–42.

Erikson, K., and Vallas, S. P. (eds.). 1990. *The Nature of Work: Sociological Perspectives.* New Haven, Conn.: Yale University Press.

Fagiano, D. 1994. Designating a leader. *Management Review* 83(3):4.

Fairholm, G. W. 1998. *Perspectives on Leadership: From the Science of Management to Its Spiritual Heart.* Westport, Conn: Quorum Books.

Farrell, G. A. 1997. Aggression in clinical settings: nurses' views. *Journal of Advanced Nursing* 29(3):532.

Fishman, C. 1998. The war for talent. *Fast Company* 16:104–8.

Flower, J. 1990. The chasm between management and leadership. *Healthcare Forum Journal* 33(4):59–62.

Flower, J. 1999. Building the idea factory: a conversation with John Kao. *Health Forum Journal* 42(2):12–15.

Flower, J. 2002. Good to great: a conversation with Jim Collins. *Health Forum Journal* 45(5):17–20.

Fredrickson, B. L. 1998. What good are positive emotions? *Review of General Psychology* 2(3):300–319.

Fredrickson, B. L. 2001. The role of positive emotions in positive psychology. *American Psychologist* 56(3):218–26.

Fredrickson, B. L. 2003. The value of positive emotions. *American Scientist* 91(7):330–35.

Frick, D., and Spears, L. (eds.). 1996. *On Becoming a Servant-Leader: The Private Writings of Robert K. Greenleaf.* San Francisco: Jossey–Bass Publishers.

Gelinas, L., and Bohlen, C. 2002. *Tomorrow's Work Force: A Strategic Approach.* 2002 Research Series, volume 1. Irving, Tex.: VHA.

George, J. M. 2000. Emotions and leadership: the role of emotional intelligence. *Human Relations* 53(8):1027–55.

Gibson, C. 1991. A concept analysis of empowerment. *Journal of Advanced Nursing* 16:354–61.

Gilligan, C. 1982. *In A Different Voice: Psychological Theory and Women's Development.* Cambridge, Mass.: Harvard University Press.

Goleman, D. 1995. *Emotional Intelligence: Why It Can Matter More than IQ.* New York City: Bantam Books.

Goleman, D., Boyatzis, R., and McKee, A. 2002. *Primal Leadership: Realizing the Power of Emotional Intelligence*. Boston: Harvard Business School Press.

Gould, S. B., Weiner, K. J., and Levin, B. R. 1997. *Free Agents: People and Organizations Creating a New Working Community*. San Francisco: Jossey–Bass Publishers.

Gowing, M. K., Kraft, J. D., and Quick, J. C. (eds.). 1998. *The New Organizational Reality: Downsizing, Restructuring and Revitalization*. Washington, D.C.: American Psychological Association.

Greiff, B. S. 1999. *Legacy: The Giving of Life's Greatest Treasures*. New York City: HarperCollins Publishers.

Grossman, H. Y. (ed.). 1990. *The Experience and Meaning of Work in Women's Lives*. Hillsdale, N.J.: Lawrence Erlbaum Associates, Publishers.

Grote, D. 1995. *Discipline without Punishment: The Proven Strategy That Turns Problem Employees into Superior Performers*. New York City: AMACOM.

Grote, D. 2002. *The Performance Appraisal Question and Answer Book*. New York City: AMACOM.

Gryskiewicz, S. S. 1999. Positive turbulence: a climate for creativity. *Health Forum Journal* 42(2):16–19.

Hammonds, K. 2004. We, incorporated. *Fast Company* 84:67–69.

Harvey, E. 1986. Discipline vs punishment. *Management Review* March [unpaged reprint].

Hattori, R. A., and Wycoff, J. 2002. Innovation DNA. *Training and Development* 56(1):24–30.

Heenan, D. A., and Bennis, W. 1999. *Co-Leaders: The Power of Great Partnerships*. New York City: John Wiley & Sons.

Helgesen, S. 1995. *The Web of Inclusion: A New Architecture of Building Great Organizations*. New York City: Currency/Doubleday.

Henry, J. D., and Henry, L. S. 2004. Caring from the inside out: strategies to enhance nurse retention and patient satisfaction. *Nurse Leader* 2(1):28–32.

Hesse-Biber, S., and Carter, G. L. 2000. *Working Women in America: Split Dreams*. New York City: Oxford University Press.

Hirschhorn, L. 1997. *Reworking Authority: Leading and Following in the Post-Modern Organization*. Cambridge, Mass.: MIT Press.

Hock, D. 1999. *Birth of the Chaordic Age*. San Francisco: Berrett-Koehler Publishers.

Houck, John. 2003. Presentation at a meeting of the Maryland Hospital Association, July 29, 2003.

Iverson, R., and Buttigieg, D. 1999. Affective, normative and continuance commitment: some methodological considerations. *Journal of Management Studies* 36:307–33.

Iyengar, S. S., and Lepper, M. R. 1999. Rethinking the value of choice: a cultural perspective on intrinsic motivation. *Journal of Personality and Social Psychology* 76(3):349–66.

Johnson, B. 1996. *Polarity Management: Identifying and Managing Unsolvable Problems*. Amherst, Mass.: HRD Press.

Josselson, R. 1996. *Revising Herself: The Story of Women's Identity from College to Midlife*. New York City: Oxford University Press.

Kalisch, B. J. 2003. Recruiting nurses: the problem is the process. *Journal of Nursing Administration* 33(9):468–77.

Kangas, S., Kee, C. C., and McKee-Waddle, R. 1999. Organizational factors, nurses' job satisfaction, and patient satisfaction with nursing care. *Journal of Nursing Administration* 29(1):32–42.

Kanter, R. M. 1972. *Commitment and Community: Communes and Utopia in Sociological Perspective*. Cambridge, Mass.: Harvard University Press.

Kanter, R. M. 1997. *On the Frontiers of Management*. Middlebury, Vt.: Soundview Executive Book Summaries.

Katzenbach, J. R. 2003. *Why Pride Matters More than Money: The Power of the World's Greatest Motivational Force*. New York City: Crown Business.

Katzenbach, J. R., and Smith, D. K. 1993. *The Wisdom of Teams: Creating the High-Performance Organization*. Boston: Harvard Business School Press.

Kaye, B., and Jordan-Evans, S. 1999. *Love 'em or Lose 'em*. San Francisco: Berrett–Koehler Publishers.

Kaye, B., and Jordan-Evans, S. 2002. Retention in tough times. *Training and Development* 56(1):32–37.

Kleinman, C. S. 2004. Leadership and retention: research needed. *Journal of Nursing Administration* 34(3):111–13.

Kouzes, J. W., and Posner, B. Z. 1993. *The Credibility Factor*. San Francisco: Jossey–Bass Publishers.

Kouzes, J. W., and Posner, B. Z. 2003. *Encouraging the Heart: A Leader's Guide to Rewarding and Recognizing Others*. San Francisco: Jossey–Bass Publishers.

LaBarre, P. 2002. Weird ideas that work. *Fast Company* 54:68–73.

Lachman, V. 2001. Personality Disorders in the Workplace: Identification and Intervention. Presentation for the Forum on Healthcare Leadership, Philadelphia, August 19, 2001.

Lanser, E. G. 2001. Leveraging your nursing resources. *Healthcare Executive* 16(4):50–51.

Larson, C. E., and LaFosta, F. 1989. *Team Work: What Must Go Right/What Can Go Wrong*. Newport Park, Calif.: Sage.

Leander, W., Shortridge, D., and Watson, P. 1996. *Patients First*. Chicago: Health Administration Press.

Lee, C. 1999. Mean streets and rude workplaces: the death of civility. *Training* 36(7):24–30.

Lencioni, P. 2002. *The Five Dysfunctions of a Team: A Leadership Fable*. San Francisco: Jossey–Bass Publishers.

Loehr, J., and Schwartz, T. 2003. *The Power of Full Engagement: Managing Energy, Not Time, Is the Key to High Performance and Personal Renewal.* New York City: Free Press.

Lorimer, W., and Manion, J. 1996. Team-based organizations: leading the essential transformation. *Patient-Focused Care Association Review* Summer, pp. 15–19.

Losada, M. 1999. The complex dynamics of high performance teams. *Mathematical and Computer Modeling* 30:179–92.

Ludema, J. D., Cooperrider, D. L., and Barrett, F. J. 2000. Appreciative inquiry: the power of the unconditional positive question. In P. Reason and H. Bradbury (eds.), *Handbook of Action Research*. London: Sage.

Lydon, J. E., and Zanna, M. P. 1990. Commitment in the face of adversity: a value-affirmation approach. *Journal of Personality and Social Psychology* 58(6):1040–47.

Lykken, D. 1999. *Happiness: What Studies on Twins Show Us about Nature, Nurture, and the Happiness Set Point.* New York City: Golden Books.

Makin, P. J., Cooper, C. L., and Cox, C. J. 1996. *Organizations and the Psychological Contract: Managing People at Work.* Westport, Conn.: Quorum Publishers.

Manion, J. 1989. Professional collaboration: more than a committee structure. *Nursing Options* 1(4):9–12.

Manion, J. 1990. *Change from Within: Nurse Intrapreneurs as Health Care Innovators.* Washington, D.C.: American Nurses Association.

Manion, J. 1993. Chaos or transformation? *Journal of Nursing Administration* 23(5):41–48.

Manion, J. 1997. Teams 101: the manager's role. *Seminars for Nurse Managers* 5(1):31–38.

Manion, J. 1998. *From Management to Leadership: Interpersonal Skills for Success in Health Care.* Chicago: AHA Press.

Manion, J. 2000. Retaining current leaders: a gold mine in your back yard. *Health Forum Journal* 43(5):24–27.

Manion, J. 2002. Joy at Work: As Experienced, As Expressed. Unpublished doctoral dissertation. Santa Barbara, Calif.: The Fielding Graduate Institute.

Manion, J. 2003. Joy at work: creating a positive workplace. *Journal of Nursing Administration* 33(12):652–59.

Manion, J. 2004a. Community in the workplace. *Journal of Nursing Administration* 34(1):46–53.

Manion, J. 2004b. Nurture a culture of retention: front-line nurse leaders share perceptions regarding what makes—or breaks—a flourishing nursing environment. *Nursing Management* 35(4):28–39.

Manion, J. 2004c. Strengthening organizational commitment: understanding the concept as a basis for creating effective workforce retention strategies. *The Health Care Manager* 23(2):167–76.

Manion, J. 2005. *From Management to Leadership: Interpersonal Skills for Success in Health Care*, second edition. San Francisco: Jossey–Bass Publishers.

Manion, J., and Bartholomew, K. 2004. Community in the workplace. *Journal of Nursing Administration* 34(1):46–53.

Manion, J., Lorimer, W., and Leander, W. 1996. *Team-Based Health Care Organizations: Blueprint for Success.* Gaithersburg, Md.: Aspen Publishers.

Manion, J., Sieg, M. J., and Watson, P. W. 1998. Managerial partnerships: the wave of the future? *Journal of Nursing Administration* 28(4):47–55.

Mayer, J. D., Salovey, P., and Caruso, D. R. 2000. Models of human intelligence. In R. J. Sternberg (ed.), *Handbook of Human Intelligence*, second edition. New York City: Cambridge University Press.

Mayer, R., and Schoorman, D. 1998. Differentiating antecedents of organizational commitment. *Journal of Organizational Behavior* 19(1):15–28.

Maxwell, J. Inspiration point. *Nurse Leader* September/October, p. 8.

McCarthy, D. 1997. *The Loyalty Link.* New York City: John Wiley & Sons.

McKenna, E. P. 1997. *When Work Doesn't Work Anymore: Women, Work, and Identity.* New York City: Delacorte Press.

McNeese-Smith, D. K. 2001. Building organizational commitment among nurses. *Journal of Healthcare Management* 46(3):173–87.

McNeese-Smith, D. K., and Crook, M. 2003. Nursing values and a changing nurse workforce: values, age, and job stages. *Journal of Nursing Administration* 33(5):260–70.

Meilaender, G. C. (ed.). 2000. *Working: Its Meaning and Its Limits.* Lafayette, Ind.: University of Notre Dame Press.

Melrose, K. 1996. Leader as servant. *Executive Excellence* 13(4):20.

Menninger, B. 2001. The sad state of healthcare staffing. *Health Leaders* August, pp. 42–50.

Meyer, J., and Allen, N. J. 1984. Testing the "side-bet theory" of organizational commitment: some methodological considerations. *Journal of Applied Psychology* 69(3):372–78.

Meyer, J., Allen, N. J., and Smith, C. A. 1993. Commitment to organizations and occupations: extensions and test of a three-component conceptualization. *Journal of Applied Psychology* 78(4):538–51.

Meyer, J., Paunonen, S., Gellatly, I., Goffin, R., and Jackson, D. 1989. Organizational commitment and job performance: it's the nature of the commitment that counts. *Journal of Applied Psychology* 74(1): 152–56.

Miller, J. B. 1976. *Toward a New Psychology of Women.* Boston: Beacon Press.

Moore, T. 1994. *Care of the Soul.* New York City: Harper Perennial.

Morgan, G. 1998. *Images of Organization: The Executive Edition*. San Francisco: Berrett–Koehler Publishers.

Murray, B. 2003. Positive discipline reaps retention. *Nursing Management* 34(6):19–22.

Mycek, S. 1998. Leadership for a healthy 21st century. *Healthcare Forum Journal* 41(4):26–30.

Myers, D. G. 1992. *The Pursuit of Happiness: Discovering the Pathway to Fulfillment, Well-being, and Enduring Personal Joy*. New York City: Avon Books.

Myers, D. G., and Diener, E. 1995. Who is happy? *Psychological Science* 6(1):10–19.

Nadler, D. A., and Tushman, M. L. 1997. *Competing by Design: The Power of Organizational Architecture*. New York City: Oxford University Press.

Naylor, T. H. 1996. The search for community in the workplace. *Business and Society Review* 97:42–48.

Naylor, T. H., Willimon, W. H., and Osterberg, R. 1996. *The Search for Meaning in the Workplace*. Nashville, Tenn.: Abingdon Press.

Noer, D. M. (1993) *Healing the Wounds: Overcoming the Trauma of Layoffs and Revitalizing Downsized Organizations*. San Francisco: Jossey–Bass Publishers.

Oster, C. 2004. Director of organizational development, General Motors Powertrain. Personal conversation. Pontiac, Mich., June.

Parker, P. 1997. Teamwork and team players. *Team Management Briefings* 5(5):8.

Patterson, L., and Deblieux, M. 1993. *Supervisor's Guide to Documenting Employee Discipline*. Carlsbad, Calif.: Parker & Sons.

Peck, M. S. 1987. *The Different Drum: Community Making and Peace*. New York City: Simon & Schuster.

Peters, T., and Austin, N. 1985. *A Passion for Excellence*. New York City: Random House.

Peterson, C., and Seligman, M. E. P. 2004. *Character Strengths and Virtues: A Classification Handbook*. Washington, D.C.: American Psychological Association.

Pfeffer, J. 1999. Practices of successful organizations. *Health Forum Journal* 42(2):55–58.

Phillips, D. 1992. *Lincoln on Leadership: Executive Strategies for Tough Times*. New York City: Warner Books.

Pinchot, G., and Pinchot, E. 1994. *The Intelligent Organization: Engaging the Talent and Initiative of Everyone in the Workplace*. San Francisco: Berrett–Koehler Publishers.

Plotkin, H. 1999. Six Sigma: what it is and how to use it. *Harvard Management Update* 4(6):6–7.

Ponte, P. R., Kruger, N., DeMarco, R., Hanley, D., and Conlin, G. 2004. Reshaping the practice environment: the importance of coherence. *Journal of Nursing Administration* 34(4):173–79.

Porter-O'Grady, T. 1992. *Implementing Shared Governance: Creating a Professional Organization.* St. Louis: Mosby.

Porter-O'Grady, T. 2001. Is shared governance still relevant? *Journal of Nursing Administration* 31(10):468–73.

Porter-O'Grady, T. 2003. Creators and dreamweavers: building conspiracies for innovation. *Nurse Leader* 1(1):30–32.

Post, N. 1989. Managing human energy: an ancient tool of change experts. *OD Practitioner* 6:14–16.

Post, N. 1993. Presentation on systems energetics, Philadelphia.

Putnam, R. 2000. *Bowling Alone.* New York City: Simon & Schuster.

Raudsepp, E. 1981. *How Creative Are You?* New York City: Putnam.

Reina, D., and Reina, M. L. 1999. *Trust and Betrayal in the Workplace: Building Effective Relationships in Your Organization.* San Francisco: Berrett–Koehler Publishers.

Reivich, K., and Shatte, A. 2002. *The Resilience Factor: Seven Essential Skills for Overcoming Life's Inevitable Obstacles.* New York City: Broadway Books.

Richards, D. 1995a. *Artful Work: Awakening Joy, Meaning, and Commitment in the Workplace.* New York City: Berkley Books.

Richards, D. 1995b. Artistry and the experience of joy. *Journal for Quality and Participation* 18(7):6–9.

Riggs, C. J., and Rantz, M. J. 2001. A model of staff support to improve retention in long-term care. *Nursing Administration Quarterly* 25(2):43–54.

Rogers, R. 1994. The psychological contract of trust. *Executive Excellence* 11(7):6.

Rousseau, M. F. 1991. *Community: The Tie That Binds.* New York City: University Press of America.

Runy, L. A. 2003. How committed are health care employees? *Hospitals & Healthcare Networks* 77(11):28.

Ryan, K. D., and Oestreich, D. K. 1991. *Driving Fear out of the Workplace: How to Overcome the Invisible Barriers to Quality, Productivity and Innovation.* San Francisco: Jossey–Bass Publishers.

Scalise, D. 2004. Shhh, quiet please! *Hospitals & Healthcare Networks* 78(5):16–17.

Scholtes, P. 1998. *The Leader's Handbook.* New York City: McGraw–Hill.

Schuster, D. T. 1990. Work, relationships, and balance in the lives of gifted women. In H. Y. Grossman and N. L. Chester (eds.), *The Experience and Meaning of Work in Women's Lives,* pp. 189–211. Hillsdale, N.J.: Lawrence Erlbaum Associates.

Schutz, W. C. 1989. *Joy: 20 Years Later.* (Revised edition of *Joy: Expanding Human Awareness,* 1967 edition.) Berkeley, Calif.: Ten Speed Press.

Schwartz, B. 2004. *The Paradox of Choice: Why More Is Less.* New York City: HarperCollins.

Searcy, B. 2003. Director of employee and labor relations for Genesys Regional Medical Center in Grand Blanc, Mich. Personal conversation.

Seashore, C. N., Seashore, E. W., and Weinberg, G. M. 1999. *What Did You Say? The Art of Giving and Receiving Feedback*. Columbia, Md.: Bingham House Books.

Seiling, J. G. (1997). *The Membership Organization: Achieving Top Performance through the New Workplace Community*. Palo Alto, Calif.: Davies–Black Publishing.

Seligman, M. E. P. 1998. *Learned Optimism: How to Change Your Mind and Your Life*. New York City: Pocket Books.

Seligman, M. E. P. 2002. *Authentic Happiness: Using the New Positive Psychology to Realize Your Potential for Lasting Fulfillment*. New York City: The Free Press.

Senge, P. M. 1990. *The Fifth Discipline: The Art and Practice of the Learning Organization*. New York City: Doubleday/Currency.

Shaffer, C. R., and Anundsen, K. 1993. *Creating Community Anywhere: Finding Support and Connection in a Fragmented World*. New York City: Jeremy P. Tarcher/Putnam.

Sherwood, G. 2003. Leadership for a healthy work environment: caring for the human spirit. *Nurse Leader* 1(5):36–40.

Sievers, B. 1993. *Work, Death, and Life Itself*. New York City: Walter de Gruyter.

Silberstang, J. 1995. Does joy in work have a place on your balance sheet? *Journal for Quality and Participation* 18(7):20–23.

Snow, C. C., Lipnack, J., and Stamps, J. 1999. The virtual organization: promises and payoffs, large and small. In C. L. Cooper and D. M. Rousseau (eds.), *Trends in Organizational Behavior: The Virtual Organization*, pp. 15–30. New York City: John Wiley & Sons.

Spencer, A. L. 1982. *Seasons: Women's Search for Self through Life's Stages*. New York City: Paulist Press.

Stacey, R. D. 1992. *Managing the Unknowable: Strategic Boundaries between Order and Chaos in Organizations*. San Francisco: Jossey–Bass Publishers.

Strachota, E., Normandin, P., O'Brien, N., Clary, M., and Krukow, B. 2003. Reasons registered nurses leave or change employment status. *Journal of Nursing Administration* 33(2):111–17.

Sutton, R. 2001. *Weird Ideas That Work: 11$^1/_2$ Practices for Promoting, Managing, and Sustaining Innovation*. New York City: Free Press.

Taylor, B. J. 2004. Improving communication through practical reflection. *Reflections on Nursing Leadership* Second Quarter, pp. 28–38.

Terez, T. 1999. Meaningful work. *Executive Excellence* 16(2):19.

Terkel, S. 1972. *Working*. New York City: Pantheon.

Thomas, K. W. 2000. *Intrinsic Motivation at Work: Building Energy and Commitment*. San Francisco: Berrett–Koehler Publishers.

Thomas, S. P. 2004. *Transforming Nurses' Stress and Anger: Steps toward Healing*, second edition. New York City: Springer Verlag.

Thompson, D. N., Wolf, G. A., and Spear, S. J. 2003. Driving improvement in patient care: lessons from Toyota. *Journal of Nursing Administration* 33(11):585–95.

Tichy, N., and Cardwell, N. 2002. *The Cycle of Leadership: How Great Leaders Teach Their Companies to Win*. New York City: HarperBusiness.

Totterdell, P. (2000). Catching moods and hitting runs: mood linkage and subjective performance in professional sport teams. *Journal of Applied Psychology* 85(6):848–59.

Totterdell, P., Kellett, S., Teuchmann, K., and Briner, R. B. 1998. Evidence of mood linkage in work groups. *Journal of Personality and Social Psychology* 74(6):1504–15.

Trigg, R. 1973. *Reason and Commitment*. Cambridge: Cambridge University Press.

Tubbs, W. 1993. Karoushi: stress-death and the meaning of work. *Journal of Business Ethics* 12:869–77.

Tushman, M. L., and O'Reilly, C. A. 1999. Building ambidextrous organizations: forming your own "skunk works." *Health Forum Journal* 42(2):20–23, 64.

Vance, M. 1982. *Creative Thinking*. Chicago: Nightingale-Conant Corporation.

Vogl, A. J. 1997. Soul searching: looking for meaning in the workplace. *Across the Board* 34(9):16–24.

Waterman, R. H. 1987. *The Renewal Factor: How the Best Get and Keep the Competitive Edge*. New York City: Bantam Books.

Waterman, R. H. 1990. *Adhocracy: The Power to Change*. New York City: W. W. Norton & Company.

Webber, A. M. 1998. Danger: toxic company. *Fast Company* 19:152–61.

Weber, D. O. 2003. Ideology. *Health Forum Journal* 47(3):21–24.

Wesorick, B. 2002. 21st century leadership challenge: creating and sustaining healthy healing work cultures and integrated service at the point of care. *Nursing Administration Quarterly* 26(5):18–32.

Wheatley, M. J. 1999. *Leadership and the New Science: Learning about Organizations from an Orderly Universe*, second edition. San Francisco: Berrett–Koehler Publishers.

Whiley, K. 2001. The nurse manager's role in creating a healthy work environment. *AACN Clinical Issues* 12(3):356–65.

Whyte, D. 2001. *Crossing the Unknown Sea: Work as a Pilgrimage of Identity*. New York City: Riverhead Books.

Wiener, Y. 1982. Commitment in organizations. *Academy of Management Review* 7(3):418–28.

Wolff, S. B. 1998. *The Role of Caring Behavior and Peer Feedback in Creating Team Effectiveness*. Unpublished thesis. Boston: Boston University.

Womack, J. P., and Jones, D. 1996. *Lean Thinking: Banish Waste and Create Wealth within Your Organization*. New York City: Simon & Schuster.

Worthington, C. H. 1994. Beyond Job Satisfaction: The Phenomenon of Joy in Work. Unpublished doctoral dissertation, Georgia State University, Atlanta.

Wycoff, J. 1991 *Mindmapping: Your Personal Guide to Exploring Creativity and Problem-Solving*. New York City: Berkley Publishing.

Zander, R. S., and Zander, B. 2000. *The Art of Possibility: Transforming Professional and Personal Life*. Boston: Harvard Business School Press.

Zemke, R. 1996. The call of community. *Training* 33(3):24–30.

Zemke, R. 1999. Problem-solving is the problem: don't fix that company. *Training* 36(6):26–33.

Index